Respiratory Medicine

Series Editors

Sharon I. S. Rounds, Brown University, Providence, RI, USA

Anne Dixon, University of Vermont, Larner College of Medicine
Burlington, VT, USA

Lynn M. Schnapp, University of Wisconsin - Madison, Madison, WI, USA

Respiratory Medicine offers clinical and research-oriented resources for pulmonologists and other practitioners and researchers interested in respiratory care. Spanning a broad range of clinical and research issues in respiratory medicine, the series covers such topics as COPD, asthma and allergy, pulmonary problems in pregnancy, molecular basis of lung disease, sleep disordered breathing, and others.

The series editors are Sharon Rounds, MD, Professor of Medicine and of Pathology and Laboratory Medicine at the Alpert Medical School at Brown University, Anne Dixon, MD, Professor of Medicine and Director of the Division of Pulmonary and Critical Care at Robert Larner, MD College of Medicine at the University of Vermont, and Lynn M. Schnapp, MD, George R. And Elaine Love Professor and Chair of Medicine at the University of Wisconsin-Madison School of Medicine and Public Health.

Christina R. MacRosty • M. Patricia Rivera
Editors

Lung Cancer

A Comprehensive Guide for the Clinician

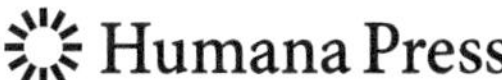 Humana Press

Editors
Christina R. MacRosty
Division of Pulmonary Diseases and
Critical Care Medicine
University of North Carolina
Chapel Hill, NC, USA

M. Patricia Rivera
Division of Pulmonary and Critical Care
Medicine
University of Rochester Medical Center
Rochester, NY, USA

ISSN 2197-7372   ISSN 2197-7380   (electronic)
Respiratory Medicine
ISBN 978-3-031-38414-1   ISBN 978-3-031-38412-7   (eBook)
https://doi.org/10.1007/978-3-031-38412-7

This Humana imprint is published by the registered company Springer Nature Switzerland AG
The registered company address is: Gewerbestrasse 11, 6330 Cham, Switzerland

Paper in this product is recyclable.

Preface

In the early twentieth century, about 374 lung cancer cases had been reported in the medical literature [1], and an association had been made between cigarette smoking and the development of lung cancer [2]. By the mid-twentieth century, tobacco smoking was described as a likely cause of lung cancer, with two landmark studies published in the United States (US) and the United Kingdom [2–4]. In 1959, the first cancer prevention study (CPSI) reported a relative risk of death from lung cancer among those who smoke of 2.69 for men and 11.3 for women [5, 6]. The US Surgeon General Report published in 1964 described a ninefold to tenfold increased risk of lung cancer in people who smoke compared to those that do not smoke and a 20-fold increased risk in people who smoke heavily. That risk increased with the duration of smoking and decreased with smoking cessation [7, 8]. The report became "a landmark first step to diminishing the impact of tobacco use on the health of the American people;" it was so monumental that it was released on a Saturday to diminish its effects on the stock market and was a lead story in many newspapers, radio, and television broadcasts in the US and worldwide [8, 9]. The widespread distribution of the US Surgeon General's report resulted in a significant increase in public awareness of the role of smoking in the development of lung cancer [8, 9].

Despite the increased awareness of tobacco smoking as a cause of lung cancer, lung cancer remains the second most common cancer in men and women in the US, and a leading cause of cancer deaths worldwide, especially in developing countries [10].

Advances in diagnosis, staging, and treatment of lung cancer have led to improved survival in the US. Siegel et al. describe a decline in the incidence of advanced-stage lung cancer and improved median survival from 8 to 13 months between 2015 and 2017 and an increase in the percentage of people living at least 3 years after a lung cancer diagnosis from 19% in 2001 to 31% through 2017 [10]. Howlader et al. describe an increase in lung cancer-specific survival in men from 26% to 35% between 2001 and 2015, respectively [11]. These improvements correlate with the approval of targeted therapies [11].

Early detection of lung cancer through screening had been fraught with challenges for decades. The National Lung Screening Trial (NLST) was a landmark study published in 2011 that demonstrated a 20% relative reduction in lung cancer mortality with low-dose computed tomography [12], leading to a 2013 update in the United States Preventive Services Task Force (USPSTF) lung cancer screening guidelines with a favorable Grade B recommendation [13]. The mortality benefit of lung cancer screening is due to a significant shift to earlier-stage diagnosis [14]. Modeling studies demonstrated that expanding eligibility for LCS to include a lower smoke exposure and broader age range demonstrated improved eligibility and benefit than the screening criteria recommended in 2013. This led to a revision of the USPSTF lung cancer screening eligibility criteria in 2021 [15, 16]. The revised criteria specifically benefit women and patients identifying as Black, Hispanic, and American Indian/Native Alaskan who may have an increased risk of lung cancer at a younger age, despite lower exposures to tobacco smoke [16].

Advances in imaging and diagnostic techniques, including positron emission tomography (PET) with fluorodeoxyglucose, endobronchial ultrasound, and peripheral navigational bronchoscopy, have transformed the approach to lung cancer diagnosis and mediastinal staging. Moreover, standardization and global implementation of tumor, node, metastasis (TNM) staging have allowed for better prognostication in non-small cell lung cancer (NSCLC) [17, 18].

A meta-analysis published in 1995 demonstrated that systemic treatment with doublet platinum-based chemotherapy had a 10% improvement in 1-year survival compared to supportive care [19]. This landmark study transformed treatment for lung cancer. It led to modern interest in studying lung cancer therapies, the development of new chemotherapeutic agents, and their use as adjuvant therapy with surgery for NSCLC. In the last two decades, advances in molecular diagnostics, which allow for identification of specific genomic and immune checkpoint targets for delivery of precision therapies, revolutionized lung cancer treatment and significantly improved survival. Future innovations focus on additional molecular targets and biomarkers that may allow diagnosing and identifying molecular targets through less invasive testing. Additionally, advances in minimally invasive surgical techniques and stereotactic body radiation therapy have decreased surgical morbidity and allowed nonsurgical therapy of early-stage lung cancers in patients ineligible for surgical resection, respectively [19].

As lung cancer diagnoses occur at earlier stages, patients are receiving treatment and surviving longer, with over 650,000 people living in the US estimated to have a history of lung cancer [20]. This patient population has unique health concerns due to the sometimes-lasting effects of lung cancer therapies. Further research is needed to discover the best way to care for patients who have survived lung cancer.

Providing a text inclusive of all innovations in lung cancer care from the early twentieth century to now would be overwhelming. *Lung Cancer: A Comprehensive Guide for the Clinician* presents a comprehensive review of the most applicable developments and information on guideline-based care across the continuum of lung cancer, written for the busy clinician. The volume begins with a discussion of the US and global epidemiology of lung cancer, including incidence rates and risk factors. Further discussions include updated information on tobacco prevalence and treatment and lung cancer screening, diagnosis, and staging. Therapeutics are discussed based on lung cancer stage and include therapies for early-stage (I–II), stage III, and stage IV non-small cell lung cancer with separate chapters on small cell lung cancer and management of malignant pleural effusions. Comprehensive information on pulmonary complications of lung cancer treatment is included as this is an integral part of lung cancer care for pulmonologists, particularly as our therapies expand and newer agents are developed. Finally, a review of multidisciplinary care and physiologic assessment are provided as these are critical components in the care of patients with lung cancer.

In editing this text, we applaud the efforts of the authors to provide the most updated information available at the time of publication. We hope this comprehensive volume encourages you to expand your knowledge further as diagnostic and therapeutic options evolve and you provide the best care possible for your patients.

References

1. Adler I. Primary malignant growths of the lungs and bronchi. New York, NY: Longmans, Green, and Company; 1912.
2. Lickint F. Tabak and Tabakrauch als aetiologischer Faktor des Carcinoms. [Tobacco and tobacco smoke as etiological factors for cancer]. Z Krebsforch 1929;30:349–65.
3. Doll R, Hill AB. Smoking and carcinoma of the lung; preliminary report. Br Med J. 1950;2:739–48.
4. Wynder EL, Graham EA. Tobacco smoking as a possible etiologic factor in bronchogenic carcinoma; a study of 684 proved cases. J Am Med Assoc. 1950;143:329–36.
5. Garfinkel L. Selection, follow up and analysis in the American Cancer Society prospective studies. Natl Cancer Inst Monogr. 1985;67:49–52.
6. American Cancer Society. History of the cancer prevention studies. n.d. https://www.cancer.org/research/population-science/cancer-prevention-and-survivorship-research-team/acs-cancer-prevention-studies/history-cancer-prevention-study.html. Accessed 8 Apr 2023.
7. Smoking and Health. United States Surgeon General's Advisory Committee on Smoking and Health. United States Public Health Service Office of the Surgeon General. 1964.
8. Centers for Disease Control and Prevention Office on Smoking and Health, National Center for Chronic Disease Prevention and Health Promotion. Surgeon general's reports on smoking and tobacco use. 2022. https://www.cdc.gov/tobacco/sgr/index.htm#:~:text=The%20first%20report%20of%20tth,health%20of%20the%20American%20people. Accessed 8 Apr 2023.
9. National Library of Medicine. Profiles in science: the 1964 Report on smoking and health. n.d. https://profiles.nlm.nih.gov/spotlight/nn/feature/smoking#. Accessed 8 Apr 2023.
10. Siegel RL, Miller KD, Fuchs HE, Jemal A. Cancer statistics 2022. CA Cancer J Clin. 2022;72(1):7–33.

11. Howlader N, Jorjaz G, Mooradian MJ, Meza R, Kong CY, et al. The effect of advance sin lung cancer treatment on population mortality. N Engl J Med. 2020;383(7):640–9.
12. Aberle DR, Adams AM, Berg CD, Black WC, Clapp JD, Fagerstrom RM, et al. Reduced lung cancer mortality with low-dose computed tomographic screening. N Engl J Med. 2011;365(5):395–409.
13. United States Preventive Services Task Force. Final recommendation statement lung cancer screening: United States Preventative Services Task Force. 2013. https://www.uspreventiveservicestaskforce.org/uspstf/recommendation/lung-cancer-screening-december-2013. Accessed 8 Sep 2022.
14. Passiglia F, Cinquini M, Bertolaccini L, et al. Benefits and harms of lung cancer screening by chest computed tomography: a systematic review and meta-analysis. J Clin Oncol. 2021;39(23):2574–85.
15. United States Preventive Services Task Force. Final recommendation statement lung cancer screening: United States Preventive Services Task Force. 2021. https://www.uspreventiveservicestaskforce.org/uspstf/recommendation/lung-cancer-screening#fullrecommendationstart. Accessed 8 Apr 2023.
16. Meza R, Jeon J, Toumazis I, ten Haaf K, et al. Evaluation of the benefits and harms of lung cancer screening with low-dose computed tomography: modeling study for the US Preventive Services Task Force. JAMA. 2021;325(10):988–97.
17. Detterbeck FC. The eighth edition TNM stage classification for lung cancer: what does it mean on main street? J Thorac Cardiovasc Surg. 2018;155(1):356–9.
18. Detterbeck F, Boffa D, Kim A, Tanoue L. The eighth edition lung cancer stage classification. Chest. 2017;151(1):193–203.
19. Chemotherapy in non-small cell lung cancer: a meta-analysis using updated data on individual patients from 52 randomized clinical trials. BMJ. 1995;311:899–909.
20. Miller KD, Nogueira L, Devasia T, Mariotto AB, Yabroff KR, Jemal A, et al. Cancer treatment and survivorship statistics 2022. CA Cancer J Clin. 2022;72(5):409–36.

Chapel Hill, NC, USA   Christina R. MacRosty
Rochester, NY, USA   M. Patricia Rivera

Contents

1 US and Global Epidemiology and Incidence Rates of Lung Cancer 1
Erin DeBiasi

2 Lung Cancer Screening 25
Christine M. Lambert and Abbie Begnaud

3 Tobacco Prevalence and Treatment 49
Joelle T. Fathi and Hasmeena Kathuria

4 Approach to Lung Nodules 71
Srikanth Vedachalam, Nichole T. Tanner, and Catherine R. Sears

5 Staging and Diagnosis of Lung Cancer 97
Ghosh Sohini, Marshall Tanya, and Baltaji Stephanie

6 Treatment of Early-Stage (Stage I and II) Non-Small Cell Lung Cancer 123
Panagiotis Tasoudis, Ashley A. Weiner, and Gita N. Mody

7 Treatment of Stage III Non-small Cell Lung Cancer 147
Shinsuke Kitazawa, Alexander Gregor, and Kazuhiro Yasufuku

8 Treatment of Stage IV Non-small Cell Lung Cancer 165
Thomas Yang Sun and Millie Das

9 Treatment of Small Cell Lung Cancer 187
Russell Hales and Khinh Ranh Voong

10 Management of Malignant Pleural Effusion 211
Benjamin DeMarco and Christina R. MacRosty

11 Pulmonary Complications of Lung Cancer Treatment 229
Kathleen A. McAvoy and Jennifer D. Possick

12 Multidisciplinary Approach to Lung Cancer Care 255
Thomas Bilfinger, Lee Ann Santore, and Barbara Nemesure

**13 Physiologic and Patient-Centered Considerations in Lung Cancer
Care** 277
Duc M. Ha

Index 297

Contributors

Abbie Begnaud Medicine, University of Minnesota Twin Cities, Minneapolis, MN, USA

Thomas Bilfinger Renaissance School of Medicine, Stony Brook University, Stony Brook, NY, USA

Stony Brook Chest Clinic, Stony Brook University Hospital, Stony Brook, NY, USA

Department of Surgery, Stony Brook University, Stony Brook, NY, USA

Millie Das Division of Oncology, Department of Medicine, Stanford University School of Medicine, Palo Alto, CA, USA

Department of Medicine, Veteran Affairs Palo Alto Healthcare System, Palo Alto, CA, USA

Erin DeBiasi Section of Pulmonary, Critical Care, and Sleep Medicine, Department of Internal Medicine, Yale University School of Medicine, New Haven, CT, USA

Benjamin DeMarco Division of Pulmonary and Critical Care Medicine, Johns Hopkins University, Baltimore, United States

Joelle T. Fathi Department of Biobehavioral Nursing and Health Informatics, University of Washington School of Nursing, Seattle, WA, USA

Alexander Gregor Division of Thoracic Surgery, Department of Surgery, Toronto General Hospital, University Health Network, Toronto, ON, Canada

Duc M. Ha Section of Pulmonary and Critical Care, Rocky Mountain Regional Veterans Affairs Medical Center, Aurora, CO, USA

Division of Pulmonary Sciences and Critical Care Medicine, University of Colorado Anschutz Medical Campus, Aurora, CO, USA

Russell Hales Johns Hopkins School of Medicine, Baltimore, MD, USA

Hasmeena Kathuria The Pulmonary Center, Boston University Chobanian and Avedisian School of Medicine, Boston, MA, USA

Shinsuke Kitazawa Division of Thoracic Surgery, Department of Surgery, Toronto General Hospital, University Health Network, Toronto, ON, Canada

Christine M. Lambert Medicine, University of Minnesota Twin Cities, Minneapolis, MN, USA

Christina R. MacRosty Division of Pulmonary Diseases and Critical Care Medicine, University of North Carolina, Chapel Hill, NC, USA

Kathleen A. McAvoy Section of Pulmonary, Critical Care, and Sleep Medicine, Yale School of Medicine, New Haven, CT, USA

Gita N. Mody Division of Cardiothoracic Surgery, Department of Surgery, University of North Carolina at Chapel Hill, Chapel Hill, NC, USA

Barbara Nemesure Renaissance School of Medicine, Stony Brook University, Stony Brook, NY, USA

Stony Brook Chest Clinic, Stony Brook University Hospital, Stony Brook, NY, USA

Department of Family, Population and Preventive, Medicine, Stony Brook University, Stony Brook, NY, USA

Jennifer D. Possick Section of Pulmonary, Critical Care, and Sleep Medicine, Yale School of Medicine, New Haven, CT, USA

Lee Ann Santore Renaissance School of Medicine, Stony Brook University, Stony Brook, NY, USA

Catherine R. Sears Division of Pulmonary, Critical Care, Sleep and Occupational Medicine, Indiana University School of Medicine, Indianapolis, IN, USA

Pulmonary/Pulmonary Oncology, Richard L. Roudebush VA Medical Center, Indianapolis, IN, USA

Ghosh Sohini Department of Pulmonary and Critical Care, Allegheny Health Network, Pittsburgh, PA, USA

Baltaji Stephanie Department of Pulmonary Disease and Critical Care, Virginia Commonwealth University, Richmond, VA, USA

Thomas Yang Sun Division of Oncology, Department of Medicine, Stanford University School of Medicine, Palo Alto, CA, USA

Nichole T. Tanner Division of Pulmonary, Department of Medicine, Critical Care, Allergy, and Sleep Medicine, Medical University of South Carolina, Charleston, SC, USA

Health Equity and Rural Outreach Innovation Center (HEROIC), Ralph H. Johnson Veterans Affairs Hospital, Charleston, SC, USA

Marshall Tanya Department of Pulmonary and Critical Care, Allegheny Health Network, Pittsburgh, PA, USA

Panagiotis Tasoudis Division of Cardiothoracic Surgery, Department of Surgery, University of North Carolina at Chapel Hill, Chapel Hill, NC, USA

Srikanth Vedachalam Division of Pulmonary, Critical Care, Sleep and Occupational Medicine, Indiana University School of Medicine, Indianapolis, IN, USA

Khinh Ranh Voong Johns Hopkins School of Medicine, Baltimore, MD, USA

Ashley A. Weiner Department of Radiation Oncology, University of North Carolina at Chapel Hill, Chapel Hill, NC, USA

Kazuhiro Yasufuku Division of Thoracic Surgery, Department of Surgery, Toronto General Hospital, University Health Network, Toronto, ON, Canada

Chapter 1
US and Global Epidemiology and Incidence Rates of Lung Cancer

Erin DeBiasi

Introduction

The global incidence of lung cancer in 2020 was 2.2 million cases [1]. It is the second most common cause of cancer, accounting for 11% of all cancer cases, and the most common cause of cancer-related death [1]. There were 1.8 million deaths from lung cancer in 2020, accounting for 18% of all cancer mortality [1].

The incidence and mortality of lung cancer mirror each other closely, with a reported mortality incidence ratio of 0.85. The 5-year survival rate is low, most recently 23% in the USA, but lower in low-income countries [2, 3]. For example, the 5-year survival is less than 10% in Brazil, Bulgaria, India, and Thailand. Relative to other malignancies, this is quite low [4]. The impact of lung cancer is severe, leading to 40 million disability-adjusted life years, 99% of which were due to years of life lost [5]. Lung cancer is consistently the number one type of malignancy with the highest years of life lost.

Globally, the overall number of lung cancer cases is still rising. Over 10 years, from 2007 to 2017, there was a 37% increase in cases [5]. However, the incidence rates for advanced disease over the past decade have steeply declined (6.5% annually) with a concurrent rise (4.5% annually) in incidence rates of localized disease, likely due to screening methods [4]. Higher incidence of localized lung cancer has led to an increase in 3-year survival rates from 21% to 31% (2004–2018). Overall in the USA, the incidence rate is declining, 3% annually in males and 1% annually in females.

E. DeBiasi (✉)
Section of Pulmonary, Critical Care, and Sleep Medicine, Department of Internal Medicine, Yale University School of Medicine, New Haven, CT, USA
e-mail: Erin.debiasi@yale.edu

© The Author(s), under exclusive license to Springer Nature Switzerland AG 2023
C. MacRosty, M. P. Rivera (eds.), *Lung Cancer*, Respiratory Medicine,
https://doi.org/10.1007/978-3-031-38412-7_1

Influential Factors of Lung Cancer Incidence

Several factors affect the incidence rate in specific populations, including age, sex, socioeconomic background, and tobacco use.

Age

Increasing DNA damage over time and shortened telomeres lead to an increase in the incidence of cancers with age. In both males and females, the median age of lung cancer diagnosis is 70 [6]. In the USA, the probability of developing lung cancer is highest in males above age 70 (1 in 17) with successively lower probability in lower age ranges (1 in 169 for ages 50–59 and 1 in 59 for ages 60–69) [4]. Figures are slightly lower in US females. Younger patients diagnosed with non-small cell lung cancer (NSCLC) are more likely to be female and/or non-white [7]. Tumors tend to be adenocarcinoma and present with larger, later-stage disease. However, younger patients are more likely to undergo treatment with an overall improved survival due to relatively less comorbid conditions than similarly staged older patients.

Sex

Globally, lung cancer remains the second most common cancer in females, following breast cancer and the second most common cause of cancer death in females [1]. The incidence in females compared to males had a later uptrend in case rates following a delayed uptake of tobacco use comparatively [8].

In a recent analysis of a Statistics, Epidemiology, and End Results database of over 450,000 lung cancer cases in the USA, the disease remains disproportionally higher in males versus females (74 per 100,000 in males versus 52 per 100,000 in females) at all disease stages [9], and males are still more likely to be diagnosed with late-stage 3–4 lung cancer [9]. However, the incidence gap is successively getting smaller. In the USA, lung cancer rates in females are falling after a peak in the late 1990s, but at a much slower pace than in males (Fig. 1.1a) [4]. In addition, in the USA and several other countries, there has been a notable increase in the female-to-male incidence rates in successively lower birth cohorts [10, 11]. Outside of the USA, sex-related incidence rates vary widely based on geographic region (Fig. 1.2). For example, the male-to-female ratio is 1.2 in Northern America but 5.6 in Northern Africa [1].

While lung cancer deaths continue to decline in both sexes, the decline is less precipitously in females versus males (Fig. 1.1b). Comparative modeling predicts lung cancer deaths will be higher in females than males by 2045 [12].

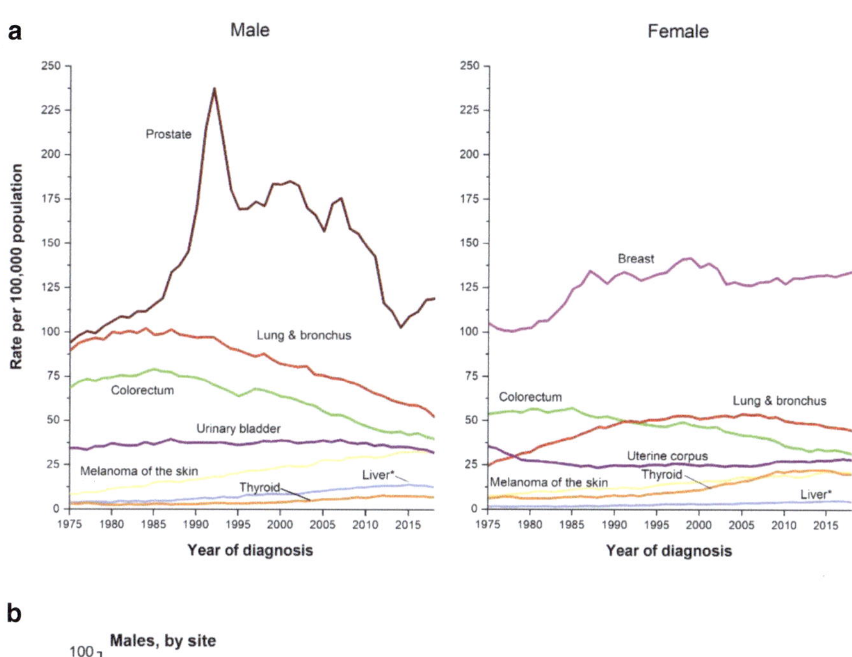

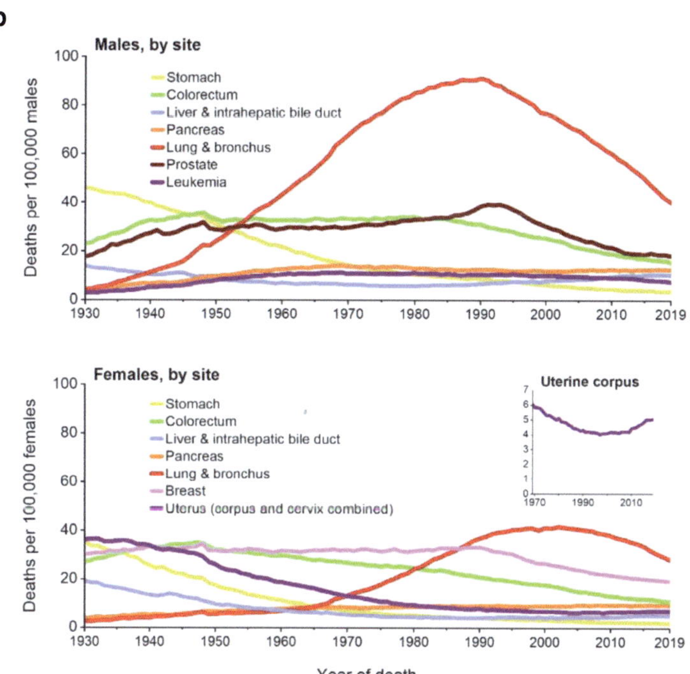

Fig. 1.1 (**a**) Trends in incidence of cancer by sex in the USA 1975–2018. (**b**) Trends in mortality rate of cancer by sex in the USA 1930–2019. (Reproduced with permission from Siegel RL, 2022)

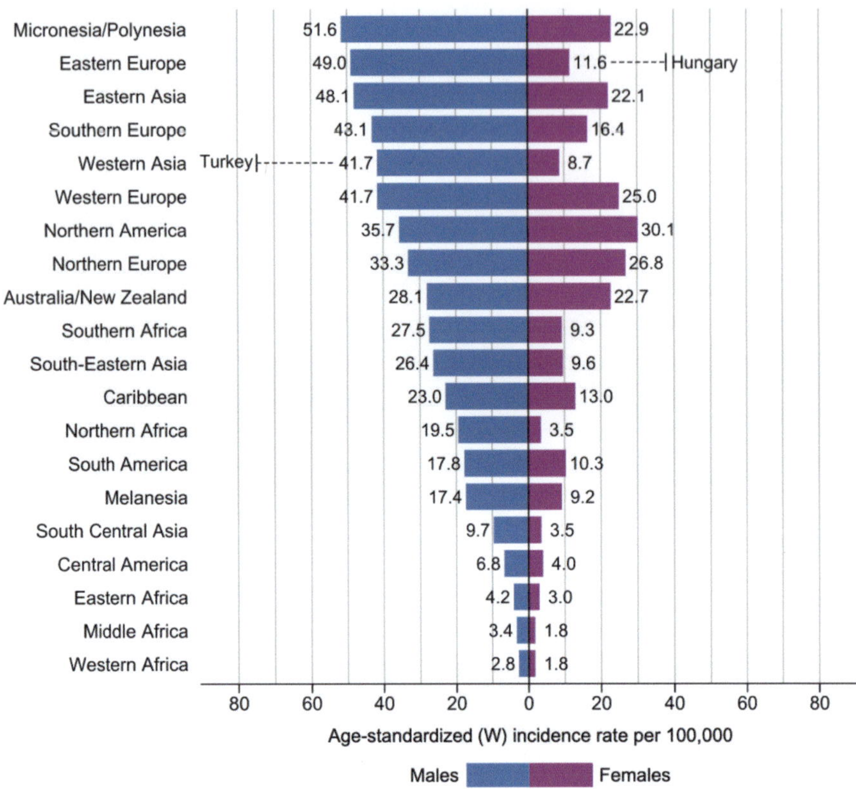

Fig. 1.2 Geographic variation in the age-standardized rates of lung cancer in males and females in 2020. (Reproduced with permission from Sung, H 2021)

Tobacco Use

As discussed above, it is expected that global trends in lung cancer incidence and death will change over time, mostly driven by trends in tobacco use. Over 80% of tobacco users currently reside in low-income countries [13]. However, tobacco use was initially highest in high-income countries such as the USA and UK, which in parallel developed a high incidence of lung cancer [14]. Subsequently, the decline in tobacco use in high-income countries has led to a decline in lung cancer deaths [15]. Tobacco smoking prevalence remains positively associated with age-adjusted incidence and mortality rates due to lung cancer [16]. Sex-specific differences in tobacco use account for a continued rise in incidence among women in many countries [17].

Socioeconomic Factors

The sociodemographic index (SDI) and human development index (HDI) can be used to stratify the global disease burden. The SDI is a composite indicator of gross national income per capita, educational attainment, and total fertility rate, whereas the HDI also incorporates life expectancy at birth. Regarding the incidence of lung cancer, it was highest in men (1 in 13), in high-middle SDI countries; highest in women (1 in 28), in high SDI countries; and lowest in men and women (1 in 45 and 1 in 142, respectively), in low SDI countries [5]. Overall, lung cancer rates are three to four times higher in high HDI countries compared to low [1]. Specifically, the rates are highest in men in Micronesia/Polynesia, Eastern and Southern Europe, and Eastern and Western Asia. In women, the highest rates are observed in Northern America, Northern and Western Europe, Micronesia/Polynesia, and Australia/New Zealand. There is a bivariate association between mortality—to—incidence ratio (MIR) and HDI; countries with higher HDI (more developed) have lower MIR (higher 5-year survival rates) [16].

Smoking-Related Risk Factors

Cigarette Smoking

In the USA, 80% to 90% of all lung cancers are caused by cigarette smoking [18, 19]. A higher proportion of lung cancer is associated with smoking in males than females. The proportion of lung cancer associated with smoking is gradually decreasing in locations where tobacco use is becoming less common; however, 72% of women and 81% of men with newly diagnosed lung cancers aged 20–49 years have a smoking history [19]. The cumulative risk of lung cancer is high in individuals who smoke up to 16% by the age of 75 years and 30% by 85 years in those with a heavy smoking history [20, 21]. This is compared to an average lifetime risk of 1% in individuals who have never smoked.

Before the twentieth century, lung cancer was rare, with only 140 published reports by 1900 [22]. However, cigarettes gained popularity at the beginning of the twentieth century due to mass production and marketing.

Tobacco smoke was first linked to lung cancer in 1912 when Issac Adler noted a marked increase of tumors in the lung and postulated that this may be due to the abuse of tobacco [23]. This theory, however, was not fully elucidated until the mid-1900s when evidence from population studies, animal experiments, cellular pathology, and the discovery of carcinogens in tobacco smoke provided additional evidence. In 1939, Franz Hermann Müller published a case-control study identifying a significantly higher rate of cancer in tobacco user [24]. Several other observational studies were published in Germany, the UK, and the USA. In 1954, Doll and Hill reported their findings regarding the incidence of lung cancer among 3093 male doctors in the UK stratified by their smoking habits [25]. Those who smoked more than 35 cigarettes/day were found to be 40 times more likely to die from lung cancer. In the same year, similar findings were confirmed in a cohort of 187,766 men in the USA, making the association between smoking and lung cancer indisputable [26]. Additionally, research regarding the changes induced in the lungs at a cellular level provided mechanistic explanations for the association of tobacco smoke and cancer; cigarette smoke caused ciliastasis and cilia cell death leading to further concentration of the carcinogenic substances within the lungs [27]. Concurrently, experiments were underway demonstrating the carcinogenesis induced by tobacco smoke and tar in animal models [28, 29]. Polycyclic aromatic hydrocarbons in coal tar had previously been identified as carcinogenic and were soon identified in tobacco smoke [30]. Soon thereafter, several dozen carcinogens were identified in cigarette smoke. In 1954, the American Cancer Society's Board of Directors announced that tobacco smoke unequivocally led to lung cancer, which was recognized by the US Surgeon General in 1964.

Smoking is still quite prevalent globally despite 70 years since tobacco smoke was implicated with lung cancer. Tobacco smoking prevalence was still 21.6% worldwide in 2016 [16]. An estimated 1.1 billion people over the age of 15 are currently smoking [13]. There is geographic variation, with tobacco smoking being more prevalent in European countries (Fig. 1.3). Five of the top ten countries with the highest smoking prevalence are in Europe. The peak of the tobacco epidemic in the USA was in the 1950s to 1960s when approximately half of the adult males smoked cigarettes, which has decreased since then (Fig. 1.4). In 2020, 12.5% of

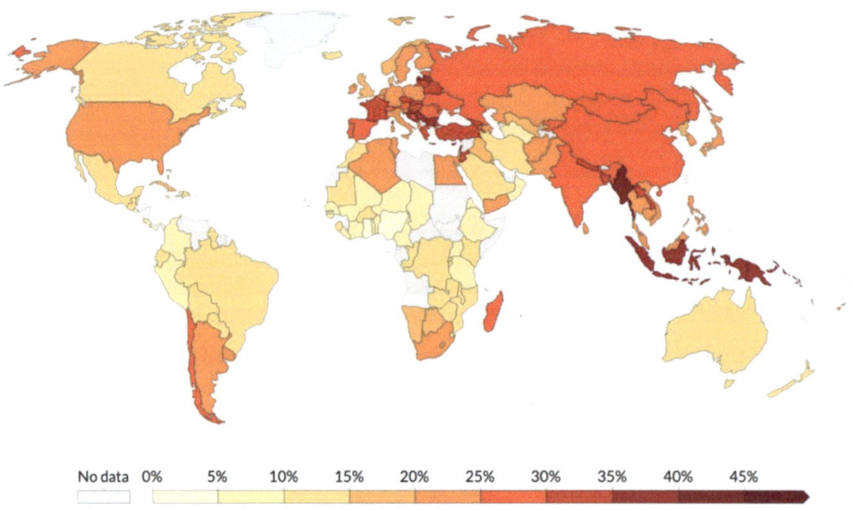

Fig. 1.3 Tobacco smoking prevalence (percent) globally in 2020 per World Health Organization Data. (Figure reproduced from Hannah Ritchie and Max Roser (2013)—"Smoking." Published online at OurWorldInData.org. Retrieved from: https://ourworldindata.org/smoking [Online Resource])

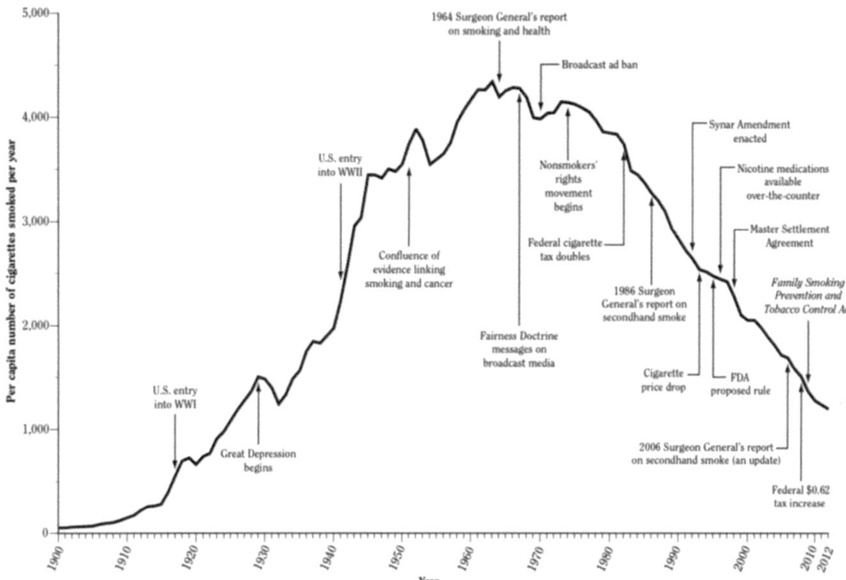

Fig. 1.4 Timeline of cigarette use in the USA. (Reproduced from US Department of Health and Human Services, The Health Consequences of Smoking-50 Years of Progress: a report of the Surgeon General, Centers for Disease Control and Prevention, National Center for Chronic Disease Prevention and Health Promotion, and Office of Smoking and Health)

adults over 18 (30.8 million people) smoked [31]. This figure is substantially less than in 2005 when 21% of American adults were currently smoking cigarettes. Tobacco use remains higher in males (14% compared to 11% of US females) and among American Indian/Alaska Natives (27%).

Secondhand Smoke

Exposure to carcinogens from burning tobacco products can also occur indirectly through secondhand smoke (SHS) or sidestream smoke. Shortly after discovering the carcinogenic properties of personal tobacco use, the effect of SHS was studied. Although exposure to the carcinogens in SHS is typically less concentrated, exposure can begin young in childhood, creating a more significant overall lifetime exposure. In the 1960s, it was demonstrated that the children of individuals who smoke were sick, primarily with respiratory illnesses, more often than those of individuals who did not smoke [32]. Later, in the 1980s, it was noted that the nonsmoking wives of heavy individuals who smoke had a higher incidence of lung cancer [33]. In 1986, SHS was recognized as a cause of lung cancer [34]. Serum cotinine can detect recent nicotine exposure and, in individuals that do not smoke, can be used as a marker of SHS exposure. From 1988 to 2014, exposure to SHS declined from 87.5% of the nonsmoking population in the USA to 25.2% but plateaued at this level (Fig. 1.5) [35]. Highest levels of exposure were seen in children aged 3–11, non-Hispanic blacks, those living in poverty and/or with someone who smoked inside the home. In 2006, the US Surgeon General released a report entitled "The Health Consequences of Involuntary Exposure to Tobacco Smoke" [36]. In this report, it was noted that despite efforts to control exposure to SHS, 43% of individuals that do not smoke still had detectable levels of cotinine, and more than 60% of children aged 3–11 were exposed to SHS. Adverse events related to SHS exposure in children and adults were noted, including development of lung cancer. Overall, 2.7% of lung cancers can be attributed to secondhand smoke [18]. Individuals that do not smoke who are exposed to SHS at home or work increase their risk of developing lung cancer by 20–30%. Compared to individuals that do not smoke not exposed to SHS, people exposed to SHS had an odds ratio of developing lung cancer of 1.31 (95% confidence interval (CI), 1.17–1.45) [37]. A recent study investigated the in utero effects of smoking and the impact on SHS during childhood in a cohort of 432,831 participants [38]. The incidence of lung cancer was significantly increased in those exposed to tobacco earlier in life (adjusted HRs for adulthood, adolescence, and childhood (vs. never tobacco users) were 6.10 (5.25–7.09), 9.56 (8.31–11.00), and 15.15 (12.90–17.79)). Additionally, compared with participants without in utero exposure, those with in utero exposure had a higher risk of both incidence of lung cancer (HR: 1.59, 95% CI, 1.44–1.76, $p < 0.001$) as well as lung cancer mortality (HR: 1.70, 95% CI, 1.54–1.87, $p < 0.001$).

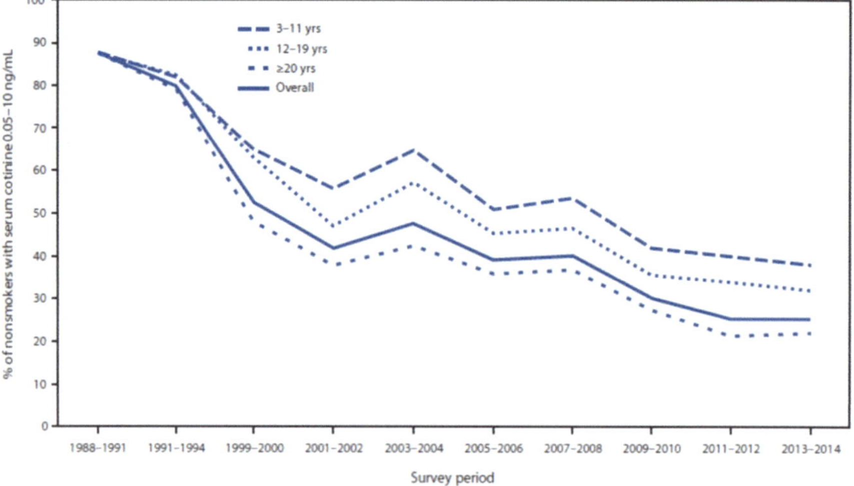

* Nonsmokers aged ≥4 years for NHANES III 1988–1994.

Fig. 1.5 Percentage of individuals that do not smoke in the USA over age 3 years with secondhand smoke exposure 21988–2014. (Reproduced from Tsai J, Homa DM, Gentzke AS, et al. Exposure to Secondhand Smoke Among Nonsmokers—United States, 1988–2014. MMWR Morb Mortal Wkly Rep 2018;67:1342–1346)

Due to the relative novelty, the effects from inhalation of secondhand vapors produced by e-electronic cigarettes (EC) are not yet well established.

Cigar Smoking

Cigar smoking and sales have increased over the past several decades due to taxation and regulation of cigarette sales and the perception that smoking cigars has fewer health consequences [39, 40]. Individuals who smoke cigars and cigarettes adjust their smoking habits by exposing themselves to similar amounts of nicotine and other components of mainstream smoke when smoking cigars [41]. However, cigar and pipe smoking increases the risk of developing lung cancer [42–45]. Exclusively smoking cigars and pipes is still associated with an increased risk of cancer-related mortality, although less compared to exclusively smoking cigarettes (HR, 1.61; 95% CI, 1.11–2.32; HR, 1.58; 95% CI, 1.05–2.38; and HR, 4.06; 95% CI, 3.84–4.29, respectively) [45]. Compared to those who do not smoke, the relative risk of lung cancer death, in particular, is high in those that smoke cigars (RR = 5.1; 95% CI 4.0–6.6) [44].

Cannabis Smoking

Frequent concomitant use of marijuana and cigarettes and the illegal status in many countries make directly studying the effects of marijuana on lung cancer risk challenging. Studies have shown a positive association between marijuana use and the development of lung cancer, especially in heavy users [46]. A meta-analysis of several studies demonstrated a biologic plausibility of lung cancer development in response to marijuana smoke but failed to identify an association between them [47].

Electronic Cigarette Smoking

Although initially designed as a harm-reduction product as an alternative to tobacco cigarettes, EC use has skyrocketed among prior nontobacco users, particularly the youth [48–51]. Containing a liquid mixture of nicotine and other flavorings dissolved in glycerin or propylene glycol, these devices produce vapor when heated. Given their relative novelty, longitudinal data regarding their safety is not yet known. However, in response to the increased use of EC as a "safer" alternative to tobacco cigarettes, the National Academies of Science, Engineering, and Medicine released a consensus statement in 2018 clearly delineating the health risks associated with EC use [52]. EC are known to contain both definite and probable carcinogens including nicotine derivatives, polycyclic aromatic hydrocarbons, heavy metals, aldehydes, and other complex organic compounds. Compared to individuals who smoke tobacco, EC users have lower levels of toxic and carcinogenic metabolites in their urine, although they are still detectable [53]. EC vapor has tumorigenic properties in the lungs of animal models [54]. Additionally, it causes DNA damage in both human and animal models [54, 55]. Ongoing, longitudinal epidemiologic studies will be needed to establish the relationship between EC use and lung cancer.

Smoking Cessation

Massive public health efforts have resulted in increasing rates of smoking cessation. Cessation of smoking results in significant lung cancer risk reduction [56–58], and sustained smoking cessation increasingly reduces the risk of lung cancer; men who quit at ages 60, 50, 40, and 30 had a cumulative risk of lung cancer by age 75 of 10%, 6%, 3%, and 2%, respectively [56]. A similar trend was noted in life expectancy after smoking cessation; those that quit smoking at age 25–34 years, 35–44 years, or 45–54 years gained about 10 years, 9 years, and 6 years of life, respectively [58]. Reductions in smoking also can result in a lower incidence of lung cancer in a dose-dependent manner [59]. Resumption of smoking following quitting, even at a lower amount, results in an increased risk of lung cancer compared to sustained quitting. However, the risk remains elevated compared to those that do not smoke [57].

Even after a diagnosis of lung cancer, smoking cessation is beneficial [60]. Ongoing smoking after a diagnosis of early-stage lung cancer can result in an increased risk of all-cause mortality (hazard ratio 2.94, 95% CI, 1.15–7.54), cancer recurrence (1.86, 95% CI, 1.01–3.41), and development of a second primary tumor (4.31, 95% CI, 1.09–16.98). Cessation after diagnosis of lung cancer resulted in increased adjusted median overall survival time compared to ongoing smoking (6.6 years vs. 4.8 years, respectively; $p = 0.001$), higher 5-year overall survival (60.6% vs. 48.6%; $p = 0.001$), and progression-free survival (54.4% vs. 43.8%; $p = 0.004$) [61]. Ongoing nicotine exposure in patients with established lung cancer can increase the incidence and progression of brain metastasis [62].

Never-Smoking

Approximately 25% of newly diagnosed lung cancer occurs in individuals who have never smoked, defined as having smoked less than 100 cigarettes in a lifetime, comprise approximately 25% of newly diagnosed lung cancer [63]. Overall, the proportion of patients with lung cancer, especially non-adenocarcinoma, that have never smoked is small [19, 64]. However, the proportion of individuals who have never smoked and are diagnosed with lung cancer is increasing, particularly in women [65, 66]. In some Asian countries, 60–80% of women with lung cancer have never smoked [63], while in the USA, women with lung cancer are much more likely to have never smoked compared with men, 19% versus 9%, respectively [67]. The highest incidence of nonsmoking-related lung cancers in the USA is among women aged 20–49 (28%) [19]. The incidence of lung cancer in individuals that have never smoked in the USA has increased from 8% in 1995 to 15% in 2013 and is independent of sex, stage at diagnosis, and ethnicity [66].

The predominant subtype of lung cancer in this group is adenocarcinoma, making up 50–60% of lung cancers. In contrast, approximately 6–8% of all cases of squamous cell carcinoma and 2.5% of small cell carcinoma are in individuals that have never smoked [68].

Driver mutations are more commonly found in lung adenocarcinomas in individuals who have never smoked. A recent study of a cohort of individuals who do not smoke with adenocarcinoma in the USA identified genetic alterations in tumors in 80% [69]. Additionally, approximately 7% of samples in individuals that never smoked had alterations in germline DNA repair genes similar to those that did smoke. Finally, several samples had genetic mutation signatures that indicated a response to passive exposure to cigarette smoke.

In the USA, epidermal growth factor receptor (EGFR) mutations are identified in approximately 40–60% of lung adenocarcinomas in individuals that never smoked, whereas this mutation is identified in only about 15% of total adenocarcinomas [70]. Low or no exposure to tobacco smoke is mainly associated with exon 19 and 21 mutations in the EGFR gene [71].

Anaplastic lymphoma kinase (ALK) mutations leading to fusion with echinoderm microtubule-associated protein-like 4 (EML4) are found in approximately 3–7% of patients with NSCLC [70]. This mutation is mutually exclusive with the EGFR and Kirsten rat sarcoma viral oncogene homolog (KRAS) mutations. Compared to both wild-type and those with EGFR mutations, ALK mutations are found more frequently in a younger population and in men [72]. Similar to those with EGFR mutations, ALK mutations are more commonly found in light and individuals that never smoked.

In contrast, the KRAS's driver mutations are found more commonly in former and active individuals that smoke [73, 74]. However, a distinct mutational profile is observed in individuals that do not smoke; a transition mutation (G → A) rather than a transversion mutation is noted in the nonsmoking population [74].

Nonsmoking-Related Risk Factors

Sex

Early studies suggested that women may be more susceptible to lung cancer due to smoking. Several have demonstrated that women tend to be diagnosed with lung cancer at relatively younger ages and with lower tobacco use [75–77]. However, other large studies have not demonstrated any increase in susceptibility to the carcinogenic effects of tobacco. In a large cohort study of over 460,000 Americans, there was no significant difference in the development of lung cancer in men and women with comparable smoking histories [78].

The rates of lung cancer in never-smoking women are higher than in men. Hormonal factors are postulated to be, at least in part, what drives these differences. There is differential expression of estrogen receptors in lung tissue individuals that do not smoke. Estrogen receptor-beta (ERB) expression in NSCLC specimens has a more favorable outcome than ER-alpha [79]. Higher rates of ERB expression have been noted in females who do not smoke compared to males [80].

Race

In the USA, there are notable racial disparities in the presenting stage and ultimate treatment regimens. According to the American Lung Association, white Americans are diagnosed with lung cancer in an early stage much more frequently than other racial minorities (25% compared to 21% black Americans, 21% Asian Americans, and 22% Latinos) [81]. Blacks and Latinos in America are also less likely than whites to undergo surgical treatment. The Latino group in America, in particular, is significantly less likely to undergo treatment (20% versus 15% of white Americans).

Diet and Supplements

Diet modifications and supplements have long been thought to play a preventative role in cancer development [82, 83]. However, in 2014, the US Preventive Services Task Force (USPSTF) recommended against the routine use of supplements, including beta-carotene and vitamin E, to prevent cancer [84]. This was primarily based on two large randomized placebo-controlled trials evaluating vitamin supplementation in high-risk lung cancer groups [85, 86]. In both the Alpha-Tocopherol Beta-Carotene Prevention and Carotene and Retinol Efficacy Trial of groups at high risk of lung cancer due to tobacco use or asbestos exposure, follow-up was terminated early due to excess cases of lung cancer and overall mortality in groups taking the supplements beta-carotene, vitamin E, and/or vitamin A. In post-intervention analysis, this increased risk persisted for several years following supplementation [87, 88]. A recent meta-analysis done by the USPSTF demonstrated an odds ratio of 1.2 (95% CI, 1.01–1.42) for lung cancer development associated with beta-carotene supplementation [89].

Weight

High body mass index (BMI) and obesity are associated with an increased risk of many cancers. Lung cancer risk, however, is inversely related to higher BMI. While it is challenging to differentiate the actual BMI effect from confounding factors such as tobacco use and preclinical wasting before an obvious manifestation of lung cancer, several studies demonstrate that low BMI is an independent risk factor for lung cancer [90, 91]. In a recent large cohort study, escalating BMI trajectories in adulthood led to reduced lung cancer risk [90]. This trend even applied when excluding patients who developed the disease during the first to fourth years of follow-up. In this study, several genetic foci involved in regulating cell growth, differentiation, and inflammation were identified and associated with these BMI trajectories, possibly identifying a causal relationship. In a study with a median follow-up of 20 years of over 770,000 individuals, the inverse relationship between BMI and lung cancer persisted after controlling variability in smoking [91].

Underlying Lung Disease

While the influence of benign lung diseases on lung cancer development is often confounded by concurrent tobacco, several underlying lung diseases are associated with an increased risk of lung cancer independent of smoking history. Chronic inflammation associated with various diseases creates a tumor-supporting microenvironment [92]. Additionally, activation of innate immunity and inflammation leads to the production of cytokines, which are critical for stimulating tumor growth [93].

One of the largest studies to evaluate the impact of underlying lung disease was performed with pooled analysis of 17 studies with 24,607 lung cancer cases and 81,829 controls in the International Lung Cancer Consortium [94]. Emphysema conferred the highest risk of lung cancer (relative risk (RR) = 2.44), followed by pneumonia (RR = 1.57), tuberculosis (RR = 1.48), and chronic bronchitis (RR = 1.47). In an analysis of individuals that never smoked, elevated risks were observed for emphysema (RR = 2.21), tuberculosis (RR = 1.50), and pneumonia (RR = 1.35) A dose-response relationship was noted as well, with an increasing number of underlying lung conditions being positively associated with a risk of lung cancer.

Several other studies confirmed that chronic obstructive pulmonary disease (COPD), including emphysema and chronic bronchitis, is positively associated with lung cancer and can be independent of smoking history [95–97]. In a cohort of 602 patients with lung cancer, 50% had COPD compared to 8% in a community control group [95]. In a 20-year prospective study of 448,600 individuals that do not smoke, the hazard ratio (HR) of lung cancer-related death was increased in those with emphysema or chronic bronchitis (2.44) [96]. Additionally, alpha(1)-antitrypsin deficiency carriers have up to a 70% higher risk of developing lung cancer than noncarriers [97]. Data from 18,473 individuals that smoke in the National Lung Screening Trial demonstrated that the severity of airflow obstruction had a linear relationship with lung cancer risk [98]. The exact mechanism by which increasing airflow limitation incurs a higher risk of lung cancer is unknown. However, it is felt that premalignant transformation, or epithelial-mesenchymal transition, is promoted by the excess of metalloproteinases and growth factors found in COPD. This is correlated with airflow limitation [99, 100].

Interstitial lung disease and idiopathic pulmonary fibrosis (IPF) are associated with increased lung cancer. In a meta-analysis, the incidence rate of lung cancer in IPF was 13% [101]. In a US population of patients with IPF, lung cancer was found to be 3.34-fold higher than in the general population [102]. In this population, cancer was more often found in the lower lobes (63% in IPF versus 26% in non-IPF) and was squamous histology. There was a significant increase in the risk of lung cancer over time in IPF patients (1.1% at 1 year, 8.7% at 3 years, 15.9% at 5 years, and 31.1% at 10 years) [103].

Bronchiectasis is also an independent risk factor for lung cancer. In a non-cystic fibrosis population, the incidence of lung cancer is significantly higher in patients with bronchiectasis (2.099 vs. 0.742 per 1000 person-years, $p < 0.001$) [104]. This difference is independent of smoking status (aHR = 1.28, 95% CI, 1.17–1.41 for individuals that never smoked; aHR = 1.26, 95% CI, 1.10–1.44 for individuals that ever smoked).

Significant inflammation associated with tuberculosis infections can lead to changes within the lung that can promote tumor growth [105]. In a cohort study in Taiwan, lung cancer incidence rate was 269 per 100,000 person-years in those with a history of tuberculosis compared to 153 per 100,000 person-years in those without [106]. The highest risk was in the years just following TB infection (incidence rate ratio (IRR) = 1.98 at 2–4 years), but the risk was persistently elevated 12 years following infection (IRR = 1.59).

Radiation Therapy

A history of prior radiation therapy for other primary cancers may lead to an increased risk of developing lung cancer. The most robust data is in those with a history of mediastinal radiation for Hodgkin's lymphoma or breast cancer. Particularly in individuals that use tobacco, the risk of developing lung cancer following chemo/radiotherapy for Hodgkin's lymphoma is 50–150 per 1000 within 10–20 years following treatment [107]. Compared to those not treated with radiation therapy, patients with breast cancer who underwent radiation therapy were significantly more likely to develop primary lung cancer (2.25% versus 0.23%) [108].

Familial Risk Factors

Several studies establish that a positive family history of lung cancer increases the risk for the disease, particularly among individuals that do not smoke [109, 110]. Both genetic and shared environmental factors may be responsible. A first-degree relative with a history of lung cancer before age 50 results in a significantly higher risk of lung cancer development in a nonsmoking population (OR 1.8, 95% CI, 1.0–3.2) [109]. Similar results were demonstrated in another study with a heterogeneous population of both those that smoke and do not smoke (OR 1.63, 95% CI 1.31–2.01) [110]. Risk was further increased with lung cancer history in more than one family member (OR 3.6, 95% CI, 1.56–8.31). This positive association resulted in the inclusion of family history of lung cancer in several lung cancer risk prediction models [111, 112].

Occupational and Environmental Factors

Many occupational and environmental exposures increase the risk of lung cancer. Radon and asbestos are the two most common and will be discussed in detail below. Still, others include arsenic, hard metal dust, beryllium, chloromethyl ether, chromium, formaldehyde, nickel, polycyclic aromatic hydrocarbons, and vinyl chloride. Concurrent tobacco use may compound the risk associated with exposures.

Asbestos

Asbestos is naturally occurring fibers that are composed of hydrated magnesium silicates. The two main types of fibers are serpentine (with the most common subtype being chrysotile) and amphibole. Serpentine fibers are the most common asbestos used commercially and are considered less toxic but can still be pathogenic [113, 114]. Asbestos exposure can cause various pulmonary diseases, including asbestosis, pleural disease, and malignancies—NSCLC, small cell lung cancer, and mesothelioma. Occupational exposure can occur in multiple ways, but most commonly, mining or milling of fibers and industrial applications, including textile, cement, shipbuilding, and insulation work. Nonoccupational exposure can occur via close contact with soiled clothing of an asbestos worker, renovation/demolition work in buildings containing asbestos, and environmental exposure. In the USA, the use of asbestos has been limited since the 1970s, with use limited to automotive brake pads and roofing products.

The most common parenchymal complication of asbestos exposure is development of asbestosis or a slowly progressive diffuse pulmonary fibrosis typically in the subpleural regions of the lower lobes. This is caused by the direct toxic effects of the fibers on the parenchyma and the release of inflammatory mediators.

Asbestos exposure is the leading occupational exposure associated with lung cancer risk accounting for up to 12% of lung cancer cases in men after adjusting for smoking status and diet [115]. In a cohort of American insulators, lung cancer was the cause of death in 19% [116]. Among individuals that do not smoke, lung cancer mortality was increased by asbestos exposure (rate ratio = 3.6) and asbestosis (rate ratio = 7.40). Cigarette smoking, in conjunction with asbestos exposure, can significantly increase the risk of lung cancer [116, 117]. In the above cohort, smoking was additive to the risk of lung cancer (rate ratio = 14.1). This risk was significantly increased in those with asbestosis (rate ratio = 36.8).

The risk of lung cancer associated with nonoccupational exposure to asbestos is debated. A study performed in a mining town in Canada judged to have an intermediate environmental exposure to asbestos showed no increased risk of lung cancer in women [118]. However, a recent study demonstrated an increased risk of lung cancer in those that live near a source of asbestos (risk estimate 1.48) [119].

Radon

Radon is a natural gas that is colorless and odorless. It results from the decay of naturally occurring uranium-238 in rock and soil. It damages the respiratory epithelium via alpha particles. Typically found in high concentrations in mines from the ore or water, it was first linked to lung cancer in miners, but it also can be found in high concentrations in the home. Radon enters homes as gas from the soil through cracks in the foundation. The association of radon with lung cancer was established in the 1960s in a mining population [120].

While concentrations in residential homes are typically less than that in mines, high concentrations can develop. Radon is the second leading cause of lung cancer in the USA, and 1 in every 15 homes in the USA has radon levels above the Environmental Protection Agency's recommended threshold [121]. The risk of lung cancer increases proportionally with the amount of residential radon, 11%, with each 100 Bq/m^3 increase [122]. In Europe, it is estimated that 2% of lung cancer deaths can be attributed to radon exposure [123].

Environmental Pollution

In approximately half of the world, unprocessed biomass fuels and coal are used for heating or cooking [124]. Emissions from indoor combustion of coal are carcinogenic to humans [125]. Emissions include polycyclic aromatic hydrocarbons (PAHs), methylated PAHs, and nitrogen-containing heterocyclic aromatic compounds [126]. These compounds and others can be found in high concentrations, especially in unvented areas. In a large cohort study of over 27,000 people in China, the absolute risk of death from lung cancer was 18–20% among users of smoky coal, compared to 0.5% among users of smokeless coal [127].

Ambient air pollution, especially particulate matter with high amounts of absorbed polycyclic aromatic hydrocarbons and other toxic chemicals, is associated with an increased risk of lung cancer [128]. In a large analysis of 17 European studies, the long-term effect of exposure to particulate matter in the air on lung cancer development was assessed [128]. With both exposure to particulate matter of aerodynamic diameters less than 10 μm and 2.5 μm (PM_{10} and $PM_{2.5}$, respectively), the hazard ratio for developing lung cancer, particularly adenocarcinoma, was increased in a combined cohort population of over 300,000 people. In the US population, for every 10 μg/m^3 increase in particulate air pollution, there was an 8% increase risk of lung cancer death [129]. Additionally, diesel motor exhaust can increase the risk of lung cancer in a dose-dependent manner [130].

Conclusion

While many factors may influence the development of lung cancer, tobacco use remains the primary etiology of lung cancer in the USA and globally. While lung cancer prognosis is overall improving with earlier detection, lung cancer remains the leading cause of cancer death. In the USA, tobacco use and associated second-hand smoke exposure have dramatically decreased due to successful public health efforts; however, tobacco use remains high globally. Nontobacco smoking is rising, particularly in the USA, where ECs are largely unregulated, and cannabis use is regionally legalized. The impact of this trend is yet to be realized.

References

1. Sung H, Ferlay J, Siegel RL, Laversanne M, Soerjomataram I, Jemal A, et al. Global cancer statistics 2020: GLOBOCAN estimates of incidence and mortality worldwide for 36 cancers in 185 countries. CA Cancer J Clin. 2021;71(3):209–49.
2. Allemani C, Matsuda T, Di Carlo V, Harewood R, Matz M, Niksic M, et al. Global surveillance of trends in cancer survival 2000-14 (CONCORD-3): analysis of individual records for 37 513 025 patients diagnosed with one of 18 cancers from 322 population-based registries in 71 countries. Lancet. 2018;391(10125):1023–75.
3. SEER. Cancer stat facts: lung and bronchus cancer. 2022. https://seer.cancer.gov/statfacts/html/lungb.html.
4. Siegel RL, Miller KD, Fuchs HE, Jemal A. Cancer statistics, 2022. CA Cancer J Clin. 2022;72(1):7–33.
5. Fitzmaurice C, Abate D, Abbasi N, Abbastabar H, Abd-Allah F, Abdel-Rahman O, et al. Global, regional, and national cancer incidence, mortality, years of life lost, years lived with disability, and disability-adjusted life-years for 29 cancer groups, 1990 to 2017: a systematic analysis for the global burden of disease study. JAMA Oncol. 2019;5(12):1749–68.

6. Torre LA, Siegel RL, Jemal A. Lung cancer statistics. Adv Exp Med Biol. 2016;893:1–19.
7. Arnold BN, Thomas DC, Rosen JE, Salazar MC, Blasberg JD, Boffa DJ, et al. Lung cancer in the very young: treatment and survival in the national cancer data base. J Thorac Oncol. 2016;11(7):1121–31.
8. Thomas L, Doyle LA, Edelman MJ. Lung cancer in women: emerging differences in epidemiology, biology, and therapy. Chest. 2005;128(1):370–81.
9. Tolwin Y, Gillis R, Peled N. Gender and lung cancer-SEER-based analysis. Ann Epidemiol. 2020;46:14–9.
10. Jemal A, Miller KD, Ma J, Siegel RL, Fedewa SA, Islami F, et al. Higher lung cancer incidence in young women than young men in the United States. N Engl J Med. 2018;378(21):1999–2009.
11. Fidler-Benaoudia MM, Torre LA, Bray F, Ferlay J, Jemal A. Lung cancer incidence in young women vs. young men: a systematic analysis in 40 countries. Int J Cancer. 2020;147(3):811–9.
12. Jeon J, Holford TR, Levy DT, Feuer EJ, Cao P, Tam J, et al. Smoking and lung cancer mortality in the united states from 2015 to 2065: a comparative modeling approach. Ann Intern Med. 2018;169(10):684–93.
13. WHO. Global report on trends in prevalence of tobacco use 2000–2025. Geneva: World Health Organization; 2019.
14. Parkin DM, Bray FI, Devesa SS. Cancer burden in the year 2000. The global picture. Eur J Cancer. 2001;37(Suppl 8):S4–66.
15. Devesa SS, Blot WJ, Fraumeni JF Jr. Declining lung cancer rates among young men and women in the United States: a cohort analysis. J Natl Cancer Inst. 1989;81(20):1568–71.
16. Sharma R. Mapping of global, regional and national incidence, mortality and mortality-to-incidence ratio of lung cancer in 2020 and 2050. Int J Clin Oncol. 2022;27(4):665–75.
17. Lortet-Tieulent J, Renteria E, Sharp L, Weiderpass E, Comber H, Baas P, et al. Convergence of decreasing male and increasing female incidence rates in major tobacco-related cancers in Europe in 1988-2010. Eur J Cancer. 2015;51(9):1144–63.
18. Islami F, Goding Sauer A, Miller KD, Siegel RL, Fedewa SA, Jacobs EJ, et al. Proportion and number of cancer cases and deaths attributable to potentially modifiable risk factors in the United States. CA Cancer J Clin. 2018;68(1):31–54.
19. Siegel DA, Fedewa SA, Henley SJ, Pollack LA, Jemal A. Proportion of never smokers among men and women with lung cancer in 7 US States. JAMA Oncol. 2021;7(2):302–4.
20. Samet JM, Wiggins CL, Humble CG, Pathak DR. Cigarette smoking and lung cancer in New Mexico. Am Rev Respir Dis. 1988;137(5):1110–3.
21. Crispo A, Brennan P, Jockel KH, Schaffrath-Rosario A, Wichmann HE, Nyberg F, et al. The cumulative risk of lung cancer among current, ex- and never-smokers in European men. Br J Cancer. 2004;91(7):1280–6.
22. Proctor RN. The history of the discovery of the cigarette-lung cancer link: evidentiary traditions, corporate denial, global toll. Tob Control. 2012;21(2):87–91.
23. Adler I. Primary malignant growth of the lung and bronchi. New York, NY: Longman, Green, Company; 1912.
24. Müller FH. Tabakmissbrauch und lungencarcinom. Zeitschrift für Krebsforschung. 1940;49(1):57–85.
25. Doll R, Hill AB. The mortality of doctors in relation to their smoking habits; a preliminary report. Br Med J. 1954;1(4877):1451–5.
26. Hammond EC, Horn D. The relationship between human smoking habits and death rates: a follow-up study of 187,766 men. J Am Med Assoc. 1954;155(15):1316–28.
27. Hilding AC. On cigarette smoking, bronchial carcinoma and ciliary action. II. Experimental study on the filtering action of cow's lungs, the deposition of tar in the bronchial tree and removal by ciliary action. N Engl J Med. 1956;254(25):1155–60.
28. Wynder EL, Graham EA, Croninger AB. Experimental production of carcinoma with cigarette tar. Cancer Res. 1953;13(12):855–64.

29. Roffo AH. Durch Tabak beim Kaninchen entwickeltes Carcinom. Zeitschrift für Krebsforschung. 1931;33(1):321–32.
30. Roffo A. Krebserzeugendes benzpyren, gewonnen aus tabakteer. Zeitschrift für Krebsforschung. 1939;49(5):588–97.
31. Cornelius ME, Loretan CG, Wang TW, Jamal A, Homa DM. Tobacco product use among adults - United States, 2020. MMWR Morb Mortal Wkly Rep. 2022;71(11):397–405.
32. Cameron P, Kostin JS, Zaks JM, Wolfe JH, Tighe G, Oselett B, et al. The health of smokers' and nonsmokers' children. J Allergy. 1969;43(6):336–41.
33. Hirayama T. Non-smoking wives of heavy smokers have a higher risk of lung cancer: a study from Japan. Br Med J (Clin Res Ed). 1981;282(6259):183–5.
34. 1986 Surgeon General's report: the health consequences of involuntary smoking. MMWR Morb Mortal Wkly Rep. 1986;35(50):769–70.
35. Tsai J, Homa DM, Gentzke AS, Mahoney M, Sharapova SR, Sosnoff CS, et al. Exposure to secondhand smoke among nonsmokers - United States, 1988-2014. MMWR Morb Mortal Wkly Rep. 2018;67(48):1342–6.
36. US Department of Health and Human Services. The health consequences of involuntary exposure to tobacco smoke. Bethesda, MD: USDHHS; 2006.
37. Kim CH, Lee YC, Hung RJ, McNallan SR, Cote ML, Lim WY, et al. Exposure to secondhand tobacco smoke and lung cancer by histological type: a pooled analysis of the International Lung Cancer Consortium (ILCCO). Int J Cancer. 2014;135(8):1918–30.
38. He H, He MM, Wang H, Qiu W, Liu L, Long L, et al. In utero and childhood/adolescence exposure to tobacco smoke, genetic risk and lung cancer incidence and mortality in adulthood. Am J Respir Crit Care Med. 2022;207(2):173–82.
39. Agaku IT, Alpert HR. Trends in annual sales and current use of cigarettes, cigars, roll-your-own tobacco, pipes, and smokeless tobacco among US adults, 2002-2012. Tob Control. 2016;25(4):451–7.
40. Consumption of cigarettes and combustible tobacco--United States, 2000-2011. MMWR Morb Mortal Wkly Rep. 2012;61(30):565–9.
41. Rosenberry ZR, Pickworth WB, Koszowski B. Large cigars: smoking topography and toxicant exposure. Nicotine Tob Res. 2018;20(2):183–91.
42. Malhotra J, Borron C, Freedman ND, Abnet CC, van den Brandt PA, White E, et al. Association between cigar or pipe smoking and cancer risk in men: a pooled analysis of five cohort studies. Cancer Prev Res (Phila). 2017;10(12):704–9.
43. Baker F, Ainsworth SR, Dye JT, Crammer C, Thun MJ, Hoffmann D, et al. Health risks associated with cigar smoking. JAMA. 2000;284(6):735–40.
44. Shapiro JA, Jacobs EJ, Thun MJ. Cigar smoking in men and risk of death from tobacco-related cancers. J Natl Cancer Inst. 2000;92(4):333–7.
45. Christensen CH, Rostron B, Cosgrove C, Altekruse SF, Hartman AM, Gibson JT, et al. Association of cigarette, cigar, and pipe use with mortality risk in the US population. JAMA Intern Med. 2018;178(4):469–76.
46. Callaghan RC, Allebeck P, Sidorchuk A. Marijuana use and risk of lung cancer: a 40-year cohort study. Cancer Causes Control. 2013;24(10):1811–20.
47. Mehra R, Moore BA, Crothers K, Tetrault J, Fiellin DA. The association between marijuana smoking and lung cancer: a systematic review. Arch Intern Med. 2006;166(13):1359–67.
48. McMillen RC, Gottlieb MA, Shaefer RMW, Winickoff JP, Klein JD. Trends in electronic cigarette use among US adults: use is increasing in both smokers and nonsmokers. Nicotine Tob Res. 2014;17(10):1195–202.
49. Corey CG, Ambrose BK, Apelberg BJ, King BA. Flavored tobacco product use among middle and high school students—United States, 2014. Morb Mortal Wkly Rep. 2015;64(38):1066–70.
50. Singh T, Arrazola RA, Corey CG, Husten CG, Neff LJ, Homa DM, et al. Tobacco use among middle and high school students--United States, 2011-2015. MMWR Morb Mortal Wkly Rep. 2016;65(14):361–7.

51. Gentzke AS, Wang TW, Jamal A, Park-Lee E, Ren C, Cullen KA, et al. Tobacco product use among middle and high school students - United States, 2020. MMWR Morb Mortal Wkly Rep. 2020;69(50):1881–8.
52. National Academies of Sciences E, Medicine, Stratton K, Kwan LY, Eaton DL. Public health consequences of E-cigarettes. Washington, DC: The National Academies Press; 2018.
53. Hecht SS, Carmella SG, Kotandeniya D, Pillsbury ME, Chen M, Ransom BW, et al. Evaluation of toxicant and carcinogen metabolites in the urine of e-cigarette users versus cigarette smokers. Nicotine Tob Res. 2015;17(6):704–9.
54. Canistro D, Vivarelli F, Cirillo S, Babot Marquillas C, Buschini A, Lazzaretti M, et al. E-cigarettes induce toxicological effects that can raise the cancer risk. Sci Rep. 2017;7(1):2028.
55. Ganapathy V, Manyanga J, Brame L, McGuire D, Sadhasivam B, Floyd E, et al. Electronic cigarette aerosols suppress cellular antioxidant defenses and induce significant oxidative DNA damage. PLoS One. 2017;12(5):e0177780.
56. Peto R, Darby S, Deo H, Silcocks P, Whitley E, Doll R. Smoking, smoking cessation, and lung cancer in the UK since 1950: combination of national statistics with two case-control studies. BMJ. 2000;321(7257):323–9.
57. Newcomb PA, Carbone PP. The health consequences of smoking. Cancer Med Clin North Am. 1992;76(2):305–31.
58. Jha P, Ramasundarahettige C, Landsman V, Rostron B, Thun M, Anderson RN, et al. 21st-century hazards of smoking and benefits of cessation in the United States. N Engl J Med. 2013;368(4):341–50.
59. Yoo JE, Han K, Shin DW, Jung W, Kim D, Lee CM, et al. Effect of smoking reduction, cessation, and resumption on cancer risk: a nationwide cohort study. Cancer. 2022;128(11):2126–37.
60. Parsons A, Daley A, Begh R, Aveyard P. Influence of smoking cessation after diagnosis of early stage lung cancer on prognosis: systematic review of observational studies with meta-analysis. BMJ. 2010;340:b5569.
61. Sheikh M, Mukeriya A, Shangina O, Brennan P, Zaridze D. Postdiagnosis smoking cessation and reduced risk for lung cancer progression and mortality: a prospective cohort study. Ann Intern Med. 2021;174(9):1232–9.
62. Tyagi A, Wu SY, Sharma S, Wu K, Zhao D, Deshpande R, et al. Exosomal miR-4466 from nicotine-activated neutrophils promotes tumor cell stemness and metabolism in lung cancer metastasis. Oncogene. 2022;41(22):3079–92.
63. Sun S, Schiller JH, Gazdar AF. Lung cancer in never smokers--a different disease. Nat Rev Cancer. 2007;7(10):778–90.
64. Ou SH, Ziogas A, Zell JA. Prognostic factors for survival in extensive stage small cell lung cancer (ED-SCLC): the importance of smoking history, socioeconomic and marital statuses, and ethnicity. J Thorac Oncol. 2009;4(1):37–43.
65. Zeng Q, Vogtmann E, Jia MM, Parascandola M, Li JB, Wu YL, et al. Tobacco smoking and trends in histological subtypes of female lung cancer at the Cancer Hospital of the Chinese Academy of Medical Sciences over 13 years. Thorac Cancer. 2019;10(8):1717–24.
66. Pelosof L, Ahn C, Gao A, Horn L, Madrigales A, Cox J, et al. Proportion of never-smoker non-small cell lung cancer patients at three diverse institutions. J Natl Cancer Inst. 2017;109(7):djw295.
67. Wakelee HA, Chang ET, Gomez SL, Keegan TH, Feskanich D, Clarke CA, et al. Lung cancer incidence in never smokers. J Clin Oncol. 2007;25(5):472–8.
68. Centers for Disease Control and Prevention. Lung cancer among people who never smoked. 2021. https://www.cdc.gov/cancer/lung/nonsmokers/index.htm.
69. Devarakonda S, Li Y, Martins Rodrigues F, Sankararaman S, Kadara H, Goparaju C, et al. Genomic profiling of lung adenocarcinoma in never-smokers. J Clin Oncol. 2021;39(33):3747–58.
70. Johnson BE, Kris MG, Berry LD, Kwiatkowski DJ, Iafrate AJ, Varella-Garcia M, et al. A multicenter effort to identify driver mutations and employ targeted therapy in patients with

lung adenocarcinomas: The Lung Cancer Mutation Consortium (LCMC). J Clin Oncol. 2013;31(15_suppl):8019.
71. Lee YJ, Shim HS, Kang YA, Hong SJ, Kim HK, Kim H, et al. Dose effect of cigarette smoking on frequency and spectrum of epidermal growth factor receptor gene mutations in Korean patients with non-small cell lung cancer. J Cancer Res Clin Oncol. 2010;136(12):1937–44.
72. Shaw AT, Yeap BY, Mino-Kenudson M, Digumarthy SR, Costa DB, Heist RS, et al. Clinical features and outcome of patients with non-small-cell lung cancer who harbor EML4-ALK. J Clin Oncol Off J Am Soc Clin Oncol. 2009;27(26):4247–53.
73. Le Calvez F, Mukeria A, Hunt JD, Kelm O, Hung RJ, Tanière P, et al. TP53 and KRAS mutation load and types in lung cancers in relation to tobacco smoke: distinct patterns in never, former, and current smokers. Cancer Res. 2005;65(12):5076–83.
74. Riely GJ, Kris MG, Rosenbaum D, Marks J, Li A, Chitale DA, et al. Frequency and distinctive spectrum of KRAS mutations in never smokers with lung adenocarcinoma. Clin Cancer Res. 2008;14(18):5731–4.
75. Donington JS, Colson YL. Sex and gender differences in non-small cell lung cancer. Semin Thorac Cardiovasc Surg. 2011;23(2):137–45.
76. Hansen MS, Licaj I, Braaten T, Langhammer A, Le Marchand L, Gram IT. Sex differences in risk of smoking-associated lung cancer: results from a cohort of 600,000 Norwegians. Am J Epidemiol. 2018;187(5):971–81.
77. Powell HA, Iyen-Omofoman B, Hubbard RB, Baldwin DR, Tata LJ. The association between smoking quantity and lung cancer in men and women. Chest. 2013;143(1):123–9.
78. Freedman ND, Leitzmann MF, Hollenbeck AR, Schatzkin A, Abnet CC. Cigarette smoking and subsequent risk of lung cancer in men and women: analysis of a prospective cohort study. Lancet Oncol. 2008;9(7):649–56.
79. Wu CT, Chang YL, Shih JY, Lee YC. The significance of estrogen receptor beta in 301 surgically treated non-small cell lung cancers. J Thorac Cardiovasc Surg. 2005;130(4):979–86.
80. Schwartz AG, Prysak GM, Murphy V, Lonardo F, Pass H, Schwartz J, et al. Nuclear estrogen receptor beta in lung cancer: expression and survival differences by sex. Clin Cancer Res. 2005;11(20):7280–7.
81. American Lung Association. State of lung cancer, racial and ethnic disparities. Chicago, IL: American Lung Association; 2021. https://www.lung.org/research/state-of-lung-cancer/racial-and-ethnic-disparities.
82. Steinmetz KA, Potter JD. Vegetables, fruit, and cancer. I. Epidemiology. Cancer Causes Control. 1991;2(5):325–57.
83. Shekelle RB, Rossof AH, Stamler J. Dietary cholesterol and incidence of lung cancer: the Western Electric Study. Am J Epidemiol. 1991;134(5):480–4.
84. Moyer VA. Vitamin, mineral, and multivitamin supplements for the primary prevention of cardiovascular disease and cancer: U.S. Preventive services Task Force recommendation statement. Ann Intern Med. 2014;160(8):558–64.
85. Alpha-Tocopherol BCCPSG. The effect of vitamin E and beta carotene on the incidence of lung cancer and other cancers in male smokers. N Engl J Med. 1994;330(15):1029–35.
86. Omenn GS, Goodman GE, Thornquist MD, Balmes J, Cullen MR, Glass A, et al. Effects of a combination of beta carotene and vitamin A on lung cancer and cardiovascular disease. N Engl J Med. 1996;334(18):1150–5.
87. Goodman GE, Thornquist MD, Balmes J, Cullen MR, Meyskens FL Jr, Omenn GS, et al. The beta-carotene and retinol efficacy trial: incidence of lung cancer and cardiovascular disease mortality during 6-year follow-up after stopping beta-carotene and retinol supplements. J Natl Cancer Inst. 2004;96(23):1743–50.
88. Virtamo J, Pietinen P, Huttunen JK, Korhonen P, Malila N, Virtanen MJ, et al. Incidence of cancer and mortality following alpha-tocopherol and beta-carotene supplementation: a postintervention follow-up. JAMA. 2003;290(4):476–85.
89. O'Connor EA, Evans CV, Ivlev I, Rushkin MC, Thomas RG, Martin A, et al. Vitamin and mineral supplements for the primary prevention of cardiovascular disease and cancer:

updated evidence report and systematic review for the US Preventive Services Task Force. JAMA. 2022;327(23):2334–47.

90. You D, Wang D, Wu Y, Chen X, Shao F, Wei Y, et al. Associations of genetic risk, BMI trajectories, and the risk of non-small cell lung cancer: a population-based cohort study. BMC Med. 2022;20(1):203.

91. Wood AM, Jonsson H, Nagel G, Häggström C, Manjer J, Ulmer H, et al. The inverse association of body mass index with lung cancer: exploring residual confounding, metabolic aberrations and within-person variability in smoking. Cancer Epidemiol Biomark Prev. 2021;30(8):1489–97.

92. Coussens LM, Werb Z. Inflammation and cancer. Nature. 2002;420(6917):860–7.

93. Lin WW, Karin M. A cytokine-mediated link between innate immunity, inflammation, and cancer. J Clin Invest. 2007;117(5):1175–83.

94. Brenner DR, Boffetta P, Duell EJ, Bickeboller H, Rosenberger A, McCormack V, et al. Previous lung diseases and lung cancer risk: a pooled analysis from the International Lung Cancer Consortium. Am J Epidemiol. 2012;176(7):573–85.

95. Young RP, Hopkins RJ, Christmas T, Black PN, Metcalf P, Gamble GD. COPD prevalence is increased in lung cancer, independent of age, sex and smoking history. Eur Respir J. 2009;34(2):380–6.

96. Turner MC, Chen Y, Krewski D, Calle EE, Thun MJ. Chronic obstructive pulmonary disease is associated with lung cancer mortality in a prospective study of never smokers. Am J Respir Crit Care Med. 2007;176(3):285–90.

97. Yang P, Sun Z, Krowka MJ, Aubry MC, Bamlet WR, Wampfler JA, et al. Alpha1-antitrypsin deficiency carriers, tobacco smoke, chronic obstructive pulmonary disease, and lung cancer risk. Arch Intern Med. 2008;168(10):1097–103.

98. Hopkins RJ, Duan F, Chiles C, Greco EM, Gamble GD, Aberle D, et al. Reduced expiratory flow rate among heavy smokers increases lung cancer risk. Results from the national lung screening trial-American College of Radiology Imaging Network Cohort. Ann Am Thorac Soc. 2017;14(3):392–402.

99. Gohy ST, Hupin C, Fregimilicka C, Detry BR, Bouzin C, Gaide Chevronay H, et al. Imprinting of the COPD airway epithelium for dedifferentiation and mesenchymal transition. Eur Respir J. 2015;45(5):1258–72.

100. Sohal SS, Reid D, Soltani A, Ward C, Weston S, Muller HK, et al. Reticular basement membrane fragmentation and potential epithelial mesenchymal transition is exaggerated in the airways of smokers with chronic obstructive pulmonary disease. Respirology. 2010;15(6):930–8.

101. Brown SW, Dobelle M, Padilla M, Agovino M, Wisnivesky JP, Hashim D, et al. Idiopathic pulmonary fibrosis and lung cancer. A systematic review and meta-analysis. Ann Am Thorac Soc. 2019;16(8):1041–51.

102. Yoon JH, Nouraie M, Chen X, Zou RH, Sellares J, Veraldi KL, et al. Characteristics of lung cancer among patients with idiopathic pulmonary fibrosis and interstitial lung disease - analysis of institutional and population data. Respir Res. 2018;19(1):195.

103. Yoo H, Jeong BH, Chung MJ, Lee KS, Kwon OJ, Chung MP. Risk factors and clinical characteristics of lung cancer in idiopathic pulmonary fibrosis: a retrospective cohort study. BMC Pulm Med. 2019;19(1):149.

104. Choi H, Park HY, Han K, Yoo J, Shin SH, Yang B, et al. Non-cystic fibrosis bronchiectasis increases the risk of lung cancer independent of smoking status. Ann Am Thorac Soc. 2022;19(9):1551–60.

105. Nalbandian A, Yan BS, Pichugin A, Bronson RT, Kramnik I. Lung carcinogenesis induced by chronic tuberculosis infection: the experimental model and genetic control. Oncogene. 2009;28(17):1928–38.

106. Wu CY, Hu HY, Pu CY, Huang N, Shen HC, Li CP, et al. Pulmonary tuberculosis increases the risk of lung cancer: a population-based cohort study. Cancer. 2011;117(3):618–24.

107. Lorigan P, Radford J, Howell A, Thatcher N. Lung cancer after treatment for Hodgkin's lymphoma: a systematic review. Lancet Oncol. 2005;6(10):773–9.

108. Huang YJ, Huang TW, Lin FH, Chung CH, Tsao CH, Chien WC. Radiation therapy for invasive breast cancer increases the risk of second primary lung cancer: a nationwide population-based cohort analysis. J Thorac Oncol. 2017;12(5):782–90.
109. Brenner DR, Hung RJ, Tsao MS, Shepherd FA, Johnston MR, Narod S, et al. Lung cancer risk in never-smokers: a population-based case-control study of epidemiologic risk factors. BMC Cancer. 2010;10:285.
110. Lissowska J, Foretova L, Dabek J, Zaridze D, Szeszenia-Dabrowska N, Rudnai P, et al. Family history and lung cancer risk: international multicentre case-control study in Eastern and Central Europe and meta-analyses. Cancer Causes Control. 2010;21(7):1091–104.
111. Spitz MR, Etzel CJ, Dong Q, Amos CI, Wei Q, Wu X, et al. An expanded risk prediction model for lung cancer. Cancer Prev Res (Phila). 2008;1(4):250–4.
112. Tammemagi CM, Pinsky PF, Caporaso NE, Kvale PA, Hocking WG, Church TR, et al. Lung cancer risk prediction: prostate, lung, colorectal and ovarian cancer screening trial models and validation. J Natl Cancer Inst. 2011;103(13):1058–68.
113. Sichletidis L, Chloros D, Spyratos D, Haidich AB, Fourkiotou I, Kakoura M, et al. Mortality from occupational exposure to relatively pure chrysotile: a 39-year study. Respiration. 2009;78(1):63–8.
114. Deng Q, Wang X, Wang M, Lan Y. Exposure-response relationship between chrysotile exposure and mortality from lung cancer and asbestosis. Occup Environ Med. 2012;69(2):81–6.
115. van Loon AJ, Kant IJ, Swaen GM, Goldbohm RA, Kremer AM, van den Brandt PA. Occupational exposure to carcinogens and risk of lung cancer: results from The Netherlands cohort study. Occup Environ Med. 1997;54(11):817–24.
116. Markowitz SB, Levin SM, Miller A, Morabia A. Asbestos, asbestosis, smoking, and lung cancer. New findings from the North American insulator cohort. Am J Respir Crit Care Med. 2013;188(1):90–6.
117. Ngamwong Y, Tangamornsuksan W, Lohitnavy O, Chaiyakunapruk N, Scholfield CN, Reisfeld B, et al. Additive synergism between asbestos and smoking in lung cancer risk: a systematic review and meta-analysis. PLoS One. 2015;10(8):e0135798.
118. Camus M, Siemiatycki J, Meek B. Nonoccupational exposure to chrysotile asbestos and the risk of lung cancer. N Engl J Med. 1998;338(22):1565–71.
119. Kwak K, Kang D, Paek D. Environmental exposure to asbestos and the risk of lung cancer: a systematic review and meta-analysis. Occup Environ Med. 2022;79(3):207–14.
120. Wagoner JK, Archer VE, Lundin FE Jr, Holaday DA, Lloyd JW. Radiation as the cause of lung cancer among uranium miners. N Engl J Med. 1965;273:181–8.
121. Surgeon General Releases National Health Advisory On Radon [press release]. Health and Human Services. 2005.
122. Krewski D, Lubin JH, Zielinski JM, Alavanja M, Catalan VS, Field RW, et al. Residential radon and risk of lung cancer: a combined analysis of 7 North American case-control studies. Epidemiology. 2005;16(2):137–45.
123. Darby S, Hill D, Auvinen A, Barros-Dios JM, Baysson H, Bochicchio F, et al. Radon in homes and risk of lung cancer: collaborative analysis of individual data from 13 European case-control studies. BMJ. 2005;330(7485):223.
124. Smith KR, Samet JM, Romieu I, Bruce N. Indoor air pollution in developing countries and acute lower respiratory infections in children. Thorax. 2000;55(6):518–32.
125. Household use of solid fuels and high-temperature frying. IARC Monogr Eval Carcinog Risks Hum. 2010;95:1–430.
126. Lan Q, Chapman RS, Schreinemachers DM, Tian L, He X. Household stove improvement and risk of lung cancer in Xuanwei, China. J Natl Cancer Inst. 2002;94(11):826–35.
127. Barone-Adesi F, Chapman RS, Silverman DT, He X, Hu W, Vermeulen R, et al. Risk of lung cancer associated with domestic use of coal in Xuanwei, China: retrospective cohort study. BMJ. 2012;345:e5414.
128. Raaschou-Nielsen O, Andersen ZJ, Beelen R, Samoli E, Stafoggia M, Weinmayr G, et al. Air pollution and lung cancer incidence in 17 European cohorts: prospective analyses

from the European Study of Cohorts for Air Pollution Effects (ESCAPE). Lancet Oncol. 2013;14(9):813–22.
129. Pope CA III, Burnett RT, Thun MJ, Calle EE, Krewski D, Ito K, et al. Lung cancer, cardiopulmonary mortality, and long-term exposure to fine particulate air pollution. JAMA. 2002;287(9):1132–41.
130. Olsson AC, Gustavsson P, Kromhout H, Peters S, Vermeulen R, Brüske I, et al. Exposure to diesel motor exhaust and lung cancer risk in a pooled analysis from case-control studies in Europe and Canada. Am J Respir Crit Care Med. 2011;183(7):941–8.

Chapter 2
Lung Cancer Screening

Christine M. Lambert and Abbie Begnaud

The History of Lung Cancer Screening

A successful screening test requires a significant disease with identifiable risk factors and a preclinical period. Screening might meaningfully impact disease outcomes if the disease can be identified before developing symptoms, and early treatment can reduce mortality. Lung cancer as we know it today meets these criteria. In the mid-twentieth century, the burden of lung cancer grew swiftly from a rare disease to surpassing all other cancer-related causes of death [1]. British scientists reported the association between cigarette smoking and lung cancer in 1950, reporting a 15-fold increase in lung cancer mortality from 1922 to 1947 in the United Kingdom [2]. This report was followed by the US Surgeon General, and Royal College of Physicians reports firmly linking cigarette smoking to lung cancer [3].

Sputum Cytology and Chest Radiography

For decades, clinicians and researchers sought effective lung cancer screening (LCS) tests. Early in the lung cancer epidemic, sputum cytology and chest radiographs were investigated as potential screening tests. When periodic chest radiographs alone [4] appeared inadequate for early detection and improved lung cancer mortality, a large collaborative trial between the Mayo Clinic, Johns Hopkins, and Memorial Sloan-Kettering enrolled men over 45 years of age who smoked at least one package of cigarettes daily for either chest radiograph with or without sputum cytology [5]. Over 30,000 patients were enrolled in the early 1980s and followed for

C. M. Lambert · A. Begnaud (✉)
Medicine, University of Minnesota Twin Cities, Minneapolis, MN, USA
e-mail: lambe143@umn.edu; abegnaud@umn.edu

C. MacRosty, M. P. Rivera (eds.), *Lung Cancer*, Respiratory Medicine,
https://doi.org/10.1007/978-3-031-38412-7_2

10 years, but the study failed to show significant benefit for sputum cytology and chest radiography to reduce lung cancer mortality. In 1996, the United States Preventive Services Task Force (USPSTF) issued its first recommendation about LCS, with a Grade D recommendation against using chest radiography or sputum cytology to screen asymptomatic individuals.

In the late 1990s, at the peak of lung cancer mortality, screening again gained interest, especially as reexamining prior trials demonstrated they might have been inadequately powered to detect an effect. Enter the Prostate, Lung, Colorectal, and Ovarian (PLCO) Cancer Screening Trial. With its 150,000-plus participants, the Prostate, Lung, Colon, and Ovarian (PLCO) trial was powered to detect a 10% difference in lung cancer mortality [6]. However, this trial definitively asserted the futility of annual chest radiographs for LCS, showing no mortality benefit for the 75,000 participants randomized to annual chest radiographs, compared to no lung screening. Furthermore, large studies in the United Kingdom and the United States failed to show a mortality benefit for LCS with the available diagnostic technologies at the time: sputum cytology in combination with chest radiography.

The United States Preventive Services Task Force is an independent national organization whose volunteer members review published literature about preventive care services. They evaluate the available evidence and recommend preventive services, including cancer screening. In 2004, the USPSTF issued a Grade I recommendation on LCS, a designation signifying insufficient evidence to recommend for or against screening [7]. Specifically, the recommendations stated: "Current data do not support screening for lung cancer with any method. These data, however, are also insufficient to conclude that screening does not work, particularly in women." The evidence reviewed to make this recommendation included some early small studies of low-dose chest computed tomography for LCS, and the broader availability of chest computed tomography offered new promise for an effective LCS modality.

Chest Computed Tomography for Lung Cancer Screening

In 2013, following the results of the landmark National Lung Screening Trial (NLST), [8] the USPSTF updated the LCS guidelines [9]. For the first time, LCS with low-dose computed tomography (LDCT) received a favorable Grade B recommendation meaning "high certainty that the net benefit is moderate or there is moderate certainty that the net benefit is moderate to substantial" Screening was recommended for those "55–80 years who have a 30 pack-year smoking history and currently smoke or have quit within the past 15 years. Screening should be discontinued once a person has not smoked for 15 years or develops a health problem that substantially limits life expectancy or the ability or willingness to have curative lung surgery." The Cancer Intervention and Surveillance Modeling Network (CISNET) conducted extensive scenario modeling of risk factor-based lung cancer screening patient selection strategies. The models, which included different thresholds for age at screening initiation, age at screening discontinuation, pack-years, and quit time, showed that the USPSTF 2013 guidelines were often the most efficient combination of risk factor thresholds [10].

Most major professional societies (including the American Cancer Society, American Thoracic Society, American College of Chest Physicians, Society for Thoracic Surgeons, and National Comprehensive Cancer Network) endorsed lung cancer screening with LDCT. The notable exception was the American Academy of Family Physicians (AAFP), whose recommendation remained ambivalent based on "insufficient evidence" [11]. Considering that Family Physicians comprise the largest proportion of primary care clinicians, this failure to endorse LCS with LDCT no doubt impacted the initial uptake of the service [12].

Preventative Care Coverage Policy in the United States

In 2010, a significant policy change conferred particular importance on the Grade B recommendation. The Affordable Care Act was passed into law in 2010 and required private insurers to cover preventive services recommended by the USPSTF with a grade of A or B and to cover these services with no cost-sharing (i.e., no deductible and no co-pay) [13, 14]. Furthermore, the Affordable Care Act authorizes Medicare to expand coverage of preventive services to include USPSTF recommendations and requires Medicaid to cover preventive services recommended by the USPSTF with a grade of A or B.

Coverage of preventive services under Medicare or Medicaid is codified using national coverage determinations. In 2014, the Centers for Medicare and Medicaid services (CMS) conducted a national coverage analysis of lung cancer screening at the request of lung cancer advocates [15]. The resulting coverage determination confirmed eligibility for individuals aged 55–77 who had smoked at least 30 pack-years with additional stipulations and unprecedented conditions for coverage [16]. One major condition of coverage was a shared decision-making visit to be performed by a credentialed independent clinician (physician or advanced practitioner) in person to confirm eligibility and discuss risks and benefits. Critics of this requirement saw it as an unnecessary barrier to receiving care, but others recognized that for a preventive service like LCS with LDCT, the risks and benefits vary based on individual patient factors, including lung cancer risk, medical comorbidities, and personal values.

Evidence for Lung Cancer Screening

The National Lung Screening Trial (NLST)

The NLST enrolled 53,454 individuals between the ages of 55–74 at randomization who had at minimum a 30-pack-year smoking history and who were currently smoking or had quit within the past 15 years. Individuals were randomized to single view (posteroanterior projection) chest radiography or LDCT, with an initial screening at the time of randomization, and annual screenings for 2 years, totaling three screening exams. Median follow-up was 6.5 years. Results were reported to participants without a specific study procedure mandated to work up suspicious findings.

The LDCT group had a higher rate of lung cancer diagnosis, 645 per 100,000 person-years, as opposed to 572 per 100,000 person-years in the chest radiography group. Of key clinical significance, the LDCT group had a higher stage I identification rate and a lower rate for stage III and IV non-small cell lung cancers (NSCLC). The rate of positive screenings was also higher in the LDCT group, which had a three times higher rate of identification of non-lung cancer abnormalities. Ultimately 96.4% of the positive results in the low-dose CT group and 94.5% in the radiography group were false positives.

The NLST was stopped when it reached the predetermined endpoint of a 20% reduction in lung cancer mortality in the LDCT screening group compared to the radiography group. For LDCT, the number needed to screen to prevent one lung cancer death was 320. For its 2013 recommendations, the USPSTF reviewed evidence from the NLST in making the recommendation for LCS, with further information provided by the CISNET models [10, 17].

Global Lung Cancer Screening Trials

In the years before and after the NLST, numerous LCS trials were conducted across Europe, including the German LCS Intervention (LUSI), Danish LCS Trial (DLCST), Multicentric Italian Lung Detection (MILD), and UK Lung Cancer Screening Trial (UKLS), each of which looked at the effect of screening CT vs. usual care [18–21]. While relatively similar in the study participants' age and smoking exposure inclusion criteria, the trials utilized various methods for identifying and recruiting participants, screening intervals, nodule management, and length of follow-up. Compared to the NLST, these trials had much smaller study populations and follow-up person-years and thus did not have the statistical power to show a mortality benefit for LCS [22, 23].

In 2020, the results of the second largest screening study, the Dutch-Belgian Randomized Lung Cancer Screening Trial (Dutch acronym: NELSON), were published [24]. The trial randomized 15,789 participants (13,195 men and 2594 women) aged 50–74 with a smoking history of 10 cigarettes daily for at least 30 years (15 pack-years) or 15 cigarettes daily for at least 25 years (18.75 pack-years). Those who formerly smoked needed to meet the required smoking history and have a quit date within the previous 10 years. For the intervention group, screening occurred at baseline, then at intervals of 1, 2, and 2.5 years for a total of four screening exams. Individuals were followed for a minimum of 10 years.

Among male participants, the LDCT screening group had a higher rate of lung cancer diagnosis, 5.58 cases per 1000 person-years, compared to 4.91 cases per 1000 person-years in the control group. Of the screen-detected cancers in the intervention group, 58.6% were stage I compared to 13.8% in the control group. Similarly, stage IV lung cancers comprised only 9.4% of screen-detected cancers in the intervention group but 45.7% in the control group. At 10 years, there was a 24% reduction in lung cancer mortality among men and a 33% reduction among women.

Notable aspects of the NELSON results that have prompted further interest and discussion include its finding of a mortality benefit despite conducting screening on less-than-annual basis and the lower rate of positive scans and follow-up studies required compared to the NLST. The NELSON trial reported an overall false-positive scan rate of 1.2%, with a baseline "indeterminate" scan rate of 19.7%. Most of these were later adjudicated as negative scans based on volume doubling time calculated at exam follow-up. By comparison, the NLST reported a baseline positive scan rate of 27.3% with an overall false-positive rate of 23.3%. The number of positive or indeterminate scans is of particular interest given the ramifications of a false-positive screening result, such as the psychological impact and potential need for invasive testing. The use of volume-based low-dose CT, with its focus on volumetric measurements and volume doubling time as opposed to the diameter-based estimates of standard LDCT, may have contributed to the lower percentage of positive or indeterminate scans, especially in later stages of screening.

Limitations in LCS Evidence

Both NELSON and the NLST have shown a mortality benefit from LCS. However, both trials have generalizability limitations, particularly regarding the study populations. The NLST population was 59% male and over 90% white, while the primary analyses in the NELSON study were conducted in a male population with race not reported but assumed to be white. The NELSON study was not powered to detect mortality benefits for women [25], but results suggest women would benefit even more than men. Furthermore, the NLST study sample was relatively young and healthy [26] and disproportionately comprised of individuals who no longer smoked and had higher educational attainment, compared to real-world screening [27, 28] populations. Studies have shown that participants and settings in the NLST and NELSON trials did not represent the general US population [29]. Small studies suggest the benefits of LCS may be even greater for participants with lower educational attainment [30], and Black individuals [31]. Analysis of lung cancer cases in the Southern Community Cohort Study [32] demonstrated that USPSTF 2013 criteria were less sensitive for Black individuals, with 67% of the lung cancer cases diagnosed in Black individuals who would not meet 2013 LCS eligibility due to insufficient smoking history. Lung cancer and screening are not unique in the disparities between the type of individuals included in large clinical trials and those most burdened by the disease [33, 34].

Beyond differences in participant characteristics, the NLST and NELSON also had study protocols that are not replicated in most real-world screening programs. For example, the NLST had more stringent requirements [35] for interpreting radiologists (LDCT interpretation experience and training) than are currently required in for interpretation of LDCT for LCS. The NELSON trial radiologists had computer-assisted detection [36] of nodules including volumetric measurement. In both the NLST and NELSON, screening was conducted primarily at highly respected academic medical centers, whose outcomes may not be achievable in all clinical settings.

2021 USPSTF LCS Recommendations

Since the 2013 LCS guidelines were published, several important trials warranted consideration when creating the revised 2021 USPSTF guidelines. Key evidence questions focused on patient selection, specifically, whether the NLST participants and settings were representative of the United States as a whole and whether the use of individualized risk calculation (risk model-based strategy) improved patient selection compared to age and pack-year smoking history (risk factor-based strategy). Synthesizing the evidence [37] from the largest RCTs powered to detect a mortality benefit for LDCT (NLST and NELSON trials) and modeling studies [38] supported expanded recommendations lowering the screening eligibility threshold to 50 years of age and smoking exposure to 20 pack-years. Women and individuals who identify as Black, Hispanic, and American Indian/Alaska Native stand to benefit from the lowered smoke exposure thresholds for screening. The 2021 recommendations remain Grade B, with a moderate certainty of moderate net benefit. The AAFP endorsed the new guidelines shortly after the 2021 USPSTF updated recommendations. Again, lung cancer advocates requested a reconsideration of national CMS coverage, prompting a new coverage determination [39]. In 2022, CMS issued its final decision to expand coverage for LCS using the new eligibility criteria while removing some of the previous conditions [40].

Lung Cancer Screening Methods

Low-Dose CT Screening Exam Technique

Per the National Comprehensive Cancer Network (NCCN) guidelines [41], LDCT screening exams should have a total radiation exposure less than or equal to 3 millisieverts (mSv), with 1 mSv being the annual average background radiation for an individual in the United States, and the worldwide average being 2–4 mSv (based on average size patient). The American College of Radiology (ACR) designates LCS Centers [42, 43] based on adherence to a similar set of technical guidelines, including the radiation dose from the CT scanner ($CTDI_{vol}$), slice thickness, and image acquisition time. The radiation exposure from LDCT scans is approximately one-fifth the amount of a conventional CT scan and may decrease further in the future as clinicians experiment with ultralow-dose CT scanning (ULDCT) [44].

The LDCT technique as described assumes patient BMI is less than 30, so total radiation dose is adjusted for body weight. The slice width should be less than or equal to 2.5 mm (1.0 mm preferred), with an acquisition time of less than or equal to 10 s or a single breath hold. No contrast agent of any kind is used for LDCT.

Nodule size is reported as the average two measurements: the longest nodule diameter and its perpendicular length on a single image. An alternative approach is volumetric analysis and volume doubling time, conducted using automated or semi-automated computer programs used in the recent NELSON trial [24]. Volumetric analysis may ultimately provide a lower rate of false-positive findings by giving more sensitive information on nodule growth over time. There are limitations as irregular nodules can still be hard to measure [45]. While commonly used in Europe, Volume CTs are not used in routine practice in the United States.

Interpretation

In the NLST, scans with 4 mm or greater diameter nodules were considered positive, and the study was marked by a high rate of false-positive scans, with 90% of positive scans not resulting in a lung cancer diagnosis [46]. To standardize reporting of screening exams and reduce the false-positive rate reported in the NLST, the ACR created the Lung Reporting and Data System (Lung-RADS) [47]. An analysis of NLST nodules in the 4–6 mm range and results from the International Early Lung Cancer Action Program (I-ELCAP) were considered when formulating the Lung-RADS criteria [48]. By using size criteria of 6 mm in diameter for solid nodules and greater than or equal to 20 mm for subsolid or ground-glass nodules as a positive LDCT, the Lung-RADS criteria showed a decrease in false-positive screenings with an increase in positive predictive value when applied retroactively to the participants included in the NLST [49, 50].

Two updates to Lung-RADS have been released by the ACR at the time of this publication. Lung-RADS Version 1.1 was published in 2019 and increased the threshold for classifying nonsolid nodules as probably benign from 20 to 30 mm and for likely benign perifissural nodules from 6 to 10 mm, recommended measurement of mean nodule diameter to one decimal point and included volumetric measurements in addition to diametric measurements to help facilitate future use of volumetric technology [51]. Lung-RADS version 2022, released in November 2022, included additional guidance on cystic pulmonary lesions and airway nodules. Although the British Thoracic Society has recommended volumetric measurement, the impact on clinical decision-making is unclear, and there are practical limitations to widespread use of volumetric analysis [52].

Lung-RADS v2022 categories are shown in Table 2.1.

Table 2.1 Lung-RADS v2022. Reprinted under Creative Commons Attribution-NoDerivatives 4.0 International Public License, from the American College of Radiology. https://creativecommons.org/licenses/by-nd/4.0/legalcode

American College of Radiology™

Lung-RADS® v2022

Release Date: November 2022

Lung-RADS	Category Descriptor	Findings	Management
0	**Incomplete** Estimated Population Prevalence: ~ 1%	Prior chest CT examination being located for comparison (see note 9)	Comparison to prior chest CT;
		Part or all oflungs cannot be evaluated	Additional lung cancer screening CT imaging needed;
		Findings suggestive of an inflammatory or infectious process (see note 10)	1-3 month LDCT
1	**Negative** Estimated Population Prevalence: 39%	No lung nodules **OR** **Nodule with benign features:** • Complete, central, popcorn, or concentric ring calcifications **OR** • Fat-containing	12-month screening LDCT
2	**Benign** - Based on imaging features or indolent behavior Estimated Population Prevalence: 45%	**Juxtapleural nodule:** • < 10 mm (524 mm³) mean diameter at baseline or new **AND** • Solid; smooth margins; and oval, lentiform, or triangular shape	
		Solid nodule: • < 6 mm (< 113 mm³) at baseline **OR** • New < 4 mm (< 34 mm³)	
		Part solid nodule: • < 6 mm total mean diameter (< 113 mm³) at baseline	
		Non solid nodule (GGN): • < 30 mm (< 14,137 mm³) at baseline, new, or growing **OR** • ≥ 30 mm (≥ 14,137 mm³) stable or slowly growing (see note 7)	
		Airway nodule, subsegmental - at baseline, new, or stable (see note 11)	
		Category 3 lesion that is stable or decreased in size at 6-month follow-up CT **OR** Category 4B lesion proven to be benign in etiology following appropriate diagnostic workup	
3	**Probably Benign** - Based on imaging features or behavior Estimated Population Prevalence: 9%	**Solid nodule:** • ≥ 6 to < 8 mm (≥ 113 to < 268 mm³) at baseline **OR** • New 4 mm to < 6 mm (34 to < 113 mm³)	6-month LDCT
		Part solid nodule: • ≥ 6 mm total mean diameter (≥ 113 mm³) with solid component < 6 mm (< 113 mm³) at baseline **OR** • New < 6 mm total mean diameter (< 113 mm³)	
		Non solid nodule (GGN): • ≥ 30 mm (≥ 14,137 mm³) at baseline or new	
		Atypical pulmonary cyst: (see note 12) • Growing cystic component (mean diameter) of a thick-walled cyst	
		Category 4A lesion that is stable or decreased in size at 3-month follow-up CT (excluding airway nodules)	
4A	**Suspicious** Estimated Population Prevalence: 4%	**Solid nodule:** • ≥ 8 to < 15 mm (≥ 268 to < 1,767 mm³) at baseline **OR** • Growing < 8 mm (< 268 mm³) **OR** • New 6 to < 8 mm (113 to < 268 mm³)	3-month LDCT; PET/CT may be considered if there is a ≥ 8 mm (≥ 268 mm³) solid nodule or solid component
		Part solid nodule: • ≥ 6 mm total mean diameter (≥ 113 mm³) with solid component ≥ 6 mm to < 8 mm (≥ 113 to < 268 mm³) at baseline **OR** • New or growing < 4 mm (< 34 mm³) solid component	
		Airway nodule, segmental or more proximal - at baseline (see note 11)	
		Atypical pulmonary cyst: (see note 12) • Thick-walled cyst **OR** • Multilocular cyst at baseline **OR** • Thin- or thick-walled cyst that becomes multilocular	
4B	**Very Suspicious** Estimated Population Prevalence: 2%	**Airway nodule,** segmental or more proximal - stable or growing (see note 11)	Referral for further clinical evaluation
		Solid nodule: • ≥ 15 mm (≥ 1767 mm³) at baseline **OR** • New or growing ≥ 8 mm (≥ 268 mm³)	Diagnostic chest CT with or without contrast; PET/CT may be considered if there is a ≥ 8 mm (≥ 268 mm³) solid nodule or solid component; tissue sampling; and/or referral for further clinical evaluation Management depends on clinical evaluation, patient preference, and the probability of malignancy (see note 13)
		Part solid nodule: • Solid component ≥ 8 mm (≥ 268 mm³) at baseline **OR** • New or growing ≥ 4 mm (≥ 34 mm³) solid component	
		Atypical pulmonary cyst: (see note 12) • Thick-walled cyst with growing wall thickness/nodularity **OR** • Growing multilocular cyst (mean diameter) **OR** • Multilocular cyst with increased loculation or new/increased opacity (nodular, ground glass, or consolidation)	
		Slow growing solid or part solid nodule that demonstrates growth over multiple screening exams (see note 8)	
4X	Estimated Population Prevalence: < 1%	Category 3 or 4 nodules with additional features or imaging findings that increase suspicion for lung cancer (see note 14)	
S	**Significant or Potentially Significant** Estimated Population Prevalence: 10%	**Modifier:** May add to category 0-4 for clinically significant or potentially clinically significant findings unrelated to lung cancer (see note 15)	As appropriate to the specific finding

Risks and Benefits

As with any clinical procedure, the risks and benefits of LCS need to be considered for each individual. The purpose of LCS, and therefore the primary benefit, is the potential to identify asymptomatic lung cancer early through stage shift instead of an advanced lung cancer presenting due to symptoms. The largest determinant of lung cancer survival is the stage at diagnosis. The current stage groupings (eighth edition) of the TNM Classification for Lung Cancer set forth by the International Association for the Study of Lung Cancer (IASLC) distinguishes between a 1 cm (stage IA1) and 2 cm (stage IA2) lung nodule [53], as shown in Fig. 2.1. This illustrates the impact of early detection through LCS.

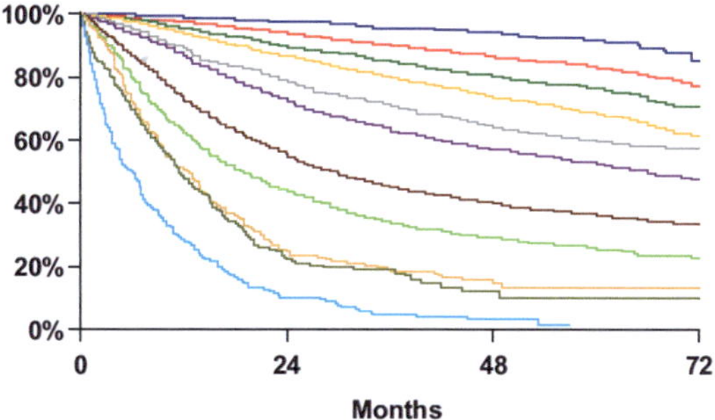

Proposed	Events / N	MST	24 Month	60 Month
IA1	68 / 781	NR	97%	92%
IA2	505 / 3105	NR	94%	83%
IA3	546 / 2417	NR	90%	77%
IB	560 / 1928	NR	87%	68%
IIA	215 / 585	NR	79%	60%
IIB	605 / 1453	66.0	72%	53%
IIIA	2052 / 3200	29.3	55%	36%
IIIB	1551 / 2140	19.0	44%	26%
IIIC	831 / 986	12.6	24%	13%
IVA	336 / 484	11.5	23%	10%
IVB	328 / 398	6.0	10%	0%

Fig. 2.1 Two- and 5-year survival by clinical stage in the eighth edition of the TNM classification for lung cancer. (Reprinted with permission from publisher)

Does Lung Cancer Screening Result in Stage Shift?

Early-stage cancer rates varied considerably among the randomized LDCT trials (Table 2.2). In all cases, LDCT screening resulted in higher earlier stage cancer rates compared to control and to average stage at diagnosis in the Surveillance, Epidemiology, and End Results (SEER) registry [58] during the same years. SEER registry reported stage at diagnosis of non-small cell lung cancer increasing from 26% to 31% stage I or II between 2006 and 2016. These findings are likely partly due to early effects of screening and partly due to incidentally detected cancers on chest CT.

Any form of cancer screening can appear beneficial when viewed through the lens of the number of cancers found or years from diagnosis to death. One must consider the possibility of lead time bias when screening leads to an earlier diagnosis and creates the appearance of a longer survival when death still occurs at the same point as it would have after a symptom-based diagnosis [59]. Overdiagnosis, the discovery of indolent cancers that will never be clinically significant, or cancer diagnosed in an individual with a life-limiting comorbid condition that causes their death before the cancer becomes clinically significant, can also impact perceptions on the effectiveness of screening [60].

The decision to pursue LCS is not without potential risk to the individual and requires discussion and consideration of these risks [60]. Annual radiation exposure, however low, potentially for decades can accumulate to significant levels [61] and increase the risk of radiation-induced cancer. Finding a suspicious nodule raises

Table 2.2 Randomized LDCT trials demonstrated stage shift to early stage lung cancer

Randomized LDCT trial (year screening concluded)	Reported proportion of early stage lung cancer (LDCT/ control)
National Lung Screening Trial (NLST) [46] 2007	50%/31% Stage I
	57%/39% Stages I + II
Italian Lung Cancer Screening Trial (ITALUNG) [54] 2009	36%/11% Stage I
	43%/18% Stages I + II
Detection and Screening of Early Lung Cancer by Novel Imaging Technology and Molecular Essays (DANTE) [55] 2010	45%/22% Stage I
	61%/41% Stages I + II
Danish Lung Cancer Screening Trial (DLST) [56] 2010	68%/21% Stage I
	68%/29% Stages I + II
Multicentric Italian Lung Detection (MILD) [57] 2011	63%/[a] Stage I
	71%/[a] Stages I + II
German Lung cancer Screening Intervention (LUSI) [18] 2011	67%/8% Stage I
	73%/22% Stages I + II
Dutch–Belgian lung-cancer screening trial (Nederlands–Leuvens Longkanker Screenings Onderzoek [NELSON]) [24] 2012	40%/13% Stage I
	49%/23% Stages I + II

[a] Group not reported

the likelihood of needing invasive diagnostic procedures such as biopsies or surgical resection, which could be curative but, for some may result in the diagnosis of a benign nodule. Incidental findings unrelated to lung cancer are also very common on LDCT, with most exams having at least one. While the NLST [62] reported 20% rate of incidental findings, real-world screening programs have reported more than half of exams to "virtually all" having incidental findings. Currently, there is no standard reporting strategy [63] for incidental findings on LDCT, leading to wide variability in reporting rates. While most of these are not clinically significant, they have the potential to impact the individual and clinician LCS experience.

Screening Strategy

A key element for maximizing LCS benefit is patient selection, individuals at high risk of lung cancer who can benefit from early detection and the possibility of surgical cure. Significant discussion and research have focused on the best way to identify these "high-risk individuals." Thus far, most lung cancer screening studies and guidelines have been based on selecting individuals for screening based on age and smoking history. So-called risk factor-based screening currently serves as the basis for screening within the United States, with individuals qualifying based on age, pack-years, or time since quitting cigarettes.

Because age and personal smoking history are not the sole determinants of lung cancer risk, considering only these factors ignores the impact of other factors (like social determinants of health and family history). Some of the NLST participants were at relatively lower risk for lung cancer but still met eligibility criteria based on risk factors, while other individuals who didn't meet the risk factor eligibility criteria are at increased risk for lung cancer. Only half of the people with lung cancer [64] in a small cohort study met the NLST or USPSTF 2013 eligibility for LCS. One approach to rectify this discordance is the use of risk model-based screening, where individuals are selected for cancer screening based on the results of risk prediction models that incorporate a variety of demographic and historical variables [65].

One example of lung cancer risk model is the $PLCOm_{2012}$, which estimates an individual's risk of developing lung cancer in the next 6 years and includes other factors that contribute to lung cancer risk besides age and smoke exposure intensity, such as family history, educational attainment, and other medical conditions [66]. Low-quality evidence including post hoc analyses and modeling studies did show that a risk model-based approach to patient selection improves performance of LCS including number needed to screen and false positives. Currently, risk prediction models are an area of active investigation, with some studies such as UK lung cancer screening trial and the International Lung Screening Trial using risk prediction models to select study populations [21, 67]. However, LCS has been difficult to implement effectively with more straightforward risk factor-based eligibility, so using a risk model-based approach requiring multiple additional pieces of information would almost certainly increase barriers to lung screening uptake.

Implementation of Lung Cancer Screening

State of Implementation

Although the recommendation and approval of LCS were heralded by many as a giant step in reducing lung cancer mortality, implementation has proved challenging. In the decade since annual low-dose chest CT scan for LCS has been demonstrated to reduce all-cause and disease-specific mortality, the proportion of eligible persons screened has progressed very slowly. Only 6% of the 8.5 million eligible persons in the United States have been screened for lung cancer [68, 69]. Compare this with breast cancer, where screening rates rose steeply just 3 years after the first USPSTF recommendation [70].

Breast cancer screening, which employs another imaging test—the mammogram–has occurred at rates consistently above 70% of eligible people since 1999 [70]. The Department of Health and Human Services Healthy People 2030 goals aim for 77% of women receiving breast cancer screening with mammograms but only 7.5% of people eligible for LCS receiving LDCT [70, 71], despite the two tests having comparable performance—the number of persons screened to save one life [72, 73]. Important distinctions between the two cancers are the public perception of the diseases and the policies governing the tests' conduct. While lessons learned from other cancer screening tests may apply to LCS, lung cancer is unique because there are additional system-level policy barriers and individual-level psychological barriers not pertinent to other cancers. Nihilism about lung cancer treatment and stigma associated with a disease attributed to a behavioral risk (cigarette smoking) are both patient- and provider-level individual barriers. Systemic barriers related to regulatory requirements of LCS coverage by payors also contribute to low LCS uptake.

System-Level Barriers

Unlike other cancers, LCS eligibility is based on historical behavior/exposure related to cigarette smoking. Estimating (and documenting) a person's "pack-year history" is time-consuming and not easily stored in most electronic health records (EHR). Recall bias and stigma toward cigarette smoking may also impact an individual's ability to accurately report their smoking history. Furthermore, the complexity of the stipulations for LCS coverage established by the CMS in their 2015 coverage determination memo was a major source of system-level barriers [16]. Identifying LCS-eligible persons is difficult because EHRs do not provide accurate estimates of smoking pack-year history [74]. As a new screening test with more complex eligibility requirements than age and/or sex, many clinicians report lack of EHR notification to aid identification of eligible candidates for LCS as a barrier [75].

The Centers for Medicare and Medicaid Services (CMS) is part of the Department of Health and Human Services and oversees the public health insurance programs Medicare and Medicaid, which cover older Americans, Americans with disabilities, and lower income, among others. CMS imposed unprecedented additional requirements for reimbursement of LCS, with implications for the ordering clinician, the screening exam order itself, the technical specifications of the images, the radiologists interpreting images, and the imaging centers conducting the exams. The most impactful of these requirements was the requirement for a face-to-face visit where shared decision-making (SDM) was conducted and documented by a physician or advanced practice provider. SDM proved to be quite a challenge for individuals eligible for LCS and healthcare systems. This contrasts with mammography for breast cancer screening, where an ordering clinician is not required—women can self-refer for mammography. A minor variation in the upper age cutoff for CMS (compared to USPSTF) also added to confusion about differing eligibility based on individual insurance coverage. Based on the NLST protocol, where participants aged 55–74 underwent three annual LDCT scans and were followed several additional years to a maximum age of 77, CMS adopted this age range [54–57, 59–77] for screening eligibility [15]. However, based on modeling data, USPSTF adopted the age range of 55–80 years for eligibility [16]. An additional CMS requirement was participation in a LCS registry. The only approved registry is hosted by the ACR in their National Radiology Data Registry. While the ACR hosts multiple imaging registries, including mammography, participation is not required for imaging centers to be reimbursed by CMS for screening mammography [76]. When CMS revisited the LCS coverage in 2021, these requirements were lightened, such that the SDM is no longer mandated to be face-to-face or conducted by a physician or advanced practice provider. Registry participation is no longer required, but the upper age limit of eligibility remains divergent from USPSTF, leading to uncertainty about eligibility for people aged 78–80 years, depending on their insurance plan.

Clinician-Level Barriers

The unprecedented complexity of eligibility and coverage for LCS contributes to clinician-level barriers. Clinicians report uncertainty about insurance coverage, lack of time, and lack of expertise to manage findings [77, 78]. Many primary care providers are family physicians, and their leading organization failed to endorse LCS until 2021, so skepticism and conflicting messages also contributed to clinician-level barriers.

Shared Decision-Making Visit and Decision Aids

Although the concept of shared decision-making (SDM) is patient-centered, the requirement to do so in a face-to-face visit places a burden on patients and clinicians alike [79, 80]. The content and quality of SDM vary widely [81]. Many decision aids have been developed to facilitate this process, with variable outcomes in terms of patient knowledge, decision conflict, and decision regret [82, 83]. The largest study to investigate the effect of decision aids on LCS uptake showed no difference in intent to screen or receipt of LDCT for LCS but did show reduced decision conflict [84]. One study showed that robust SDM, including discussion of risks, impacted patients' confidence in making the same decision again and returning for annual follow-up exams [85]. This study also demonstrated that some patients prefer to defer the decision to their healthcare provider. Other studies have shown low levels of decisional conflict when LCS knowledge was lower and no decision aid was used [80]. Most decision aids rely upon individual risk calculators based on one of two risk models, Bach or $PLCO_{m2012}$ [66, 86] and provide the user with a comparison of the risks and benefits for someone with their level of lung cancer risk. Another decision aid provides projections of how many screened persons will experience certain benefits and harms while encouraging patients to consider their own values [87].

LCS Program Structure

LCS programs can be described as centralized, decentralized, or hybrid [88]. Centralized programs accept referrals for potentially eligible patients, conduct SDM, order LDCT if appropriate, and manage follow-up of abnormal findings. Centralized programs have been shown to have higher annual adherence and concordance with screening eligibility guidelines [89, 90]. Presumably, decentralized programs increase patient access by avoiding the additional barrier of referral to another clinician and/or clinic. One hybrid program offered screening by PCPs or referral to specialists and found that most PCPs habitually behaved in consistent ways, either doing all the screening or referring all their patients for specialist-driven screening [91].

Adherence to Screening

While rates of baseline LCS exams are dismally low, with a national average [68] of 5%, annual adherence has proven to be equally challenging. A pooled analysis found 55% annual adherence rate, which is much lower than what was seen in the NLST [92]. In one study, program structure (centralized) was the greatest independent predictor of annual adherence [89]. In that study, the centralized program's annual adherence rate was 70%, compared with 41% of decentralized programs. Another study [93] reported similar findings of lower annual adherence in decentralized programs and among Black persons with normal baseline LCS. A systematic review and meta-analysis [92] concluded that patient factors like educational attainment, White race, and former smoking status also predicted higher annual adherence rates. However, to realize the full benefit of LCS, annual adherence must be higher than has been seen thus far. Microsimulation modeling showed [94] that the benefit of screening is reduced directly as adherence to annual screening is reduced.

In addition to annual adherence to LCS, adherence to recommended follow-up of abnormal LDCT is certainly required to realize the benefit of screening. A recent cohort study [95] showed that less than half of positive screening exams resulted in follow-up adherence to recommendations. More suspicious findings were associated with higher rates of positive screen adherence, but even after extending follow-up timelines, 20% of suspicious exams did not appear to have appropriate follow-up. Adherence to follow-up for positive screens appears to be higher [93] in centralized LCS programs.

Patient-Level Barriers

Some barriers at the patient level are associated with social determinants of health. That is, individuals who have smoked heavily and might benefit most from LCS are also more likely to have lower levels of educational attainment and experience systemic racism [96]. Patient access barriers include tangible considerations like insurance coverage and transportation [97]. Transportation is particularly relevant because there has been an inverse relationship between where most LCS-eligible persons are and where LCS is available, especially under 2015 CMS requirements [98]. Psychological barriers like fear, stigma, and nihilism also impact patients because of the historically low survival of lung cancer and internal and external stigma experienced by people who smoke [77].

Lung Cancer Screening and Smoking Cessation

Cigarette smoking remains the most significant risk factor for lung cancer. LCS mortality benefit is magnified to the extent that the process also leads to smoking cessation. Some studies have shown a positive effect of LCS on efforts at smoking cessation. The Italian Lung Cancer Screening Trial (ITALUNG) found higher smoking quit rates among patients in the screening arm than usual care arm [99]. A cross-sectional study using Behavioral Risk Factor Surveillance System (BRFSS) data found participants receiving lung cancer screening were less likely to be current smokers and more likely to have attempted quitting in the prior year [100].

Counseling and interventions to promote smoking cessation are included in the USPSTF recommendations and CMS decision memo on lung cancer screening [40, 101]. While the importance of smoking cessation is widely recognized, counseling on smoking cessation is often limited during the shared decision-making process. Even less often are patients referred for specific services or provided with prescriptions for pharmacologic therapy [102, 103]. Several NIH-funded studies are underway to understand how LCS can be used to maximize smoking cessation [104].

Emerging Issues in Lung Cancer Screening

Future Directions for Lung Cancer Screening Tests

A screening test for lung cancer that doesn't involve the harm of ionizing radiation or the requirement for going to an imaging center would help to improve risks of and access to LCS. A screening test with fewer false positives and incidental findings might make screening feasible for people with lower risk for lung cancer, such as people who quit smoking long ago or never smoked cigarettes but have radon exposure or a family history of lung cancer. One might imagine population screening with such a test that, if abnormal, could be followed up with a LDCT. As of 2022, no such tests LCS are available, but some new technologies being tested may hold promise.

Blood tests are available to improve risk stratification in people with indeterminate lung nodules, including techniques such as proteomics or DNA methylation. A commercially available blood test measuring relative quantities of two plasma proteins was shown to perform better than positron emission tomography (PET) for indeterminate lung nodules [105]. Another blood test is in multisite clinical trials for early detection of lung cancer among high-risk individuals, looking at methylation patterns in circulating DNA. Emerging technologies of metabolomic analysis of blood samples are being tested as well [106]. Multiple reports of dogs detecting lung cancer likely demonstrate that volatile organic compounds are emitted from people with the disease [107]. Thus, several clinical trials are underway to test exhaled breath analysis with machine learning analysis of exhaled compounds for early and noninvasive detection of lung cancer. At least one has been published with promising results [108]. These technologies are not ready for routine screening use but expand the possibilities for future screening approaches.

Lung Cancer Screening for Other High-Risk individuals

While cigarette smoking is the dominant cause of lung cancer [109], there are other environmental or occupational exposures known to cause lung cancer for which the guidelines are less clear. In addition, studies of certain high-risk groups, such as individuals with proven environmental or occupational exposure to asbestos, show a benefit from early implementation of lung cancer screening [110, 111].

The NCCN guidelines, noting that risk assessment is based on age and smoking history, suggest considering other possible risk factors for lung cancer, such as occupational exposures, radon exposure, family history of lung cancer, and personal history of lung disease (chronic obstructive pulmonary disease or pulmonary fibrosis) during the shared decision-making process [41]. However, most insurance does not routinely cover LCS for individuals who do not meet USPSTF criteria. Discussions to ascertain whether an individual meets the criteria for LCS based on age and smoking history provide an opportunity to assess and educate about other causes of lung cancer, such as possible radon exposure. In addition, it can be a significant opportunity to counsel on smoking cessation given the known synergistic effect of smoking and radon or asbestos exposure [109].

Lung Cancer Screening During the COVID-19 Pandemic

At the start of the COVID-19 pandemic in March 2020, enrollment in lung, breast, and other routine cancer screenings was deferred based on expert recommendations [112, 113]. Many screening programs resumed operations in 2020, with some reporting an increase in suspicious nodules that required further invasive workup [114]. The rate of lung cancer screening nationally appears to have remained stable from 2019 to 2020, with some significant differences at the state level, perhaps driven by lockdown procedures, infection rates, or differences in screening infrastructure [69]. The low use of LCS before the pandemic is thought to have led to smaller changes in LCS utilization compared to other types of cancer screening, such as breast or colon [115]. In the case of lung cancer, many patients at highest risk of lung cancer are also at highest risk for severe complications from COVID 19 due to their underlying lung health.

Concerns that COVID-19 may cause an exacerbation of disparities within LCS have prompted studies examining rates of LCS by sex, race, and other demographic factors. Screening rates did not differ by race or urban/rural status in one state-wide study [116]; another study did note differences by race and gender when examining "no-show" rates [114]. Ongoing attention to lung cancer incidence and mortality rates will provide additional insight into the effect of the pandemic on lung cancer screening behaviors over time.

Conclusions

Lung cancer is the deadliest cancer in the world. Screening with LDCT has shown promise in reducing lung cancer mortality. However, implementation of LCS in the United States has been relatively slow, likely due to many factors including system-level barriers such as inequitable access to health care, complicated Centers for Medicare and Medicaid reimbursement stipulations, and psychological factors like stigma and nihilism about lung cancer. Groups who potentially stand to gain the most from LCS like Black Americans, those with lower educational attainment, people who still smoke cigarettes, and women, are disproportionately behind in the race to offer screening to all eligible persons. In the future, other screening tests for lung cancer might expand access without increasing harm and cost, but these have yet to be identified. The most significant risk factor for lung cancer is cigarette smoke exposure, but there are other known risk factors, including radon, air pollution and asbestos exposure and family history. Furthermore, individuals without identifiable risk factors do develop lung cancer, so this remains an important area of study.

References

1. Sharma D, Newman TG, Aronow WS. Lung cancer screening: history, current perspectives, and future directions. Arch Med Sci. 2015;11(5):1033–43.
2. Doll R, Hill AB. Smoking and carcinoma of the lung; preliminary report. Br Med J. 1950;2(4682):739–48.
3. Ridge CA, McErlean AM, Ginsberg MS. Epidemiology of lung cancer. Semin Interv Radiol. 2013;30(2):93–8.
4. Weiss W, Boucot KR, Cooper DA. The Philadelphia pulmonary neoplasm research project. Survival factors in bronchogenic carcinoma. JAMA. 1971;216(13):2119–23.
5. Berlin NI, Buncher CR, Fontana RS, Frost JK, Melamed MR. The National Cancer Institute Cooperative Early Lung Cancer Detection Program. Results of the initial screen (prevalence). Early lung cancer detection: introduction. Am Rev Respir Dis. 1984;130(4):545–9.
6. Oken MM, Hocking WG, Kvale PA, Andriole GL, Buys SS, Church TR, et al. Screening by chest radiograph and lung cancer mortality: the Prostate, Lung, Colorectal, and Ovarian (PLCO) randomized trial. JAMA. 2011;306(17):1865–73.
7. United States Preventive Services Task Force. Final recommendation statement lung cancer: screening, May 2004: United States Preventive Services Task Force; 2004. https://www.uspreventiveservicestaskforce.org/uspstf/recommendation/lung-cancer-screening-2004. Accessed 8 Sep 2022.
8. Aberle DR, Adams AM, Berg CD, Black WC, Clapp JD, Fagerstrom RM, et al. Reduced lung-cancer mortality with low-dose computed tomographic screening. N Engl J Med. 2011;365(5):395–409.
9. United States Preventive Services Task Force. Final recommendation statement lung cancer screening: United States Preventative Services Task Force. 2013. https://www.uspreventiveservicestaskforce.org/uspstf/recommendation/lung-cancer-screening-december-2013. Accessed 8 Sep 2022.

10. de Koning HJ, Meza R, Plevritis SK, ten Haaf K, Munshi VN, Jeon J, et al. Benefits and harms of computed tomography lung cancer screening strategies: a comparative modeling study for the U.S. Preventive Services Task Force. Ann Intern Med. 2014;160(5):311–20.
11. Gates TJ. Screening for cancer: concepts and controversies. Am Fam Physician. 2014;90(9):625–31.
12. Bazemore A, Wilkinson E, Petterson S, Green LA. Proportional erosion of the primary care physician workforce has continued since 2010. Am Fam Physician. 2019;100(4):211–2.
13. Seiler N, Malcarney MB, Horton K, Dafflitto S. Coverage of clinical preventive services under the Affordable Care Act: from law to access. Public Health Rep. 2014;129(6):526–32.
14. United States Preventive Services Task Force. Procedure manual Appendix I. Congressional mandate establishing the U.S. Preventive Services Task Force. 2019. https://uspreventi-veservicestaskforce.org/uspstf/about-uspstf/methods-and-processes/procedure-manual/procedure-manual-appendix-i. Accessed 28 Feb 2022.
15. Centers for Medicare & Medicaid Services. National coverage analysis; Tracking sheet; Screening for lung cancer with low dose computed tomography (LDCT) CAG-00439N. 2015. https://www.cms.gov/medicare-coverage-database/view/ncacal-tracking-sheet.aspx?NCAI d=274&bc=AiAAAAAAgAAAA%3d%3d&. Accessed 17 Aug 2022.
16. Centers for Medicare & Medicaid Services. National coverage analysis; Decision memo; Screening for lung cancer with low dose computed tomography (LDCT) CAG-00439N. 2015. https://www.cms.gov/medicare-coverage-database/view/ncacal-decision-memo.aspx?propos ed=N&ncaid=274&bc=0. Accessed 30 Aug 2022.
17. de Koning HJ, Meza R, Plevritis SK, ten Haaf K, Munshi VN, Jeon J, Erdogan SA, Kong CY, Han SS, van Rosmalen R, Choi SE, Miller M, Moolgavkar S, Pinsky PF, Berg CD, de Gonzalez AB, Black WC, Tammemagi CM, Hazelton WD, Feuer EJ, McMahon PM. Benefits and harms of computed tomography lung cancer screening programs for high-risk populations. Rockville, MD: Agency for Healthcare Research and Quality; 2013. Contract No.: AHRQ Publication 13-05196-EF-2.
18. Becker N, Motsch E, Trotter A, Heussel CP, Dienemann H, Schnabel PA, et al. Lung cancer mortality reduction by LDCT screening-results from the randomized German LUSI trial. Int J Cancer. 2020;146(6):1503–13.
19. Wille MM, Dirksen A, Ashraf H, Saghir Z, Bach KS, Brodersen J, et al. Results of the randomized Danish lung cancer screening trial with focus on high-risk profiling. Am J Respir Crit Care Med. 2016;193(5):542–51.
20. Pastorino U, Rossi M, Rosato V, Marchianò A, Sverzellati N, Morosi C, et al. Annual or biennial CT screening versus observation in heavy smokers: 5-year results of the MILD trial. Eur J Cancer Prev. 2012;21(3):308–15.
21. Baldwin DR, Duffy SW, Wald NJ, Page R, Hansell DM, Field JK. UK Lung Screen (UKLS) nodule management protocol: modelling of a single screen randomised controlled trial of low-dose CT screening for lung cancer. Thorax. 2011;66(4):308–13.
22. Silva M, Pastorino U, Sverzellati N. Lung cancer screening with low-dose CT in Europe: strength and weakness of diverse independent screening trials. Clin Radiol. 2017;72(5):389–400.
23. van der Aalst CM, Ten Haaf K, de Koning HJ. Lung cancer screening: latest developments and unanswered questions. Lancet Respir Med. 2016;4(9):749–61.
24. de Koning HJ, van der Aalst CM, de Jong PA, Scholten ET, Nackaerts K, Heuvelmans MA, et al. Reduced lung-cancer mortality with volume CT screening in a randomized trial. N Engl J Med. 2020;382(6):503–13.
25. van Iersel CA, de Koning HJ, Draisma G, Mali WP, Scholten ET, Nackaerts K, et al. Risk-based selection from the general population in a screening trial: selection criteria, recruitment and power for the Dutch-Belgian randomised lung cancer multi-slice CT screening trial (NELSON). Int J Cancer. 2007;120(4):868–74.

26. National Lung Screening Trial Research T, Aberle DR, Adams AM, Berg CD, Clapp JD, Clingan KL, et al. Baseline characteristics of participants in the randomized national lung screening trial. J Natl Cancer Inst. 2010;102(23):1771–9.
27. Majeed H, Zhu H, Williams SA, Hamann HA, Natchimuthu VS, Lee J, et al. Prevalence and impact of medical comorbidities in a real-world lung cancer screening population. Clin Lung Cancer. 2022;23(5):419–27.
28. Melzer AC, Begnaud A, Lindgren BR, Schertz K, Fu SS, Vock DM, et al. Self-reported exercise capacity among current smokers eligible for lung cancer screening: distribution and association with key comorbidities. Cancer Treat Res Commun. 2021;28:100443.
29. Jonas DE, Reuland DS, Reddy SM, Nagle M, Clark SD, Weber RP, et al. U.S. Preventive Services Task Force Evidence Syntheses, formerly Systematic Evidence Reviews. Screening for lung cancer with low-dose computed tomography: an evidence review for the US Preventive Services Task Force. Rockville, MD: Agency for Healthcare Research and Quality (US); 2021.
30. Guichet PL, Liu BY, Desai B, Surani Z, Cen SY, Lee C. Preliminary results of lung cancer screening in a socioeconomically disadvantaged population. AJR Am J Roentgenol. 2018;210(3):489–96.
31. Prosper AE, Inoue K, Brown K, Bui AAT, Aberle D, Hsu W. Association of inclusion of more black individuals in lung cancer screening with reduced mortality. JAMA Netw Open. 2021;4(8):e2119629.
32. Aldrich MC, Mercaldo SF, Sandler KL, Blot WJ, Grogan EL, Blume JD. Evaluation of USPSTF lung cancer screening guidelines among African American adult smokers. JAMA Oncol. 2019;5(9):1318–24.
33. Haddad DN, Sandler KL, Henderson LM, Rivera MP, Aldrich MC. Disparities in lung cancer screening: a review. Ann Am Thorac Soc. 2020;17(4):399–405.
34. Siegel RL, Miller KD, Jemal A. Cancer statistics, 2019. CA Cancer J Clin. 2019;69(1):7–34.
35. National Lung Screening Trial Research T, Aberle DR, Berg CD, Black WC, Church TR, Fagerstrom RM, et al. The National Lung Screening Trial: overview and study design. Radiology. 2011;258(1):243–53.
36. Ru Zhao Y, Xie X, de Koning HJ, Mali WP, Vliegenthart R, Oudkerk M. NELSON lung cancer screening study. Cancer Imaging. 2011;11 Spec No A(1A):S79–84.
37. Jonas DE, Reuland DS, Reddy SM, Nagle M, Clark SD, Weber RP, et al. Screening for lung cancer with low-dose computed tomography: updated evidence report and systematic review for the US Preventive Services Task Force. JAMA. 2021;325(10):971–87.
38. Meza R, Jeon J, Toumazis I, Ten Haaf K, Cao P, Bastani M, et al. Evaluation of the benefits and harms of lung cancer screening with low-dose computed tomography: modeling study for the US Preventive Services Task Force. JAMA. 2021;325(10):988–97.
39. Centers for Medicare & Medicaid Services. National coverage analysis; Tracking sheet; Screening for lung cancer with low dose computed tomography (LDCT) CAG-00439R. 2022. https://www.cms.gov/medicare-coverage-database/view/ncacal-tracking-sheet.aspx?ncaid=304. Accessed 17 Aug 2022.
40. Centers for Medicare & Medicaid Services. National coverage analysis; Decision memo; Screening for lung cancer with low dose computed tomography (LDCT) CAG-00439R. 2022. https://www.cms.gov/medicare-coverage-database/view/ncacal-decision-memo.aspx?proposed=N&ncaid=304. Accessed 28 Feb 2022.
41. National Comprehensive Cancer Network. NCCN guidelines version 2.2022 lung cancer screening 2022. 2022. https://www.nccn.org/professionals/physician_gls/pdf/lung_screening.pdf. Accessed 2 Aug 2022.
42. American College of Radiology. Adult lung cancer screening technical specifications. https://www.acraccreditation.org/-/media/ACRAccreditation/Documents/LCS/Lung-Cancer-Screening-Technical-Specifications.pdf. Accessed 5 Jul 2022.

43. American College of Radiology. ACR–STR practice parameter for the performance and reporting of lung cancer screening thoracic computed tomography (CT). 2019. https://www.acr.org/-/media/ACR/Files/Practice-Parameters/CT-LungCaScr.pdf. Accessed 5 Jul 2022.
44. Vonder M, Dorrius MD, Vliegenthart R. Latest CT technologies in lung cancer screening: protocols and radiation dose reduction. Transl Lung Cancer Res. 2021;10(2):1154–64.
45. Chelala L, Hossain R, Kazerooni EA, Christensen JD, Dyer DS, White CS. Lung-RADS version 1.1: challenges and a look ahead, from the AJR special series on radiology reporting and data systems. AJR Am J Roentgenol. 2021;216(6):1411–22.
46. National Lung Screening Trial Research T, Aberle DR, Adams AM, Berg CD, Black WC, Clapp JD, et al. Reduced lung-cancer mortality with low-dose computed tomographic screening. N Engl J Med. 2011;365(5):395–409.
47. American College of Radiology. Lung-RADS version 1.0. 2014.
48. Henschke CI, Yip R, Yankelevitz DF, Smith JP. Definition of a positive test result in computed tomography screening for lung cancer: a cohort study. Ann Intern Med. 2013;158(4):246–52.
49. McKee BJ, Regis SM, McKee AB, Flacke S, Wald C. Performance of ACR lung-RADS in a clinical CT lung screening program. J Am Coll Radiol. 2015;12(3):273–6.
50. Pinsky PF, Gierada DS, Black W, Munden R, Nath H, Aberle D, et al. Performance of lung-RADS in the national lung screening trial: a retrospective assessment. Ann Intern Med. 2015;162(7):485–91.
51. Dyer SC, Bartholmai BJ, Koo CW. Implications of the updated lung CT screening reporting and data system (lung-RADS version 1.1) for lung cancer screening. J Thorac Dis. 2020;12(11):6966–77.
52. Devaraj A, van Ginneken B, Nair A, Baldwin D. Use of volumetry for lung nodule management: theory and practice. Radiology. 2017;284(3):630–44.
53. Goldstraw P, Chansky K, Crowley J, Rami-Porta R, Asamura H, Eberhardt WE, et al. The IASLC lung cancer staging project: proposals for revision of the TNM stage groupings in the forthcoming (eighth) edition of the TNM classification for lung cancer. J Thorac Oncol. 2016;11(1):39–51.
54. Paci E, Puliti D, Lopes Pegna A, Carrozzi L, Picozzi G, Falaschi F, et al. Mortality, survival and incidence rates in the ITALUNG randomised lung cancer screening trial. Thorax. 2017;72(9):825–31.
55. Infante M, Cavuto S, Lutman FR, Brambilla G, Chiesa G, Ceresoli G, et al. A randomized study of lung cancer screening with spiral computed tomography: three-year results from the DANTE trial. Am J Respir Crit Care Med. 2009;180(5):445–53.
56. Saghir Z, Dirksen A, Ashraf H, Bach KS, Brodersen J, Clementsen PF, et al. CT screening for lung cancer brings forward early disease. The randomised Danish Lung Cancer Screening Trial: status after five annual screening rounds with low-dose CT. Thorax. 2012;67(4):296–301.
57. Pastorino U, Rossi M, Rosato V, Marchiano A, Sverzellati N, Morosi C, et al. Annual or biennial CT screening versus observation in heavy smokers: 5-year results of the MILD trial. Eur J Cancer Prev. 2012;21(3):308–15.
58. Flores R, Patel P, Alpert N, Pyenson B, Taioli E. Association of stage shift and population mortality among patients with non-small cell lung cancer. JAMA Netw Open. 2021;4(12):e2137508.
59. Szklo M, Neito FJ. Epidemiology beyond the basics. 2nd ed. Sudbury, MA: Jones and Bartlett Publishers; 2007.
60. Mazzone PJ, Silvestri GA, Souter LH, Caverly TJ, Kanne JP, Katki HA, et al. Screening for lung cancer: CHEST guideline and expert panel report. Chest. 2021;160(5):e427–e94.
61. McCunney RJ, Li J. Radiation risks in lung cancer screening programs: a comparison with nuclear industry workers and atomic bomb survivors. Chest. 2014;145(3):618–24.
62. Nguyen XV, Davies L, Eastwood JD, Hoang JK. Extrapulmonary findings and malignancies in participants screened with chest CT in the national lung screening trial. J Am Coll Radiol. 2017;14(3):324–30.

63. Tanoue LT, Sather P, Cortopassi I, Dicks D, Curtis A, Michaud G, et al. Standardizing the reporting of incidental, non-lung cancer (category S) findings identified on lung cancer screening low-dose CT imaging. Chest. 2022;161(6):1697–706.
64. Pu CY, Lusk CM, Neslund-Dudas C, Gadgeel S, Soubani AO, Schwartz AG. Comparison between the 2021 USPSTF lung cancer screening criteria and other lung cancer screening criteria for racial disparity in eligibility. JAMA Oncol. 2022;8(3):374–82.
65. Ten Haaf K, Jeon J, Tammemägi MC, Han SS, Kong CY, Plevritis SK, et al. Risk prediction models for selection of lung cancer screening candidates: a retrospective validation study. PLoS Med. 2017;14(4):e1002277.
66. Tammemägi MC, Katki HA, Hocking WG, Church TR, Caporaso N, Kvale PA, et al. Selection criteria for lung-cancer screening. N Engl J Med. 2013;368(8):728–36.
67. Lim KP, Marshall H, Tammemägi M, Brims F, McWilliams A, Stone E, et al. Protocol and rationale for the international lung screening trial. Ann Am Thorac Soc. 2020;17(4):503–12.
68. Fedewa SA, Kazerooni EA, Studts JL, Smith RA, Bandi P, Sauer AG, et al. State variation in low-dose computed tomography scanning for lung cancer screening in the United States. J Natl Cancer Inst. 2021;113(8):1044–52.
69. Fedewa SA, Bandi P, Smith RA, Silvestri GA, Jemal A. Lung Cancer Screening Rates During the COVID-19 Pandemic. Chest. 2022;161(2):586–9.
70. National Cancer Institute. Cancer trends progress report; breast cancer screening: National Institutes of Health. 2022. https://progressreport.cancer.gov/detection/breast_cancer. Accessed 25 Jul 2022.
71. National Cancer Institute. Cancer trends progress report; lung cancer screening. National Institutes of Health. 2022. https://progressreport.cancer.gov/detection/lung_cancer. Accessed 25 Jul 2022.
72. Hendrick RE, Helvie MA. Mammography screening: a new estimate of number needed to screen to prevent one breast cancer death. AJR Am J Roentgenol. 2012;198(3):723–8.
73. Tammemägi MC, Church TR, Hocking WG, Silvestri GA, Kvale PA, Riley TL, et al. Evaluation of the lung cancer risks at which to screen ever- and never-smokers: screening rules applied to the PLCO and NLST cohorts. PLoS Med. 2014;11(12):e1001764.
74. Tarabichi Y, Kats DJ, Kaelber DC, Thornton JD. The impact of fluctuations in pack-year smoking history in the electronic health record on lung cancer screening practices. Chest. 2018;153(2):575–8.
75. Coughlin JM, Zang Y, Terranella S, Alex G, Karush J, Geissen N, et al. Understanding barriers to lung cancer screening in primary care. J Thorac Dis. 2020;12(5):2536–44.
76. Centers for Medicare & Medicaid Services. National coverage determination mammograms 220.4. 1978. https://www.cms.gov/medicare-coverage-database/view/ncd.aspx?NCDId=186. Accessed 26 Jul 2022.
77. Wang GX, Baggett TP, Pandharipande PV, Park ER, Percac-Lima S, Shepard JO, et al. Barriers to lung cancer screening engagement from the patient and provider perspective. Radiology. 2019;290(2):278–87.
78. Carter-Harris L, Gould MK. Multilevel barriers to the successful implementation of lung cancer screening: why does it have to be so hard? Ann Am Thorac Soc. 2017;14(8):1261–5.
79. Melzer AC, Golden SE, Ono SS, Datta S, Crothers K, Slatore CG. What exactly is shared decision-making? A qualitative study of shared decision-making in lung cancer screening. J Gen Intern Med. 2020;35(2):546–53.
80. Eberth JM, Zgodic A, Pelland SC, Wang SY, Miller DP. Outcomes of shared decision-making for low-dose screening for lung cancer in an academic medical center. J Cancer Educ. 2022;38:522.
81. Brenner AT, Malo TL, Margolis M, Elston Lafata J, James S, Vu MB, et al. Evaluating Shared Decision Making for Lung Cancer Screening. JAMA Intern Med. 2018;178(10):1311–6.
82. Nishi SPE, Lowenstein LM, Mendoza TR, Lopez Olivo MA, Crocker LC, Sepucha K, et al. Shared decision-making for lung cancer screening: how well are we "sharing"? Chest. 2021;160(1):330–40.

83. Kaufman M, Schnure N, Nicholson A, Leone F, Guerra C. A lung cancer screening personalized decision-aid improves knowledge and reduces decisional conflict among a diverse population of smokers at an urban academic medical center. J Health Disparit Res Pract. 2020;13(2):3.
84. Volk RJ, Lowenstein LM, Leal VB, Escoto KH, Cantor SB, Munden RF, et al. Effect of a patient decision aid on lung cancer screening decision-making by persons who smoke: a randomized clinical trial. JAMA Netw Open. 2020;3(1):e1920362.
85. Tan NQP, Nishi SPE, Lowenstein LM, Mendoza TR, Lopez-Olivo MA, Crocker LC, et al. Impact of the shared decision-making process on lung cancer screening decisions. Cancer Med. 2022;11(3):790–7.
86. Bach PB, Kattan MW, Thornquist MD, Kris MG, Tate RC, Barnett MJ, et al. Variations in lung cancer risk among smokers. J Natl Cancer Inst. 2003;95(6):470–8.
87. Agency for Healthcare Research and Quality. Is lung cancer screening right for me? A decision aid for people considering lung cancer screening with low-dose computed tomography. 2016. https://effectivehealthcare.ahrq.gov/sites/default/files/pdf/lung-cancer-about-160226.pdf. Accessed 25 Aug 2022.
88. Alishahi Tabriz A, Neslund-Dudas C, Turner K, Rivera MP, Reuland DS, Elston Lafata J. How health-care organizations implement shared decision-making when it is required for reimbursement: the case of lung cancer screening. Chest. 2021;159(1):413–25.
89. Sakoda LC, Rivera MP, Zhang J, Perera P, Laurent CA, Durham D, et al. Patterns and factors associated with adherence to lung cancer screening in diverse practice settings. JAMA Netw Open. 2021;4(4):e218559.
90. Smith HB, Ward R, Frazier C, Angotti J, Tanner NT. Guideline-recommended lung cancer screening adherence is superior with a centralized approach. Chest. 2022;161(3):818–25.
91. Hirsch EA, New ML, Brown SL, Barón AE, Sachs PB, Malkoski SP. Impact of a hybrid lung cancer screening model on patient outcomes and provider behavior. Clin Lung Cancer. 2020;21(6):e640–e6.
92. Lopez-Olivo MA, Maki KG, Choi NJ, Hoffman RM, Shih YT, Lowenstein LM, et al. Patient adherence to screening for lung cancer in the US: a systematic review and meta-analysis. JAMA Netw Open. 2020;3(11):e2025102.
93. Kim RY, Rendle KA, Mitra N, Saia CA, Neslund-Dudas C, Greenlee RT, et al. Racial disparities in adherence to annual lung cancer screening and recommended follow-up care: a multicenter cohort study. Ann Am Thorac Soc. 2022;19(9):1561–9.
94. Han SS, Erdogan SA, Toumazis I, Leung A, Plevritis SK. Evaluating the impact of varied compliance to lung cancer screening recommendations using a microsimulation model. Cancer Causes Control. 2017;28(9):947–58.
95. Rivera MP, Durham DD, Long JM, Perera P, Lane L, Lamb D, et al. Receipt of recommended follow-up care after a positive lung cancer screening examination. JAMA Netw Open. 2022;5(11):e2240403.
96. Rivera MP, Katki HA, Tanner NT, Triplette M, Sakoda LC, Wiener RS, et al. Addressing disparities in lung cancer screening eligibility and healthcare access. An Official American Thoracic Society Statement. Am J Respir Crit Care Med. 2020;202(7):e95–e112.
97. Schiffelbein JE, Carluzzo KL, Hasson RM, Alford-Teaster JA, Imset I, Onega T. Barriers, facilitators, and suggested interventions for lung cancer screening among a rural screening-eligible population. J Prim Care Community Health. 2020;11:2150132720930544.
98. Niranjan SJ, Opoku-Agyeman W, Carroll NW, Dorsey A, Tipre M, Baskin ML, et al. Distribution and geographic accessibility of lung cancer screening centers in the United States. Ann Am Thorac Soc. 2021;18(9):1577–80.
99. Pistelli F, Aquilini F, Falaschi F, Puliti D, Ocello C, Lopes Pegna A, et al. Smoking cessation in the ITALUNG lung cancer screening: what does "Teachable Moment" mean? Nicotine Tob Res. 2020;22(9):1484–91.
100. Heiden BT, Engelhardt KE, Cao C, Meyers BF, Puri V, Cao Y, et al. Association between lung cancer screening and smoking cessation. Cancer Epidemiol. 2022;79:102194.

101. Krist AH, Davidson KW, Mangione CM, Barry MJ, Cabana M, Caughey AB, et al. Screening for lung cancer: US Preventive Services Task Force Recommendation Statement. JAMA. 2021;325(10):962–70.
102. Shen J, Crothers K, Kross EK, Petersen K, Melzer AC, Triplette M. Provision of smoking cessation resources in the context of in-person shared decision-making for lung cancer screening. Chest. 2021;160(2):765–75.
103. Lowenstein LM, Nishi SPE, Lopez-Olivo MA, Crocker LC, Choi N, Kim B, et al. Smoking cessation services and shared decision-making practices among lung cancer screening facilities: a cross-sectional study. Cancer. 2022;128(10):1967–75.
104. Joseph AM, Rothman AJ, Almirall D, Begnaud A, Chiles C, Cinciripini PM, et al. Lung Cancer Screening and Smoking Cessation Clinical Trials. SCALE (Smoking Cessation within the Context of Lung Cancer Screening) Collaboration. Am J Respir Crit Care Med. 2018;197(2):172–82.
105. Silvestri GA, Tanner NT, Kearney P, Vachani A, Massion PP, Porter A, et al. Assessment of plasma proteomics biomarker's ability to distinguish benign from malignant lung nodules: results of the PANOPTIC (Pulmonary Nodule Plasma Proteomic Classifier) trial. Chest. 2018;154(3):491–500.
106. Schult TA, Lauer MJ, Berker Y, Cardoso MR, Vandergrift LA, Habbel P, et al. Screening human lung cancer with predictive models of serum magnetic resonance spectroscopy metabolomics. Proc Natl Acad Sci U S A. 2021;118(51):e2110633118.
107. Feil C, Staib F, Berger MR, Stein T, Schmidtmann I, Forster A, et al. Sniffer dogs can identify lung cancer patients from breath and urine samples. BMC Cancer. 2021;21(1):917.
108. Meng S, Li Q, Zhou Z, Li H, Liu X, Pan S, et al. Assessment of an exhaled breath test using high-pressure photon ionization time-of-flight mass spectrometry to detect lung cancer. JAMA Netw Open. 2021;4(3):e213486.
109. Alberg AJ, Brock MV, Ford JG, Samet JM, Spivack SD. Epidemiology of lung cancer: diagnosis and management of lung cancer, 3rd ed. American College of Chest Physicians evidence-based clinical practice guidelines. Chest. 2013;143(5 Suppl):e1S–e29S.
110. Loewen G, Black B, McNew T, Miller A. Lung cancer screening in patients with Libby amphibole disease: high yield despite predominantly environmental and household exposure. Am J Ind Med. 2019;62(12):1112–6.
111. Markowitz SB, Manowitz A, Miller JA, Frederick JS, Onyekelu-Eze AC, Widman SA, et al. Yield of low-dose computerized tomography screening for lung cancer in high-risk workers: the case of 7189 US Nuclear Weapons Workers. Am J Public Health. 2018;108(10):1296–302.
112. Mazzone PJ, Gould MK, Arenberg DA, Chen AC, Choi HK, Detterbeck FC, et al. Management of lung nodules and lung cancer screening during the COVID-19 pandemic: CHEST expert panel report. Chest. 2020;158(1):406–15.
113. Davenport MS, Bruno MA, Iyer RS, Johnson AM, Herrera R, Nicola GN, et al. ACR statement on safe resumption of routine radiology care during the coronavirus disease 2019 (COVID-19) pandemic. J Am Coll Radiol. 2020;17(7):839–44.
114. Van Haren RM, Delman AM, Turner KM, Waits B, Hemingway M, Shah SA, et al. Impact of the COVID-19 pandemic on lung cancer screening program and subsequent lung cancer. J Am Coll Surg. 2021;232(4):600–5.
115. Joung RH, Nelson H, Mullett TW, Kurtzman SH, Shafir S, Harris JB, et al. A national quality improvement study identifying and addressing cancer screening deficits due to the COVID-19 pandemic. Cancer. 2022;128(11):2119–25.
116. Henderson LM, Benefield T, Bosemani T, Long JM, Rivera MP. Impact of the COVID-19 pandemic on volumes and disparities in lung cancer screening. Chest. 2021;160(1):379–82.

Chapter 3
Tobacco Prevalence and Treatment

Joelle T. Fathi and Hasmeena Kathuria

Introduction

Since the first Surgeon General's report on smoking, *Smoking and Health: Report of the Advisory Committee to the Surgeon General of the Public Health Service* in 1964, recognizing the proven link between smoking and lung cancer [1], the prevalence of cigarette smoking has significantly declined from 42.4% in 1965 to 12.5% in 2020 among US adults [2]. Tobacco prevention, cessation, and policy control efforts have aimed to protect the public from the harms of smoking and have been critical contributors to the falling smoking rates. Yet, this decline has not been equal across populations [3–5], highlighted in the most recent Surgeon General's report in 2020 [6]. As data on the harms of smoking have accumulated, smoking prevalence shifted to communities impacted by social determinants of health such as low education level, unemployment, and poverty [7]. Thus, it is crucial to target the social factors that lead to chronic tobacco use and health inequities. A goal of the National and State Tobacco Control Program of the Center for Disease Control (CDC) is to "Advance health equity by identifying and eliminating commercial tobacco product-related inequities and disparities" [8].

J. T. Fathi (✉)
Department of Biobehavioral Nursing and Health Informatics, University of Washington School of Nursing, Seattle, WA, USA
e-mail: thirsk@uw.edu

H. Kathuria
The Pulmonary Center, Boston University Chobanian and Avedisian School of Medicine, Boston, MA, USA
e-mail: hasmeena@bu.edu

Disparities in Tobacco Use Patterns

Not surprisingly, populations with a high prevalence of tobacco use, lower quit rates, and higher secondhand smoke exposure experience tobacco-related health disparities [2, 9, 10]. Socioeconomically disadvantaged populations and certain minority groups, including (1) black, indigenous people of color (BIPOC); (2) people who have a high school education or less; (3) those with an annual household income at the federal poverty level or below; (4) belong to the LGBTQ+ community: (5) uninsured, underinsured, or on state Medicaid coverage; and (6) having any level of generalized anxiety disorder or other serious mental health disorder, suffer disproportionately high rates of smoking, nicotine dependence, and tobacco-related health disparities, including lung cancer [2, 11, 12]. Black people who do not smoke are exposed to more secondhand smoke, a known risk factor for lung cancer [13], than White people who do not smoke [14]. Even though Black people are more likely to express interest in stopping smoking, they are less likely to use approved treatments and stop smoking [15]. Forty-four percent of people who smoke cigarettes and are uninsured receive advice to quit smoking compared to 57% of those who have commercial or employer-based insurance, and 21.4% of uninsured people receive guideline-recommended cessation treatment, compared to 32.1% of people who are privately insured [11, 16]. Clinicians and healthcare systems must address these factors to reduce tobacco-related health disparities to avoid variation in the quality of care based on gender, race, ethnicity, sexual or gender identity, geographic location, and socioeconomic status [17].

Carcinogenesis of Tobacco Smoke and the Development of Lung Cancer

Genetic predisposition and environmental exposures predominantly affect whether people develop or circumvent disease. Identification of genes, molecules, and physiologic pathways influencing the risk of disease development from tobacco smoke exposure and its linkage to lung cancer have been underway for decades [18].

Constituents of combustible cigarettes have continued to rise to an all-time high of 7000, with 70 of those being known carcinogens. The primary carcinogenic components of cigarettes, known to have direct effects on the development of lung cancer, include polyaromatic hydrocarbons (PAHs), N-nitrosamines, aromatic amines, aldehydes, and volatile organic hydrocarbons. These ingredients must undergo conversion through cytochrome P-450 enzyme activation to have carcinogenic effects. Cigarette smoke triggers this metabolic activation and the chemicals' carcinogenic properties, whereby they more readily bind to DNA (DNA adduction) [19–21]. DNA adducts (segments of human DNA bound to carcinogens) can contribute to

DNA miscoding during replication leading to the mutation of certain oncogenes directly implicated in the development of lung cancer [22]. The concentration and prevalence of DNA adducts, as a result of tobacco smoke exposure, correlate with the development of lung cancer. Nicotine, while not known to be carcinogenic, does promote the survival and proliferation of malignant cells through reduced apoptosis and increased angiogenesis [19]. Humans possess DNA repair capability that can mitigate DNA adduct harm and reduce the risk of developing lung cancer. This partly explains why some people develop lung cancer while others do not [23].

Lung Cancer Continuum: An Opportunity to Promote Smoking Cessation

Lung cancer is the leading cause of cancer death among men and women, accounting for 18% of cancer deaths worldwide. Smoking is implicated in about 90% of all lung cancers [24, 25]. Substantial evidence demonstrates the benefits of stopping smoking along the lung cancer continuum, including before, at the time, and after a lung cancer diagnosis. Thus, healthcare providers have multiple opportunities and teachable moments to proactively address and motivate smoking cessation in an individual's health journey. Healthcare providers specifically trained in tobacco treatment improve the provision of smoking cessation services [26].

Lung Cancer Screening

Among individuals enrolled in lung cancer screening (LCS), about 50% smoke cigarettes [27]. Individuals eligible for LCS who currently smoke cigarettes can achieve a three- to fivefold mortality reduction if they quit smoking and stay quit [28]. To receive reimbursement for LCS, the Centers for Medicare and Medicaid Services National Coverage Determination for LCS requires that providers offer both tobacco treatment and shared decision-making (SDM), during which patients and providers discuss the benefits and harms of LCS, the patient's preferences and values, and make a decision together about whether to proceed with LCS [29, 30]. Notably, the SDM visit provides an opportunity to initiate a conversation about patients' tobacco use and offer tobacco treatment. Lung cancer screening is not a one-time scan, with the cumulative benefit of screening appreciated by subsequent low-dose CT scans over time. Annual or more frequent follow-up screening intervals are excellent opportunities for critical touchpoints to maintain the cessation conversation with people currently smoking and to provide ongoing opportunities for cessation treatment.

Lung Cancer Care

In individuals who continue to smoke after a lung cancer diagnosis, the mortality risk is twice that of those who stop smoking [31]. A systematic review with meta-analysis that examined the effects of smoking cessation after a primary lung cancer diagnosis demonstrated that quitting smoking following early-stage lung cancer diagnosis resulted in at least a 30% increased 5-year survival for people who stopped smoking compared to those who continued to smoke [31]. Furthermore, quitting smoking increases the therapeutic response to cancer treatment, decreases treatment-related toxicities, and decreases the likelihood of disease progression, developing a second primary cancer, and cancer recurrence [32–34].

Informed by Ongoing Research

The National Institutes of Health and National Cancer Institute have dedicated research funding to examine how best to integrate tobacco treatment into routine cancer care through the Cancer Center Cessation Initiative (3CI): NCI Cancer Moonshot Project and in the LCS setting through the Smoking Cessation at Lung Examination: The SCALE Collaboration; the results of these trials are expected shortly.

Understanding Nicotine Addiction

The brain's neurochemical response to nicotine and resulting neurohormonal alterations are directly implicated in the development of nicotine addiction [35]. Circulating nicotine in the brain attaches to nicotinic acetylcholine receptors (nAChRs) located throughout the brain, causing a cascade of reactions, including the expression of neurohormones [35]; the main effectors of nicotine addiction are in sites that are important to basic survival functions [36, 37]. Nicotine stimulates nAChRs on dopaminergic neurons in the ventral tegmental area (VTA), leading to increased dopamine levels within the striatum and nucleus accumbens [38, 39]. Increased dopamine creates a false safety signal and improved mood, arousal, and cognition disrupted by nicotine withdrawal. In addition, nicotine stimulates other neurotransmitters, including norepinephrine, acetylcholine, serotonin, gamma-aminobutyric acid (GABA), glutamate, and endorphins [40]. Nicotine also promotes long-term learned associations that trigger strong behavioral compulsions to smoke, placing people at lifelong risk for relapse. Furthermore, brain circuits undergo neuroadaptations with repeated exposure to nicotine (e.g., an increase in nAChRs), reinforcing continued nicotine use [41–43].

When people with tobacco use disorder are faced with the possibility of absti-nence, they experience a threat to survival [44]. Discontinuation of nicotine can lead to withdrawal symptoms that include emotional, behavioral, and cognitive disrup-tions that can begin within 1 h, peak at 48–72 h, and gradually decline in most people over the next 6 months [45–47]. As discussed below, starting pharmaco-therapy before quit attempts and extending treatment duration to more than 3 months circumvent the constellation of complex withdrawal symptoms and may facilitate abstinence and prevent relapse.

Dismantling Stigma through Healthcare Provider Self-Awareness and Proactive Work

Understanding the mechanism of nicotine addiction and how to manage tobacco use disorder therapeutically is one step closer to helping people quit smoking. Developing awareness and directing attention to understanding how healthcare pro-viders' life experiences and resources contribute to success and social privilege, and how this privilege leads to power and implicit bias is equally critical to helping people succeed in their cessation journey [48]. Implicit biases and stigmatizing beliefs that people are responsible for their tobacco use disorder lead to discrimina-tion and poor health outcomes for marginalized people [49] who are at higher risk for developing or currently smoking. Furthermore, these stigmatizing beliefs pro-voke self-stigmatization (self-blame) and even nihilism (no value in treatment) for people who smoke cigarettes [50–52], with adverse effects on health-seeking behav-iors [53] and worse quality of life with more psychological distress [54]. Understanding the detrimental effects of provider privilege, implicit biases, and resulting stigma and poor health outcomes points to the criticality of addressing these issues straight on. This begins with a call to action for healthcare providers to examine how they may proactively dismantle stigma to transform the healthcare delivery system.

Taking a Structured and Comprehensive Tobacco Use History

Assessing Nicotine Dependency

Nicotine dependence can be measured by the Fagerstrom test for nicotine depen-dence (FTND); scores range from 0 to 10, with higher scores indicating higher nico-tine dependence [55]. Time to first cigarette (TTFC) is also used to measure nicotine dependence, with shorter TTFC after waking correlated with greater nicotine depen-dency [56]. Data from FTND and TTFC measurements can be instrumental when initiating cessation work. Taking this history opens an opportunity to explore further the struggle patients have had in their cessation journey and, perhaps more important, bolster an understanding of the intensity of the therapeutic interventions that may be necessary for successful cessation.

Motivational Interviewing for Behavior Change

Motivational interviewing (MI) for behavior change is a patient-centered practice that acknowledges the patient as an expert in their story, values, and beliefs [57]. Centered on the patient and healthcare provider partnership, provider acceptance and empathy are foundational. MI is leveraged as a conceptual framework to help patients identify perceived barriers and build their confidence to quit [57]. This communication technique allows providers to express compassion for patients to help them resolve their ambivalence in smoking cessation. It may be adopted and adapted by almost anyone interested in helping patients with behavior change and quitting smoking.

Leveraging the 5As Model for Behavior Change in Cessation Work

The 5As Model for Behavior Change reaches the end-to-end landscape of nicotine addiction, is simple to implement when helping people to quit smoking, is strongly recommended by the US Preventive Services Task Force [58], and is effective in promoting smoking cessation [59–61]. Developed to be applied sequentially, this model is initiated by (1) *Asking* all patients about tobacco use (this is where FTND and TTFC could be assessed); (2) *Advising* those who use tobacco products to stop; and (3) *Assessing* willingness to make a quit attempt. This third step could be facilitated by motivational interviewing, including determining the patient's motivation to quit and their confidence in quitting. The transtheoretical Model of Behavior Change, aka Stages of Change [62], may also be helpful in this *Assess* step to identify a patient's readiness to quit and meet them where they are. (4) *Assisting* the patient interested in quitting includes counseling and developing a personalized combination of pharmacotherapy and behavior change cessation plan. For the patient who is not ready to quit at this time, the MI strategies may help patients move forward in the Readiness to Change stages; (5) finally, *Arrange* for the patient to have a clinical follow-up, even and especially if they express they are not ready to quit [63]. While "Asking" and "Advising" are commonly performed in the clinic, the more complex steps, particularly "Arranging" follow-up, occur less frequently [64] due to barriers including lack of knowledge, training, or confidence in intervention delivery, time constraints, or uncertainty about insurance coverage [65].

Taking a Comprehensive Tobacco History and Examination for Success

The strategies and frameworks discussed above facilitate taking a comprehensive tobacco history that further enhances an opportunity to collect an accurate history of the intensity and duration of tobacco use. This includes the onset (date) of regular smoking and other tobacco products, the frequency (daily, weekly, etc.) of use, intake quantity (number of cigarettes or packs per day), and the duration of use (how many years). It is essential to also inquire about where they have been in their tobacco use and cessation journey, where they are now, their goals for the future, what has and has not worked in their efforts to quit, and what has led to relapse. Reconciling current medication use, taking a medical and psychiatric history, and a thorough social history will provide critical information to support the patient's efforts to quit and design a personalized pharmacologic and non-pharmacologic therapeutic management plan. Physical examination findings related to the effects of smoking (e.g., claudication, hypertension, wheezing) may provide teachable moments to proactively address and motivate smoking cessation.

Counseling

Opt-out approaches to offering tobacco treatment to all individuals who smoke regardless of readiness to quit and allowing patients to decline treatment have been shown to have both a high acceptance rate and increased smoking abstinence compared to opt-in approaches, where tobacco treatment is only offered to individuals who are ready to stop smoking [66–68].

Behavioral interventions confer skills for managing behavioral and psychological factors that may undermine quitting [69], including behavioral counseling, motivational interviewing, and cognitive therapy. Behavioral counseling addresses the processes by which cigarette use becomes associated with social and environmental contexts by providing practical tools to avoid triggering situations and manage urges [70]. Individuals who smoke frequently experience conflict between their motivation to stop smoking and their confidence in quitting based on previous attempts and abstinence experiences. Healthcare providers can elicit behavior change by resolving ambivalence through motivational strategies, such as motivational interviewing [71]. Brief motivational interventions using the "5Rs" have been shown to positively affect abstinence [72]. The "5Rs" include (1) discussing the personal "Relevance" of smoking cessation; (2) articulating the "Risks" of continued smoking; (3) developing the anticipated "Rewards" of quitting; (4) preconceiving the "Roadblocks" to stopping smoking; and (5) addressing these issues on a "Repeated" basis [73]. Cognitive therapy addresses maladaptive cognitions that underlie compulsive smoking behaviors due to environmental and emotional triggers and the emotional distress that accompanies such experiences that often place people at high risk for relapse [74, 75].

Both individual and group counseling that emphasizes problem-solving skills are effective [76, 77]. Outcomes improve with greater intensity of counseling and when accompanied by pharmacotherapy [77], and all patients should be encouraged to use available support services [73]. Printed self-help materials only slightly increase quit rates compared to no intervention [78]. Telephone-based counseling may be effective in promoting smoking cessation. Quitlines (800-QUIT-NOW) are available in all 50 states and the District of Columbia, Guam, and Puerto Rico at no cost, with many offering free supplemental nicotine replacement products. Although current utilization is low, Quitlines can increase access to tobacco cessation counseling and treatment for people with limited resources, including those who experience low SES and rurality [69, 79–82]. Proactive telephone counseling increases the likelihood of quitting with three to five telephone calls yielding a 27% increased successful cessation compared to a minimal intervention (one call) [83]. In the LCS setting, telephone-based counseling was feasible and effective in improving 3-month biochemically verified abstinence [84]. Interactive text-messaging services that deliver motivational messages and education about smoking and cessation increase 6-month quit rates [79, 85].

Pharmacotherapy

Pharmacotherapy effectively reduces withdrawal symptoms and improves control over the desire to smoke [36, 44]. The combination of counseling and pharmacotherapy is more effective than either intervention alone. There are seven FDA-approved medications for tobacco treatment (Table 3.1): (1) five forms of nicotine replacement therapy (nicotine lozenges, gum, and patches can be purchased over the counter; nicotine nasal inhalers and spray are available by prescription only); (2) bupropion (Wellbutrin; Zyban); and (3) varenicline (Chantix). All FDA-approved pharmacotherapies for tobacco cessation have some action that mimics or inhibits the effects of nicotine use while also stimulating dopamine. The table provides strategies, dosing considerations, and side effect management for busy clinicians initiating pharmacotherapy for tobacco dependence.

A recent American Thoracic Society clinical guideline established varenicline as the optimal controller compared to bupropion and nicotine patches for both long-term abstinence and serious adverse events [86]. Other practical considerations include initiating combination therapy (e.g., varenicline plus nicotine patch; nicotine patch plus nicotine inhaler or gum; bupropion plus nicotine patch) since combination therapy can increase abstinence compared to monotherapy [86] and extending pharmacotherapy for up to 6 months since pharmacotherapy that extends beyond 12 weeks can improve abstinence and reduce the likelihood of relapses [86]. Guidelines also recommend starting varenicline before a patient is ready to abstain since pretreatment increases the likelihood of eventual abstinence, with an

Table 3.1 FDA-approved medications for tobacco treatment

	Medication and formulation	Equivalent of 1 cigarette	Available strengths	Dose and frequency
Prescription only	Varenicline	Not applicable	0.5 mg 1.0 mg	Initiate treatment 1 week before quit date Take 0.5 mg once daily (days 1–3), then take 0.5 mg BID (days 4–7), then on day 8, take 1 mg BID For patients not ready to set a quit date, consider a flexible quit date during days 8–35 of treatment
	Bupropion	Not applicable	Immediate release 75 mg, 100 mg Sustained release 100 mg, 150 mg, and 200 mg Extended release 150 mg & 300 mg	Take 150 mg PO QD for 3 days then increase to 150 mg BID
	Oral nicotine inhaler	1/4 cartridge = 1 cigarette 1 cartridge = 4-mg nicotine or 4 cigarettes	4 mg/cartridge	Frequent or continuous puffing until craving subsides Max dose: 16 cartridges/day Initially use 1 cartridge every 1–2 h PRN and at least 6 cartridges per day
	Nicotine nasal spray	2 sprays (actuations) = 1 cigarette	0.5 mg/spray (actuation) One dose = 2 sprays (one in each nostril) Approximately 50 mg (100 sprays) per bottle	1–2 doses every hour as needed Max daily dose is 40 mg (80 sprays/day) Can use up to 5 doses (10 sprays) per hour

(continued)

Table 3.1 (continued)

	Medication and formulation	Equivalent of 1 cigarette	Available strengths	Dose and frequency
Over the counter	Nicotine transdermal patch	Goal of nicotine replacement patch is to match the total daily dose of nicotine consumption (see dose and frequency column)	7 mg/day 14 mg/day 21 mg/day	21 mg for >20 cigarettes per day 14 mg for <20 cigarettes per day 7 mg for <10 cigarettes per day
	Nicotine gum and lozenge	2 mg piece of gum or lozenge (only ~1 mg available/absorbed orally)	2 mg 4 mg	Time to first cigarette ≥30 min start at 2 mg Time to first cigarette ≤30 min start at 4 mg Max 20 pieces/day

Pharmacokinetics	Dosing considerations	Side effects management
Mechanism: Partial agonist and antagonist at the $\alpha 4\beta 2$nAChR and dopamine release **Half-life:** ~ 24 h **Metabolism:** Minimal, <10% metabolized **Excretion:** Urine (92% excreted unchanged)	Dose adjustment needed with renal impairment and end-stage renal disease No dose adjustment needed with hepatic impairment Lowers seizure threshold; precautions advised accordingly Treatment duration is 12 weeks but can be up to 6 months and even longer in certain patients	**GI symptoms =** take with food and full glass of water **Activation and agitation =** avoid concurrent cigarette smoking or reduce cigarette intake, consider reducing the dose **Vivid dreams and nocturnal wakefulness =** reduce dose **Mood changes =** severe agitation, depression = discontinue medication if severe
Mechanism: Partial $\alpha 4\beta 2$nAChR antagonist and reuptake of dopamine and norepinephrine **Half-life:** 8–24 h for immediate release; 21 h (extended release) **Metabolism:** Hepatic, via CYP2B6 **Excretion:** Urine (87%); feces (10%)	Initiate treatment 1 week before quit date and continue treatment for 7–12 weeks Can be taken in combination with nicotine replacement therapy Lowers seizure threshold; precautions advised accordingly Avoid in hepatic impairment	Same as above **Anorexia =** suppresses appetite, avoid in people who have appetite suppression (e.g. anorexia and bulimia) **MAOIs =** avoid using with MAOIs

Pharmacokinetics	Dosing considerations	Side effects management
Mechanism: α4β2nAChR agonist with dopamine release **Half-life:** 1–2 h **Metabolism:** Primarily liver and minor metabolism in kidney **Excretion:** Urine	Should take short puffs, not inhale Do not eat or drink 15 min before or during use Remove dentures before using	**Nausea** = avoid smoking when using NRT, reduce amount of nicotine replacement when taking varenicline, avoid drinking liquids when using gum or lozenge (avoid swallowing nicotine) **Activation and agitation** = avoid drinking with short acting NRT, consider reducing the dose
Mechanism: α4β2nAChR agonist with dopamine release **Half-life:** 1–2 h **Metabolism:** Primarily liver and minor metabolism in kidney **Excretion:** Urine: (10–30% unchanged)	Spray toward septum; do *not* sniff or snort Commonly burns or stings	**Vivid dreams and nocturnal wakefulness** = take patch off at bedtime **Skin rash** = rotate patch on body **Mood changes** = severe agitation, depression = discontinue medication if severe
Mechanism: α4β2nAChR agonist with dopamine release **Half-life:** 3–4 h **Metabolism:** Primarily liver and minor metabolism in kidney **Excretion:** Urine	Apply to clean and dry skin Apply new patch each day Rotate location of patch daily Do not cut patch Strongly consider using in combination with short-acting nicotine replacement therapy	
Mechanism: α4β2nAChR agonist with dopamine release **Half-life:** 3–4 h **Metabolism:** Primarily liver and minor metabolism in kidney **Excretion:** Urine	Absorbed through oral mucosa Do not eat or drink 15 min before or during use Remove dentures before using Gum: Chew and tuck, repeat, until flavor diminishes Lozenge: Tuck in cheek until melted; do not bite, chew, or swallow	

estimated 308 more patients achieving abstinence per 1000 patients treated and only a small increase in SAEs [86]. In addition, a study by Hartwell and colleagues showed that starting varenicline before a quit attempt was associated with increased memory and attentiveness and reduced cravings [87].

Nicotine Replacement Therapy

NRT is a nonselective agonist of nAChRs. NRT generally provides a much slower release and absorption of nicotine into the blood than the immediate peak from smoking a cigarette, making it a nonaddictive and safe alternative to smoking [36, 44].

Combining a "controller" that provides continuous dosing to produce steady levels of nicotine (transdermal nicotine patch) with a "reliever" that allows for "as needed" dosing in response to acute cravings (nasal spray, inhaler, gum, or lozenge) is more effective in achieving prolonged abstinence than either alone.

The transdermal nicotine patch (available in 21 mg, 14 mg, and 7 mg doses) reaches peak blood levels of nicotine 1–4 h after application and provides the longest and most constant delivery rate. The side effects of transdermal nicotine patches include abnormal dreams and skin irritation at the application site.

Blood levels of nicotine peak about 10 min after using the nasal spray or inhaler and 20 min after using the gum or lozenge; they are, therefore, often used as "as needed" adjuncts to the nicotine patch. Both nicotine gum and lozenge are available in 2 mg and 4 mg doses. For the gum, patients are instructed to chew until the gum releases a "peppery" taste or tingling sensation, at which point they should place it between the gum and cheek to allow for absorption. When the "peppery" taste or tingling stops, they should rechew the gum until the sensation is released again, at which point they should place the gum on the alternate side of the cheek. This process is repeated for about 30 min or until the "peppery" taste or tingling sensation no longer occurs. For the lozenge, patients are instructed to place the lozenge against the cheek to allow for mucosal absorption. The lozenge can be rotated side to side to minimize discomfort if left in one place for too long. Side effects can include hiccups, heartburn, nausea, mouth sores, and mouth soreness when used incorrectly.

The nicotine inhaler consists of a cartridge that can deliver approximately 4 mg of nicotine placed inside a plastic mouthpiece. Patients take short puffs, and when used continuously, last about 20 min. Patients use a minimum of 6 cartridges and up to 16 cartridges per day. Side effects can include cough and mouth and throat irritation. The nicotine nasal spray can also rapidly deliver a high dose of nicotine and may be especially useful if patients have high nicotine dependence. However, common side effects of nasal irritation, runny nose, watery eyes, sneezing, and coughing are frequently limiting. Finally, it is important to note that these oral nicotine replacement medications will not be effective in patients who wear dentures. However, these short-acting nicotine replacement medications may be safely and effectively used when dentures are removed.

Varenicline

Varenicline is a selective partial agonist of nAChRs and competes with nicotine for nAChR binding, thus acting as a mixed agonist/antagonist at these receptors [88, 89]. Individuals are often started on varenicline at 0.5 mg daily and titrated to a target dose of 1 mg twice daily. Instructing the patient to delay attempts at quitting during the first week is often recommended and safe since the onset of action is delayed [90]. Dosing is reduced for individuals with creatinine clearance of less than 30 ml/min to 0.5 mg twice daily. Patients on hemodialysis are prescribed 0.5 mg daily. Taking varenicline with food decreases common side effects of nausea and vomiting. Other side effects include abnormal dreams and headaches, which can be managed by dose reduction with little impact on the outcome [91]. It is important to note that nausea is a common side effect when the nAChRs are over-stimulated and saturated by nicotine. Because of the mechanism of action of vareni-cline at this receptor and its high affinity for the nAChRs, people may experience significant nausea when taking varenicline and smoking cigarettes. Therefore, it is prudent to advise patients taking varenicline and smoking to reduce their cigarette intake or, ideally, quit altogether to avoid this overstimulation (flooding) of the nAChRs and nausea.

Findings from pooled clinical trial data, several large observational studies, and a large prospective randomized trial (EAGLES) have assuaged concern over the link between varenicline and suicidal ideation and suicidal behavior [92]. The Boxed Warning for serious mental health side effects was removed from the drug label in December 2016.

Bupropion Sustained Release

Bupropion sustained release (S.R.), a non-tricyclic antidepressant, acts partially as a dopamine/norepinephrine reuptake inhibitor [88, 93]. Bupropion likely alleviates tobacco withdrawal via its dopamine/norepinephrine-stimulating properties. Since it can nonselectively antagonize nAChRs, bupropion may also block nicotine rein-forcement and cue-induced craving [94]. Bupropion S.R. is most effective in achiev-ing abstinence and controlling withdrawal symptoms when combined with NRT [95, 96]. Patients with tobacco use disorder should begin bupropion S.R. 7 days before the anticipated quit date, though a longer pretreatment may be needed to see the full effect. Bupropion S.R. is started at 150 mg once daily for the first 3 days, then increased to twice daily dosing on day 4 to treatment completion. Commonly described side effects may include insomnia, abnormal dreams, dizziness, xerosto-mia, nausea, agitation, and anxiety. Bupropion should not be combined with other medications or conditions (e.g., alcohol use disorder) that lower the seizure thresh-old [97]. Based on the EAGLES trial [92], the Boxed Warning for serious mental health side effects was removed from the drug label in December 2016.

Extended Duration of Cessation Therapy

The neurohormonal alterations of the brain from chronic nicotine use are known to cause ongoing and long-term cravings for nicotine placing people vulnerable to triggers that previously led to tobacco use. The current recommendation for a treatment course for NRT is 12 weeks, but research has shown even better outcomes with a longer duration of treatment, with people being twice as likely to quit smoking with a 24-week treatment compared to a 12-week course of treatment and less likely to relapse [98].

Examining the Role of Electronic Cigarettes in Promoting Smoking Cessation

Evidence suggests that electronic cigarettes (e-cigarettes) may aid in smoking cessation when used as a therapeutic intervention with counseling [99–101]. A Cochrane review found that quit rates were higher with nicotine e-cigarettes than with NRT and non-nicotine e-cigarettes. E-cigarettes, however, are not associated with a reduction in nicotine dependency [102] and may lead to dual use of e-cigarettes and cigarettes. On the other hand, a recent meta-analysis of observational studies that provide evidence on how e-cigarette devices are used in actual practice found that e-cigarette consumer product use was not significantly associated with smoking cessation [101]. In the American Thoracic Society Clinical Practice Guideline, varenicline, rather than e-cigarettes, is recommended for smoking cessation [86]. The US Preventive Services Task Force concludes that there is insufficient evidence to evaluate the harms and benefits of e-cigarettes for smoking cessation [103].

Relapse Prevention

The complex neurochemistry and neurohormonal alterations in the brain and behavioral components of nicotine dependence often lead to a chronic relapsing condition [104]. Helping people quit smoking is the first giant leap forward in living tobacco-free, but assisting people to maintain abstinence from smoking is equally if not more important. In 2021, the US Preventive Services Task Force issued a Grade A recommendation for combined pharmacotherapy and behavioral therapy to optimize the opportunity for sustained abstinence [58]. Pharmacotherapy prevents withdrawal from nicotine and the resulting unpleasant symptoms that provoke relapse. In addition, ongoing behavioral counseling and cessation coaching are critical to avoiding succumbing to associated behavioral changes and environmental cues that reinforce tobacco use [105].

Conclusion

Routine lung cancer screening or a lung cancer diagnosis avails a series of encounters to deliver discussions and treatment on tobacco use. Healthcare providers and multidisciplinary teams are positioned to provide life-saving tobacco cessation services to all people accessing the healthcare system and seeking care. Patient-centered and nonjudgmental approaches to providing tobacco treatment at each clinical encounter must be tailored to each person's unique attributes and address unmet social needs. A comprehensive tobacco treatment plan combined with pharmacotherapy and behavioral counseling yields the best opportunity for people to quit smoking and the health benefits of long-term success. Addressing provider and structural and systemic contributors to implicit bias and stigma is critical and imperative to the success of reaching the most vulnerable and at-risk populations who have the most to benefit from cessation services.

Conflict of Interest Statement Hasmeena Kathuria is a section editor for UpToDate (Tobacco Dependence Treatment). Joelle T. Fathi reports no conflict of interest

References

1. United States Public Health Service. Smoking and health: report of the advisory committee to the surgeon general of the public health service. Washington, DC: U.S. Department of Health, Education, and Welfare; 1964.
2. Cornelius ME, Loretan CG, Wang TW, Jamal A, Homa DM. Tobacco product use among adults - United States, 2020. MMWR Morb Mortal Wkly Rep. 2022;71(11):397–405. https://doi.org/10.15585/mmwr.mm7111a1.
3. Garrett BE, Dube SR, Winder C, Caraballo RS. Cigarette smoking—United States, 2006-2008 and 2009-2010. MMWR Suppl. 2013;62(3):81–4.
4. Martell BN, Garrett BE, Caraballo RS. Disparities in adult cigarette smoking—United States, 2002-2005 and 2010-2013. MMWR Morb Mortal Wkly Rep. 2016;65(30):753–8. https://doi.org/10.15585/mmwr.mm6530a1.
5. Jamal A, Agaku IT, O'Connor E, King BA, Kenemer JB, Neff L. Current cigarette smoking among adults—United States, 2005–2013. MMWR Morb Mortal Wkly Rep. 2014;63(47):1108–12.
6. Graham H. Why social disparities matter for tobacco-control policy. Am J Prev Med. 2009;37(2 Suppl):S183–4. https://doi.org/10.1016/j.amepre.2009.05.007.
7. Department of Health and Human Services. Smoking cessation: a report of the surgeon general. Washington, DC: U.S. Department of Health and Human Services, Centers for Disease Control and Prevention, National Center for Chronic Disease Prevention and Health Promotion, Office on Smoking and Health; 2020.
8. Cdcgov: National and State Tobacco Control Program | Smoking & Tobacco Use | CDC. 2021. https://www.cdc.gov/tobacco/stateandcommunity/tobacco-control/index.htm. Accessed Dec 17 2021.
9. Drope J, Liber AC, Cahn Z, Stoklosa M, Kennedy R, Douglas CE, et al. Who's still smoking? Disparities in adult cigarette smoking prevalence in the United States. CA Cancer J Clin. 2018;68(2):106–15. https://doi.org/10.3322/caac.21444.
10. Tobacco use among U.S. racial/ethnic minority groups; African Americans, American Indians and Alaska Natives, Asian Americans and Pacific Islanders, Hispanics: a report of the

Surgeon General. In: National Center for Chronic Disease P, Health Promotion OoS, Health, editors. Dept. of Health and Human Services, Center for Disease Control and Prevention, National Center for Chronic Disease Prevention and Health Promotion, Office on Smoking and Health 1998.

11. Babb S, Malarcher A, Schauer G, Asman K, Jamal A. Quitting smoking among adults—United States, 2000–2015. MMWR Morb Mortal Wkly Rep. 2017;65(52):1457–64.

12. Smith PH, Mazure CM, McKee SA. Smoking and mental illness in the U.S. population. Tob Control. 2014;23(e2):e147–53. https://doi.org/10.1136/tobaccocontrol-2013-051466.

13. Eriksen MP, LeMaistre CA, Newell GR. Health hazards of passive smoking. Annu Rev Public Health. 1988;9:47–70. https://doi.org/10.1146/annurev.pu.09.050188.000403.

14. Truth Initiative—Inspiring Tobacco-Free Lives. 2020.

15. Cdcgov: D.C. Best practices for comprehensive tobacco control programs, 2014. Atlanta, GA: U.S. Department of Health and Human Services, CDC; 2014. https://www.cdc.gov/tobacco/stateandcommunity/guides/index.htm?CDC_AA_refVal=https%3A%2F%2Fwww.cdc.gov%2Ftobacco%2Fstateandcommunity%2Fbest_practices%2Findex.htm. Accessed 3 Jan 2022.

16. Kaiser Family Foundation: Key Facts about the Unisnured Population. 2020. https://www.kff.org/uninsured/issue-brief/key-facts-about-the-uninsured-population/. Accessed 1 Dec 2021.

17. Institute of Medicine (U.S.). Committee on quality of health Care in America., National Academies Press (U.S.). crossing the quality chasm: a new health system for the 21st century. Washington, DC: National Academy Press; 2001.

18. Stepanov I. Carcinogens and toxicants in combusted tobacco products and related cancer risks. In: Hecht SSH, editor. Tobacco and cancer: the science and the story. New Jersey: World Scientific; 2022. p. 101–27.

19. U.S. Department of Health & Human Services. Cancer. How tobacco smoke causes disease: the biology and behavioral basis for smoking-attributable disease. Rockville, MD: U.S. Department of Health and Human Services; 2010. p. 221–305.

20. O'Connor RJ. Tobacco. In: DeVita VT, Lawrence TS, Rosenberg SA, editors. Cancer: principles & practice of oncology. Philadelphia: Wolters Kluwer; 2019. p. 90–8.

21. Guengerich FP. Common and uncommon cytochrome P450 reactions related to metabolism and chemical toxicity. Chem Res Toxicol. 2001;14(6):611–50. https://doi.org/10.1021/tx0002583.

22. Boyle P. Tobacco and public health: science and policy. Oxford: Oxford University Press; 2004.

23. Nishikawa A, Mori Y, Lee IS, Tanaka T, Hirose M. Cigarette smoking, metabolic activation and carcinogenesis. Curr Drug Metab. 2004;5(5):363–73. https://doi.org/10.2174/1389200043335441.

24. Hecht SS, Szabo E. Fifty years of tobacco carcinogenesis research: from mechanisms to early detection and prevention of lung cancer. Cancer Prev Res (Phila). 2014;7(1):1–8. https://doi.org/10.1158/1940-6207.CAPR-13-0371.

25. U.S. Department of Health & Human Services. The health consequences of smoking—50 years of Progress: a report of the surgeon general 2014. Executive Summary 2014. https://www.hhs.gov/surgeongeneral/reports-and-publications/tobacco/index.html.

26. Carson K, Verbiest ME, Crone MR, Brin MP, Esterman AJ, Assendelft WJ, Smith BJ. Training health professionals in smoking cessation. Cochrane Database Syst Rev. 2012;2012(5):CD000214. Accessed 1 Dec 2021.

27. Aberle DR, Adams AM, Berg CD, Black WC, Clapp JD, Fagerstrom RM, et al. Reduced lung-cancer mortality with low-dose computed tomographic screening. N Engl J Med. 2011;365(5):395–409. https://doi.org/10.1056/NEJMoa1102873.

28. Pastorino U, Boffi R, Marchiano A, Sestini S, Munarini E, Calareso G, et al. Stopping smoking reduces mortality in low-dose computed tomography screening participants. J Thorac Oncol. 2016;11(5):693–9. https://doi.org/10.1016/j.jtho.2016.02.011.

29. Wiener RS, Gould MK, Arenberg DA, Au DH, Fennig K, Lamb CR, et al. An official American Thoracic Society/American College of Chest Physicians policy statement: implementation of low-dose computed tomography lung cancer screening programs in clinical practice. Am J Respir Crit Care Med. 2015;192(7):881–91. https://doi.org/10.1164/rccm.201508-1671ST.
30. Centers for Medicare & Medicaid Services: Screening for Lung Cancer with Low Dose Computed Tomography (LDCT). 2021. https://www.cms.gov/medicare-coverage-database/view/ncacal-decision-memo.aspx?proposed=N&ncaid=304. Accessed 23 Aug 2022.
31. Parsons A, Daley A, Begh R, Aveyard P. Influence of smoking cessation after diagnosis of early stage lung cancer on prognosis: systematic review of observational studies with meta-analysis. BMJ. 2010;340:b5569. https://doi.org/10.1136/bmj.b5569.
32. Warren GW, Alberg AJ, Cummings KM, Dresler C. Smoking cessation after a cancer diagnosis is associated with improved survival. J Thorac Oncol. 2020;15(5):705–8. https://doi.org/10.1016/j.jtho.2020.02.002.
33. Toll BA, Brandon TH, Gritz ER, Warren GW, Herbst RS, ASO T, et al. Assessing tobacco use by cancer patients and facilitating cessation: an American Association for Cancer Research policy statement. Clin Cancer Res. 2013;19(8):1941–8. https://doi.org/10.1158/1078-0432.CCR-13-0666.
34. Aredo JV, Luo SJ, Gardner RM, Sanyal N, Choi E, Hickey TP, et al. Tobacco smoking and risk of second primary lung cancer. J Thorac Oncol. 2021;16(6):968–79. https://doi.org/10.1016/j.jtho.2021.02.024.
35. Benowitz NL. Nicotine addiction. N Engl J Med. 2010;362(24):2295–303. https://doi.org/10.1056/NEJMra0809890.
36. Leone FT, Evers-Casey S. Developing a rational approach to tobacco use treatment in pulmonary practice: a review of the biological basis of nicotine addiction. Clin Pulm Med. 2012;19(2):53–61. https://doi.org/10.1097/CPM.0b013e318247cada.
37. Subramaniyan M, Dani JA. Dopaminergic and cholinergic learning mechanisms in nicotine addiction. Ann N Y Acad Sci. 2015;1349:46–63. https://doi.org/10.1111/nyas.12871.
38. Zhang T, Zhang L, Liang Y, Siapas AG, Zhou FM, Dani JA. Dopamine signaling differences in the nucleus accumbens and dorsal striatum exploited by nicotine. J Neurosci. 2009;29(13):4035–43. https://doi.org/10.1523/JNEUROSCI.0261-09.2009.
39. Exley R, Clements MA, Hartung H, McIntosh JM, Cragg SJ. Alpha6-containing nicotinic acetylcholine receptors dominate the nicotine control of dopamine neurotransmission in nucleus accumbens. Neuropsychopharmacology. 2008;33(9):2158–66. https://doi.org/10.1038/sj.npp.1301617.
40. Benowitz NL. Neurobiology of nicotine addiction: implications for smoking cessation treatment. Am J Med. 2008;121(4 Suppl 1):S3–10. https://doi.org/10.1016/j.amjmed.2008.01.015.
41. Mukhin AG, Kimes AS, Chefer SI, Matochik JA, Contoreggi CS, Horti AG, et al. Greater nicotinic acetylcholine receptor density in smokers than in nonsmokers: a PET study with 2-18F-FA-85380. J Nucl Med. 2008;49(10):1628–35. https://doi.org/10.2967/jnumed.108.050716.
42. Nashmi R, Xiao C, Deshpande P, McKinney S, Grady SR, Whiteaker P, et al. Chronic nicotine cell specifically upregulates functional alpha 4* nicotinic receptors: basis for both tolerance in midbrain and enhanced long-term potentiation in perforant path. J Neurosci. 2007;27(31):8202–18. https://doi.org/10.1523/JNEUROSCI.2199-07.2007.
43. Cosgrove KP, Batis J, Bois F, Maciejewski PK, Esterlis I, Kloczynski T, et al. beta2-nicotinic acetylcholine receptor availability during acute and prolonged abstinence from tobacco smoking. Arch Gen Psychiatry. 2009;66(6):666–76. https://doi.org/10.1001/archgenpsychiatry.2009.41.
44. Leone FT, Carlsen KH, Folan P, Latzka K, Munzer A, Neptune E, et al. An official American Thoracic Society research statement: current understanding and future research needs in tobacco control and treatment. Am J Respir Crit Care Med. 2015;192(3):e22–41. https://doi.org/10.1164/rccm.201506-1081ST.

45. Schultz W. Dopamine reward prediction error coding. Dialogues Clin Neurosci. 2016;18(1):23–32.
46. Hughes JR. Tobacco withdrawal in self-quitters. J Consult Clin Psychol. 1992;60(5):689–97. https://doi.org/10.1037//0022-006x.60.5.689.
47. Hughes JR, Hatsukami DK, Pickens RW, Svikis DS. Consistency of the tobacco withdrawal syndrome. Addict Behav. 1984;9(4):409–12. https://doi.org/10.1016/0306-4603(84)90043-1.
48. Ellis C, Jacobs M, Kendall D. The impact of racism, power, privilege, and positionality on communication sciences and disorders research: time to Reconceptualize and seek a pathway to equity. Am J Speech Lang Pathol. 2021;30(5):2032–9. https://doi.org/10.1044/2021_AJSLP-20-00346.
49. FitzGerald C, Hurst S. Implicit bias in healthcare professionals: a systematic review. BMC Med Ethics. 2017;18(1):19. https://doi.org/10.1186/s12910-017-0179-8.
50. Volkow ND. Stigma and the Toll of addiction. N Engl J Med. 2020;382(14):1289–90. https://doi.org/10.1056/NEJMp1917360.
51. Hamann HA, Ostroff JS, Marks EG, Gerber DE, Schiller JH, Lee SJ. Stigma among patients with lung cancer: a patient-reported measurement model. Psychooncology. 2014;23(1):81–92. https://doi.org/10.1002/pon.3371.
52. Rigney M, Rapsomaniki E, Carter-Harris L, King JC. A 10-year cross-sectional analysis of public, oncologist, and patient attitudes about lung cancer and associated stigma. J Thorac Oncol. 2021;16(1):151–5. https://doi.org/10.1016/j.jtho.2020.09.011.
53. Carter-Harris L. Lung cancer stigma as a barrier to medical help-seeking behavior: practice implications. J Am Assoc Nurse Pract. 2015;27(5):240–5. https://doi.org/10.1002/2327-6924.12227.
54. Chambers SK, Dunn J, Occhipinti S, Hughes S, Baade P, Sinclair S, et al. A systematic review of the impact of stigma and nihilism on lung cancer outcomes. BMC Cancer. 2012;12:184. https://doi.org/10.1186/1471-2407-12-184.
55. Heatherton TF, Kozlowski LT, Frecker RC, Fagerstrom KO. The Fagerstrom test for nicotine dependence: a revision of the Fagerstrom tolerance questionnaire. Br J Addict. 1991;86(9):1119–27.
56. Branstetter SA, Muscat JE, Mercincavage M. Time to first cigarette: a potential clinical screening tool for nicotine dependence. J Addict Med. 2020;14(5):409–14. https://doi.org/10.1097/ADM.0000000000000610.
57. Miller WR, Rollnick S. Motivational interviewing: helping people change. 3rd ed. New York: The Guilford Press; 2013.
58. United States Preventive Services Task Force: Tobacco Smoking Cessation in Adults, Including Pregnant Persons: Interventions. 2021. https://www.uspreventiveservicestaskforce.org/uspstf/recommendation/tobacco-use-in-adults-and-pregnant-women-counseling-and-interventions. Accessed 1 Nov 2021.
59. Carr AB, Ebbert J. Interventions for tobacco cessation in the dental setting. Cochrane Database Syst Rev. 2012;2012(6):CD005084. https://doi.org/10.1002/14651858.CD005084.pub3.
60. Rice VH, Heath L, Livingstone-Banks J, Hartmann-Boyce J. Nursing interventions for smoking cessation. Cochrane Database Syst Rev. 2017;12:CD001188. https://doi.org/10.1002/14651858.CD001188.pub5.
61. Stead LF, Buitrago D, Preciado N, Sanchez G, Hartmann-Boyce J, Lancaster T. Physician advice for smoking cessation. Cochrane Database Syst Rev. 2013;2013(5):CD000165. https://doi.org/10.1002/14651858.CD000165.pub4.
62. Prochaska JO, DiClemente CC. Stages and processes of self-change of smoking: toward an integrative model of change. J Consult Clin Psychol. 1983;51(3):390–5.
63. Fiore M, Jaen C, Baker T, Bailey W, Benowitz N, Curry S, et al. Treating tobacco use and dependence: 2008 update. Rockville, MD: U.S. Department of Health and Human Services; 2008.

64. King B, Dube S, Babb S, McAfee T. Patient-reported recall of smoking cessation interventions from a health professional. Prev Med. 2013;57:715–7.
65. Sheffer MA, Baker TB, Fraser DL, Adsit RT, McAfee TA, Fiore MC. Fax referrals, academic detailing, and tobacco quitline use: a randomized trial. Am J Prev Med. 2012;42(1):21–8. https://doi.org/10.1016/j.amepre.2011.08.028.
66. Fu SS, Van Ryn M, Sherman SE, Burgess DJ, Noorbaloochi S, Clothier B, et al. Proactive tobacco treatment and population-level cessation: a pragmatic randomized clinical trial. JAMA Intern Med. 2014;174:671–7.
67. Haas J, Linder J, Park E, Gonzalez I, Rigott N, Klinger E, et al. Proactive tobacco cessation outreach to smokers of low socioeconomic status: a randomized clinical trial. JAMA Intern Med. 2015;175:218–26.
68. Herbst N, Wiener R, Helm E, O'Donnell C, Fitzgerald C, Wong C, et al. Effectiveness of an opt-out electronic helath record-based tobacco treatment consult service at an urban safety net hospital. Chest. 2020;158:1734–41.
69. U.S. Department of Health and Human Services. Smoking cessation: a report of the surgeon general. Rockville, MD: Public Health Service, Office of the Surgeon General; 2020.
70. Webb MS, Rodriguez-Esquivel D, Baker EA. Smoking cessation interventions among Hispanics in the United States: a systematic review and mini meta-analysis. Am J Health Promot. 2010;25(2):109–18. https://doi.org/10.4278/ajhp.090123-LIT-25.
71. Bhattacharya A, Vilardaga R, Kientz JA, Munson SA. Lessons from practice: designing tools to facilitate individualized support for quitting smoking. ACM Trans Comput Hum Interact. 2017;2017:3057–70. https://doi.org/10.1145/3025453.3025725.
72. Klemperer EM, Hughes JR, Solomon LJ, Callas PW, Fingar JR. Motivational, reduction and usual care interventions for smokers who are not ready to quit: a randomized controlled trial. Addiction. 2017;112(1):146–55. https://doi.org/10.1111/add.13594.
73. 2008 PHS Guideline Update Panel La, and Staff. Treating tobacco use and dependence: 2008 update U.S. Public Health Service clinical practice guideline executive summary. Respir Care. 2008;53(9):1217–22.
74. Beck A. Cognitive therapy: nature and relation to behavior therapy. Behav Ther. 1970;1:184–200.
75. Butler AC, Chapman JE, Forman EM, Beck AT. The empirical status of cognitive-behavioral therapy: a review of meta-analyses. Clin Psychol Rev. 2006;26(1):17–31. https://doi.org/10.1016/j.cpr.2005.07.003.
76. Stead LF, Carroll AJ, Lancaster T. Group behaviour therapy programmes for smoking cessation. Cochrane Database Syst Rev. 2017;3:CD001007. https://doi.org/10.1002/14651858.CD001007.pub3.
77. Lancaster T, Stead LF. Individual behavioural counselling for smoking cessation. Cochrane Database Syst Rev. 2017;3:CD001292. https://doi.org/10.1002/14651858.CD001292.pub3.
78. Hartmann-Boyce J, Lancaster T, Stead LF. Print-based self-help interventions for smoking cessation. Cochrane Database Syst Rev. 2014;(6):CD001118. https://doi.org/10.1002/14651858.CD001118.pub3.
79. Whittaker R, McRobbie H, Bullen C, Rodgers A, Gu Y. Mobile phone-based interventions for smoking cessation. Cochrane Database Syst Rev. 2016;4:CD006611. https://doi.org/10.1002/14651858.CD006611.pub4.
80. Sherman SE, Krebs P, York LS, Cummins SE, Kuschner W, Guvenc-Tuncturk S, et al. Telephone care co-ordination for tobacco cessation: randomised trials testing proactive versus reactive models. Tob Control. 2018;27(1):78–82. https://doi.org/10.1136/tobaccocontrol-2016-053327.
81. Hirko KA, Kerver JM, Ford S, Szafranski C, Beckett J, Kitchen C, et al. Telehealth in response to the COVID-19 pandemic: implications for rural health disparities. J Am Med Inform Assoc. 2020;27(11):1816–8. https://doi.org/10.1093/jamia/ocaa156.

82. Merianos AL, Fevrier B, Mahabee-Gittens EM. Telemedicine for tobacco cessation and prevention to combat COVID-19 morbidity and mortality in rural areas. Front Public Health. 2020;8:598905. https://doi.org/10.3389/fpubh.2020.598905.
83. Matkin W, Ordonez-Mena J, Hartmann-Boyce J. Telephone counseling for smoking cessation. Cochrane Database Syst Rev. 2019;5(5):CD002850.
84. Taylor KL, Hagerman CJ, Luta G, Bellini PG, Stanton C, Abrams DB, et al. Preliminary evaluation of a telephone-based smoking cessation intervention in the lung cancer screening setting: a randomized clinical trial. Lung Cancer. 2017;108:242–6. https://doi.org/10.1016/j.lungcan.2017.01.020.
85. Cobos-Campos R, Fernández A, de Larrinoa A, de Lafuente S, Moriñigo A, Parraza Diez N, Aizpuru BF. Effectiveness of text messaging as an adjuvant to health advice in smoking cessation programs in primary care. A randomized clinical trial. Nicotine Tob Res. 2017;19(8):901–7. https://doi.org/10.1093/ntr/ntw300.
86. Leone FT, Zhang Y, Evers-Casey S, Evins AE, Eakin MN, Fathi J, et al. Initiating pharmacologic treatment in tobacco-dependent adults. An official American Thoracic Society clinical practice guideline. Am J Respir Crit Care Med. 2020;202(2):e5–e31. https://doi.org/10.1164/rccm.202005-1982ST.
87. Hartwell KJ, Lematty T, McRae-Clark AL, Gray KM, George MS, Brady KT. Resisting the urge to smoke and craving during a smoking quit attempt on varenicline: results from a pilot fMRI study. Am J Drug Alcohol Abuse. 2013;39(2):92–8. https://doi.org/10.3109/00952990.2012.750665.
88. Gómez-Coronado N, Walker AJ, Berk M, Dodd S. Current and emerging pharmacotherapies for cessation of tobacco smoking. Pharmacotherapy. 2018;38(2):235–58. https://doi.org/10.1002/phar.2073.
89. de Moura FB, McMahon LR. The contribution of α4β2 and non-α4β2 nicotinic acetylcholine receptors to the discriminative stimulus effects of nicotine and varenicline in mice. Psychopharmacology. 2017;234(5):781–92. https://doi.org/10.1007/s00213-016-4514-4.
90. Hajek P, McRobbie HJ, Myers KE, Stapleton J, Dhanji AR. Use of varenicline for 4 weeks before quitting smoking: decrease in ad lib smoking and increase in smoking cessation rates. Arch Intern Med. 2011;171(8):770–7. https://doi.org/10.1001/archinternmed.2011.138.
91. Niaura R, Hays JT, Jorenby DE, Leone FT, Pappas JE, Reeves KR, et al. The efficacy and safety of varenicline for smoking cessation using a flexible dosing strategy in adult smokers: a randomized controlled trial. Curr Med Res Opin. 2008;24(7):1931–41. https://doi.org/10.1185/03007990802177523.
92. Anthenelli RM, Benowitz NL, West R, St Aubin L, McRae T, Lawrence D, et al. Neuropsychiatric safety and efficacy of varenicline, bupropion, and nicotine patch in smokers with and without psychiatric disorders (EAGLES): a double-blind, randomised, placebo-controlled clinical trial. Lancet. 2016;387(10037):2507–20. https://doi.org/10.1016/S0140-6736(16)30272-0.
93. Stahl SM, Pradko JF, Haight BR, Modell JG, Rockett CB, Learned-Coughlin S. A review of the neuropharmacology of bupropion, a dual norepinephrine and dopamine reuptake inhibitor. Prim Care Companion J Clin Psychiatry. 2004;6(4):159–66.
94. Fryer JD, Lukas RJ. Noncompetitive functional inhibition at diverse, human nicotinic acetylcholine receptor subtypes by bupropion, phencyclidine, and ibogaine. J Pharmacol Exp Ther. 1999;288(1):88–92.
95. Stead LF, Koilpillai P, Fanshawe TR, Lancaster T. Combined pharmacotherapy and behavioural interventions for smoking cessation. Cochrane Database Syst Rev. 2016;3:CD008286. https://doi.org/10.1002/14651858.CD008286.pub3.
96. Windle SB, Filion KB, Mancini JG, Adye-White L, Joseph L, Gore GC, et al. Combination therapies for smoking cessation: a hierarchical Bayesian meta-analysis. Am J Prev Med. 2016;51(6):1060–71. https://doi.org/10.1016/j.amepre.2016.07.011.

97. Silverstone PH, Williams R, McMahon L, Fleming R, Fogarty S. Alcohol significantly lowers the seizure threshold in mice when co-administered with bupropion hydrochloride. Ann General Psychiatry. 2008;7:11. https://doi.org/10.1186/1744-859X-7-11.
98. Schnoll RA, Patterson F, Wileyto EP, Heitjan DF, Shields AE, Asch DA, Lerman C. Efficacy of extended duration transdermal nicotine therapy: a randomized trial. Ann Intern Med. 2010;152(3):144–51.
99. Hajek P, Phillips-Waller A, Przulj D, Pesola F, Myers Smith K, Bisal N, et al. A randomized trial of E-cigarettes versus nicotine-replacement therapy. N Engl J Med. 2019;380(7):629–37. https://doi.org/10.1056/NEJMoa1808779.
100. Hartmann-Boyce J, McRobbie H, Lindson N, Bullen C, Begh R, Theodoulou A, et al. Electronic cigarettes for smoking cessation. Cochrane Database Syst Rev. 2021;4:CD010216. https://doi.org/10.1002/14651858.CD010216.pub5.
101. Wang RJ, Bhadriraju S, Glantz SA. E-cigarette use and adult cigarette smoking cessation: a meta-analysis. Am J Public Health. 2021;111(2):230–46. https://doi.org/10.2105/AJPH.2020.305999.
102. Hanewinkel R, Niederberger K, Pedersen A, Unger JB, Galimov A. E-cigarettes and nicotine abstinence: a meta-analysis of randomised controlled trials. Eur Respir Rev. 2022;31(163):210215. https://doi.org/10.1183/16000617.0215-2021.
103. Krist AH, Davidson KW, Mangione CM, Barry MJ, Cabana M, Caughey AB, et al. Interventions for tobacco smoking cessation in adults, including pregnant persons: U.S. preventive services task force recommendation statement. JAMA. 2021;325(3):265–79. https://doi.org/10.1001/jama.2020.25019.
104. Steinberg MB, Schmelzer AC, Richardson DL, Foulds J. The case for treating tobacco dependence as a chronic disease. Ann Intern Med. 2008;148(7):554–6.
105. Chaiton M, Diemert L, Cohen JE, Bondy SJ, Selby P, Philipneri A, et al. Estimating the number of quit attempts it takes to quit smoking successfully in a longitudinal cohort of smokers. BMJ Open. 2016;6(6):e011045. https://doi.org/10.1136/bmjopen-2016-011045.

Chapter 4
Approach to Lung Nodules

Srikanth Vedachalam, Nichole T. Tanner, and Catherine R. Sears

Introduction

Pulmonary nodules are identified incidentally on imaging performed for patient symptoms or through low-dose computed tomography (LDCT) lung cancer screening. Pulmonary nodules are identified incidentally in ~29% of diagnostic chest CTs and 23–60% of LDCTs for lung cancer screening [1–3]. Clinicians are challenged to manage these nodules, which can be difficult given that these can represent a wide range of diseases, from benign infectious and inflammatory diseases to primary lung and secondary metastatic malignancies. Many professional societies have provided expert recommendations on diagnostic evaluation, and numerous

S. Vedachalam
Division of Pulmonary, Critical Care, Sleep and Occupational Medicine, Indiana University School of Medicine, Indianapolis, IN, USA
e-mail: svedacha@iu.edu

N. T. Tanner
Division of Pulmonary, Department of Medicine, Critical Care, Allergy, and Sleep Medicine, Medical University of South Carolina, Charleston, SC, USA

Health Equity and Rural Outreach Innovation Center (HEROIC), Ralph H. Johnson Veterans Affairs Hospital, Charleston, SC, USA
e-mail: tripici@musc.edu

C. R. Sears (⊠)
Division of Pulmonary, Critical Care, Sleep and Occupational Medicine, Indiana University School of Medicine, Indianapolis, IN, USA

Pulmonary/Pulmonary Oncology, Richard L. Roudebush VA Medical Center, Indianapolis, IN, USA
e-mail: crufatto@iu.edu

C. MacRosty, M. P. Rivera (eds.), *Lung Cancer*, Respiratory Medicine,
https://doi.org/10.1007/978-3-031-38412-7_4

validated models that integrate patient demographics, behaviors, and nodule characteristics can be used to predict probability of malignancy. Diagnostic evaluation of pulmonary nodules requires both considerations of individualized risks of malignancy and of diagnostic workup in an attempt to optimize the benefit-to-risk ratio. Evaluating pulmonary nodules balances the need to diagnose early-stage lung cancer with risks of invasive evaluations for benign nodules and the possible risks of delayed diagnosis. Diagnostic evaluations are rarely ideal, requiring multidisciplinary input, consideration of patient preference, available resources, and individual comorbidities. Understanding the approach to pulmonary nodules, including current techniques and future directions, is essential to providing the best personalized care for patients.

In this chapter, we discuss the subtypes and classifications of pulmonary nodules, imaging techniques to detect nodules, landmark trials, society recommendations for management, diagnostic approaches currently available, and future directions of the field, including promising diagnostic biomarkers for pulmonary nodules.

Etiology

Pulmonary nodules are defined as distinct foci of radiographic density surrounded by lung parenchyma measuring < 3 cm in diameter [4]. Pulmonary nodules can exist in isolation, referred to as a solitary pulmonary nodule (SPN), or can be multiple, which occur in more than half of patients with pulmonary nodules found on chest CT [5, 6]. When multiple nodules are seen on lung imaging, the largest is referred to as the *dominant* nodule.

Pulmonary nodules are incidentally found on approximately 30% of all CT chest scans, the majority representing benign disease [1]. In a high-risk cohort, such as those imaged by LDCT in the National Lung Screening Trial (NLST), ~25% were identified as having a pulmonary nodule. In some populations, such as those included in the Veterans Affairs (VA) Demonstration Project, ~60% of those undergoing LDCT were identified as having a pulmonary nodule [2, 3]. In each of these studies, only 2.4% and 2.5% of nodules were malignant, respectively [2, 3]. The incidental pulmonary nodule identification rate increases with advancing age and is similar in men and women [1]. Pulmonary nodules have numerous potential etiologies, including neoplasm, infection, inflammatory conditions, and congenital diseases (Fig. 4.1) [7, 8]. The first steps in determining the management of pulmonary nodules include obtaining a thorough history, physical exam, and evaluation of radiologic characteristics.

Category/Disease	Imaging or clinical findings*
Malignant Neoplasms	
Primary bronchopulmonary lung cancer	Growing, irregular, spiculated, sunburst, corona radiata. Solid, mixed solid-ground glass or necrotizing.
Carcinoid	Smooth walled, growing
Lung metastasis	Multiple smooth walled, peripheral, growing
Pulmonary lymphoma	B-symptoms
Sarcoma	Known bone/muscle sarcoma
Chondroid lesion (enchondroma,chrondrosarcoma)	Popcorn calcification
Benign Growth	
Hamartoma	Intralesional fat attenuation, possible calcifications
Neurofibroma/neurofibromatosis	Characteristics skin lesions
Chondroma	Popcorn calcification
Lipoma	Fat attenuation, rounded, homogeneous
Papilloma/Papillomatosis	HPV infection, polypoid
Thoracic endometriosis	Catamenial hemoptysis, CP, SOB; pneumo-/hemothorax
Benign metastasizing leiomyoma of the lung	Smooth-walled, uterine leiomyomas
Pleomorphic adenoma	Smooth/round. Larger tumors heterogenous
Inflammatory	
Rheumatoid nodules	Seropositive RA, severe disease, subcutaneous nodules
Nummular sarcoidosis	Characteristic bilateral hilar lymphadenopathy
Granulomatosis with polyanglitis	Concurrent kidney involvement
Organizing pneumonia (cryptogenic, secondary)	Characteristic exposures, recurrent pneumonia with transient infiltrates
Intrapulmonary lymph node	Near/on fissure; round, oval or polygonal
Pulmonary inflammatory pseudotumor	Lower lobe, no invasion
Mucoid impaction	Bronchiectasis, "finger in glove" sign
Vascular	
Arteriovenous malformation	Feeding artery and draining vein on contrasted images
Pulmonary embolism/infarct	PE on contrasted study; peripheral, wedge-shaped
Infectious	
Granuloma	Diffuse, central or laminar/concentric calcification
Endemic fungi- histoplasmosis, blastomycosis, coccidioidomycosis, aspergillosis, etc.	Known exposure/locale increasing risk of endemic mycoses
Mycobacterium (tuberculosis and non-TB)	History of mycobacterium tuberculosis
Other atypical infections	Indolent/progression of productive cough and dyspnea
Lung abscess	Necrotizing, fevers or clinical symptoms of infection
Septic embolic	Clinical symptoms of infection, endocarditis, IV drug abuse
Nocardia species	Immunosuppressed, DM, chronic lung disease (PAP)
Actinomyces	Poor dentition
Mucormycosis	Immunosuppression
Localized Pneumonia	Acute infectious symptoms, rapid development of nodule
Parasitic disease/Echinococcosis (hydatid cyst)	Hypodense cyst w/ hyperdense smooth rim, multiseptated
Cryptococcus species	Immunocompromised, DM, imaging non-specific/various
Congenital	
Bronchogenic cysts	Round/oval, smooth, fluid-density
Pulmonary sequestration	Multiple based on variant
Tuberous sclerosis/perivascular epitheloid cell neoplasms	Characteristic skin, nail and neurologic findings
Miscellaneous	
Rounded atelectasis	Round/oval pleural based, "comet tail"
Nodular pulmonary amyloidosis	Systemic findings of amyloidosis
Silicotic nodules/Progressive massive fibrosis	Occupational exposure
Post-radiation fibrosis/late post-SBRT nodular fibrosis	Radiation treatment
Lipoid pneumonia	Exogenous sources of oil inhalation, history of aspiration
Pulmonary pseudotumor	Loculated effusion in pleural fissure, fluid density

Fig. 4.1 Causes and characteristics of pulmonary nodules *Characteristic clinical and/or radiologic findings have been described for many of these causes of pulmonary nodule and can help with differential diagnosis, but their absence should not rule out the possibility of nonspecific or atypical presentations. *DM* diabetes mellitus, *RA* rheumatoid arthritis, *SOB* shortness of breath, *CP* chest pain, *IV* intravenous

Evaluation

The initial assessment of pulmonary nodules should include identification of age and a history of substance use, particularly cigarette smoking. Lung cancer risk increases with advancing age independent of other risk factors, with the median age at diagnosis 70 years [9]. Cigarette smoking is the primary cause of lung cancer in the United States and is implicated in up to 90% of all lung cancer deaths in the United States [10]. The risk of lung cancer from cigarette smoking is cumulative and dose-dependent, increasing with the number of cigarettes smoked and duration of cigarette smoking [10]. Cessation of cigarette smoking decreases the risk of lung cancer over time, but the risk remains elevated at three times compared to people who never smoked, even 25 years after cessation [11]. Although lower than cigarette smoking, pipe, cigar, and hookah smoking, as well as secondhand cigarette smoke exposure, have also been linked to lung cancer development [12–14]. Long-duration epidemiologic studies linking e-cigarettes to lung cancer are lacking; however, in vivo and in vitro studies which find carcinogens in e-cigarette vapor, increased DNA damage, and development of lung cancer in mouse models suggest a potential link [15, 16]. Approximately 25% of all patients with lung cancer globally and 10–15% in the United States never smoked cigarettes, highlighting the potential peril of relying on this risk factor alone in pulmonary nodule evaluation [17]. Patients should also be assessed for other exposures, including secondhand smoke, indoor wood, coal, and cooking fire use, all of which have been implicated in increasing the risks of lung cancer, particularly in never-smoking women [17, 18].

A detailed occupational and carcinogen exposure history is also critical in evaluating pulmonary nodules. Prior asbestosis, known asbestos exposure, or occupations known to have high asbestos exposure are associated with an increased risk of

Non-Modifiable Factors
  Advancing Age
  Strong family history
  Prior lung cancer

Smoking
  Cigarettes
    Current > Former > Never
  Secondhand smoke
  Cigar and pipe
  E-cigarettes (probable)

Other Exposures
  Asbestos
  Radon
  Biomass fuels/wood burning stoves
  Herbicides/Agent Orange (probable)
  Radiation Exposure (medical, cosmic)
  Inhaled dusts/metals/fumes
   Beryllium
   Chromium
   Cadmium
   Nickel
   Arsenic

Lung Diseases
  COPD/emphysema
  Interstitial Lung Diseases
  Prior lung infections

Other Diseases
  HIV
  HPV (squamous cell histology)

Pulmonary Nodule Characteristics
  Larger size
  Spiculation > Lobulation
  Upper lobe location > Lower/middle
lobe

Fig. 4.2 Clinical and pulmonary risk factors for nodule malignancy risk

lung cancer, particularly when combined with cigarette smoking which may increase lung cancer risk ninefold [19, 20]. Occupational exposures to other carcinogens, dust, metals, and toxic inhalants have also been associated with lung cancer development either directly or through development of chronic inflammation, pulmonary fibrosis, or other lung diseases that increase lung cancer risk (Fig. 4.2) [21]. Because they may point to other causes of nonmalignant nodules, a history of inhaled drug use, and other environmental, pet/bird, and occupational exposures should be included. Based on geographic considerations, areas high in endemic mycoses, nodules caused by histoplasmosis and coccidioidomycosis should be considered, particularly if there is a recent illness after characteristic exposure or travel, confirmatory antibody testing (such as positivity for both histoplasmosis IgG and IgM), or, in the case of blastomycosis, recent regional outbreak [22, 23]. A detailed review of systems should be explored, including questions regarding signs of autoimmune conditions, particularly rheumatoid arthritis, and sarcoidosis, in which pulmonary nodules are common.

The physical exam can prove helpful in the assessment of pulmonary nodules. In addition, it can provide clues of concomitant lung disorders associated with pulmonary nodules, such as interstitial lung diseases and sarcoidosis. Extrathoracic evaluations, including a thorough lymph node exam to evaluate for metastatic malignancy or infection and evaluating for signs of autoimmune disease, can help focus one investigation, which will involve a comprehensive exam as well as obtaining an extensive medical history.

Imaging

Approximately 1.6 million pulmonary nodules are incidentally detected in the United States each year, and that number has likely grown with increasing use and implementation of lung cancer screening [1]. The initial approach to nodule management is a comparison to previous radiographs. Pulmonary nodules present for 18–24 months or greater without change have a high probability of being benign, and most recommendations do not require further evaluation or radiologic follow-up [5, 24]. However, most nodules are new or without comparative imaging available, found incidentally on chest radiographs (CXR) or chest CT, and require further evaluation. For many clinicians, pulmonary nodules pose a diagnostic dilemma and can cause significant patient distress [25]. This section will describe common imaging techniques and recommendations.

Chest X-ray and Chest CT

Pulmonary nodules can be identified by CXR or chest CT. Chest CT is often needed to confirm and characterize a pulmonary nodule seen on CXR, as up to 20% of nodules identified on CXR represent artifacts from extrathoracic, chest wall, or pleural findings [7]. The National Lung Cancer Screening Trial, the largest randomized lung cancer screening study, enrolled more than 15,000 US participants at high risk for lung cancer and showed a more than threefold higher detection rate with CT over CXR [2]. This is consistent with numerous prior studies, which also supported the increased sensitivity of chest CT to CXR for detecting pulmonary nodules [26–28]. Several recommendations have been made to standardize chest CT imaging for pulmonary nodule identification and assessment. The American College of Radiology and the Society of Thoracic Radiology (ACR-STR) practice parameters recommend that multi-detector CT techniques in a single breath hold at full inspiration be used for nodule detection. Axial image reconstruction should be with a slice thickness of 2.5 mm or less with reconstruction intervals equal or less than the slice thickness used. 1 mm or less reconstruction intervals are ideal for minimizing volume averaging effects to detect small nodules. Radiation dose should be as low as possible, and the low dose of 3 mSv for most patients is adequate for nodule detection [29].

There is no consensus on the best method for measuring nodules on CT. One common approach is to use the long and the perpendicular short axis diameter on a single axial CT image, with the average of these diameters recommended by Fleischner Society based on better correlation with malignancy risk compared to maximum diameter [30]. A difference of at least 1.5 mm between interval scans is considered true growth [2, 31]. Applying a two-dimensional measurement to a three-dimensional nodule limits this approach. Volume-based measures can be used to classify nodule risk based on size (i.e., volumes of $50mm^3$ or less denoting likely benign findings, 50–500 mm^3 sized nodules are classified as indeterminate, and $500mm^3$ are high-risk nodules requiring further management). A volume change of $\geq 25\%$ is an often-accepted cutoff to delineate actual growth between scans [32]. Volumetric assessment allows for calculation of volume double timing (VDT), with a VDT of <400 days or development of a new solid component in a ground-glass nodule between short intervals, as early as 6 weeks after the initial CT, indicating a change that needs further investigation [33, 34]. There is debate on the superior method of nodule measurement among societies, with measurement of diameter more commonly practiced in the United States and volumetric analysis having gained traction in Europe, including a European position statement recommending volumetric assessment for lung cancer screening [35]. Some studies suggest volumetry may be more reproducible between measurements compared to diameter, decreasing the time to growth detection and subsequently the number or frequency of LDCT imaging, particularly automated or semiautomated assessments [33, 36–38]. Many factors can diminish reliability of volumetric measurements, including variations between volumetry software packages and CT scanners, slice thickness, the presence of IV contrast material, irregularities in shape, subsolid nodule density, nodule location, and decreasing pulmonary nodule size [32]. Advances in technology, including automated radiomics, and radiogenomics approaches, may dramatically impact CT chest image interpretation and subsequent pulmonary nodule management [39].

Classification of Pulmonary Nodules by Imaging

Evaluation of pulmonary nodules seen on chest CT must start with assessing the probability of malignancy. Guidelines for pulmonary nodule management have aimed to simplify this risk assessment by considering clinical risk factors (high risk denoting any clinical risk factors increasing the risk of malignancy) and nodule features, including nodule characteristics, size, number (solitary vs. multiple), and density (solid vs. subsolid vs. mixed). These are briefly discussed below and in Fig. 4.1.

Specific Morphologic Features

A nodule can be classified by its morphological characteristics as seen on CT imaging, characterized as solid, semisolid (solid component among ground-glass density), and nonsolid (or pure ground-glass). Nodule contour terms are also described with some (e.g., rounded, smooth, tentacle/polygonal) more often considered benign, while others (e.g., lobulated, spiculated, ragged, pleural tags/retractions, vessel sign, "sunburst" or "corona radiata" sign, cavitary/thick walled) are more concerning for likely malignancy [7, 40, 41]. Calcification is a common finding in nodules and can similarly suggest etiology. Diffuse, central, laminar (concentric), or popcorn calcification patterns suggest benign etiologies (e.g., granulomas or chondroid lesions) and do not require further evaluation [42, 43]. Stippled, eccentrically calcified, and noncalcified nodules may be malignant and require further diagnostic evaluation [7]. Hamartomas are benign, characteristically show fat hypoattenuation (-40 to -120 Hounsfield units on soft tissue chest CT windows), and do not require further diagnostic evaluation. Pulmonary nodules resulting from arteriovenous malformations are seen with feeding and draining vessels on either side. Other benign nodular lesions include infectious and inflammatory causes, pulmonary infarct, rounded atelectasis (presence of "comet tail" or "hurricane sign"), loculated effusion, and congenital and sequestered lung. Close collaboration with radiologists trained in interpretation of chest imaging is highly useful to avoid invasive evaluation of clearly benign nodules.

Locations of nodules within the lung can help risk stratify these lesions. Upper lobe location is associated with higher risk of lung cancer, but malignancy can occur in any lung field [5]. Nodules identified in the perifissural region often represent benign lymph nodes and can be identified by trained radiologists by their location and triangular, ovoid, or lentiform shape [44, 45]. Several small (<6 mm) bilateral nodules can many times also be seen in benign states such as endemic fungal exposure, acute inflammatory, infectious, and autoimmune diseases [30]. The presence of multiple pulmonary nodules larger than 6 mm in diameter may be associated with similar or even higher risk of malignancy. The Nederlands-Leuvens Longkanker Screenings Onderzoek (NELSON) study found an increased risk of malignancy when two to four pulmonary nodules were identified; the presence of five or more was associated with a lower risk of malignancy compared to a solitary pulmonary nodule [46]. Other studies of screen detected pulmonary nodules did not show a difference in the likelihood of malignancy in patients with multiple pulmonary nodules compared to solitary pulmonary nodules [5, 47].

Nodule Size: Solid Pulmonary Nodules

Solid pulmonary nodules (SPN) are the most commonly found nodules on chest imaging and may represent both benign and malignant diseases [48]. Unless clearly benign by characteristic calcification patterns, several societies, including the Fleischner Society, British Thoracic Society (BTS), and American College of Chest Physicians (CHEST), have provided recommendations on follow-up of incidentally diagnosed pulmonary nodules (Table 4.1) [30, 41, 49]. Very small SPN, classified by size <5–6 mm in diameter, or by volumes <80mm^3 (BTS) or < 100 mm^3 (Fleischner Society), are typically considered very low risk of malignancy. The

Table 4.1 Society recommendations for incidental pulmonary nodule radiologic follow-up by size and density

Guidelines for management of incidental nodules					
	Very small nodules (diameter)	Small nodules (diameter)	Intermediate nodules (diameter)	Nonsolid (pure ground-glass) (diameter)	Partial solid nodules (diameter)
Fleischner Society*	Solitary nodule				
	<6 mm*[a] Low risk: No follow-up needed High risk: +/− CT chest −12 mo	6-8 mm*[a] CT chest at 6–12 mo, then at 18–24 mo	>8 mm*[a] CT at 3 month vs. PET/CT vs. tissue biopsy vs. surgical excision	≥6 mm*[a] CT at 6–12 month and then every 2 year until 5 year	≥6 mm*[a] CT at 3–6 months and then annually for 5 year until growth/solid component ≥6 mm
	Multiple nodules				
	< 6 mm*[a] Low risk: No follow-up High risk: +/− CT chest at 12 mo	6–8 mm*[a] CT chest at 3–6 month then at 18–24 month	> 8 mm*[a] CT chest at 3–6 month, then at 18–24 months	< 6 mm*[a] Typically benign. CT at 3–6 month; if high risk, consider repeat at 2 and 4 year ≥ 6 mm CT 3–6 month; management based on most suspicious nodule	
ACCP/ CHEST	≤ 4 mm Low risk: +/− CT chest[b] at 12 mo High risk: CT chest[b] at 12 month	>4–8 mm >4–6 mm Low risk: CT chest[b] at 12 month High risk: CT chest[b] at 6–12 month, then at 18–24 month >6–8 mm Low risk: CT chest[b] at 6–12 month then 18–24 month High risk: CT chest[b] at 3–6 month, then 9–12 month, then at 24 month	> 8 mm Risk-based evaluation including CT surveillance (very low risk) vs PET or nonsurgical biopsy (intermediate risk) vs. diagnostic wedge resection (high risk)	>5 mm Annual CT chest[b] for 3 year >10 mm – Consider CT chest at 3 months, and biopsy (surgical vs nonsurgical) if persistent	≤8 mm CT chest[b] at 3, 12, and 24 month, then annually for another 1–3 year >8–15 mm CT chest[b] at 3 months followed by PET/CT or biopsy/ resection if persistent ≥15 mm Proceed directly to PET/CT vs. biopsy/ resection)

Table 4.1 (continued)

Guidelines for management of incidental nodules					
BTS	<5 mm No follow-up	≥5–6 mm CT at 12 months. If stable on volumetry, can discharge. If stable on diameter repeat at 24 months ≥6-8 mm CT at 3 month and if stable or VDT >400 days, then repeat at 12 months	≥8 mm/≥300 mm³ CT surveillance vs. biopsy vs. surgical excision dependent on risk calculators	≥5 mm CT at 3 months and then further CT surveillance vs. nonsurgical vs. surgical excision based on risk assessment calculators	≥5 mm CT at 3 months and then further CT surveillance vs. nonsurgical vs surgical excision based on risk assessment calculators

CT computed tomography, *SBRT* stereotactic body radiation therapy, *RFA* radiofrequency ablation, *PET/CT* positron emission tomography/computed tomography, *VDT* volume doubling time, *BTS* British Thoracic Society

[a] Fleischner Society measurements are based on average diameter of largest pulmonary nodule. They also provide volumetric equivalents to average diameter sizes: 6 mm = 100 mm³, 8 mm = 250 mm³. BTS measurements are based on maximum diameter. Evaluation of growth is recommended by calculation of >25% volume doubling time (VDT), diagnostic evaluation for VDT < 400 days

[b] Noncontrasted, low-dose CT chest recommended. Low risk = no lung cancer risk factors. High risk = at least one lung cancer risk factor. Recommendations for subsequent CT chest imaging are based on no change in size or appearance from initial scan

[*] Non-contrasted, low-dose CT chest recommended. Low Risk = no lung cancer risk factors. High Risk = at least one lung cancer risk factor. Recommendations for subsequent CT chest imaging is based on no change in size or appearance from initial scan

prevalence of malignancy in incidentally discovered SPN < 5 mm is very low, ranging from 0 to 1% [50]. Even the NLST, which included only patients typically considered higher risk for lung cancer, found that only 0.5% of nodules with diameters 4–6 mm were ultimately malignant [2]. Most guidelines recommend no further radiologic follow-up for low-risk individuals, while no radiologic follow-up or consideration of an optional CT chest at 6–12 months can be considered in those with high-risk clinical features.

SPN 6–8 mm in diameter (or 100–250 mm³) are associated with a slightly higher risk of malignancy ranging from 0.5 to 2% [21, 30]. Guidelines vary slightly but typically include an initial CT chest in 6–12 months, and, if showing stability in size, a second CT chest at 18–24 months from the initial CT to assess for long-term stability, after which subsequent imaging is not recommended. BTS advocates for the use of volume doubling time (VDT) to avoid missing slow growing tumors [49]. Enlarging nodules during this follow-up period should be assessed with further diagnostic testing depending on the size or rate of growth. A clinical trial to determine the best radiologic surveillance for these nodules is ongoing [51].

Intermediate pulmonary nodules (~8–15 mm diameter) and larger (>15 mm) SPNs are associated with a higher risk of malignancy, estimated at 5–15% and > 15%, respectively [52]. Because of the higher likelihood of malignancy, these nodules necessitate a more aggressive diagnostic approach. Fleischner Society, BTS, and CHEST recommend short-term CT chest (~3 months), PET/CT scan, or surgical or nonsurgical biopsy (i.e., resection, CT-guided percutaneous biopsy, bronchoscopic biopsy, etc.) to further evaluate and/or empirically treat these nodules. Additional factors including patient preference, ability to tolerate invasive testing/treatment, and technical feasibility of invasive procedures may guide management.

Subsolid Pulmonary Nodules

Subsolid pulmonary nodules fall into pure ground-glass and semisolid pulmonary nodules. Ground-glass or subsolid appearance refers to nodules with low attenuation in which densities do not obscure the underlying lung architecture [31]. While pure ground-glass nodules may be benign in nature, persistent growing lesions >5–6 mm are very likely to represent premalignant or early malignant lung findings such as atypical adenomatous hyperplasia, minimally invasive lung adenocarcinoma, or lipidic predominant adenocarcinoma [53–56]. When malignant, these tend to grow at a slower pace than solid lung cancers and are typically of lung adenocarcinoma histology [4]. Monitoring of subsolid nodules is based on size and is summarized in Table 4.1.

Pure Ground-Glass Nodules

Those measuring 5–6 mm are very unlikely to be malignant, and most guidelines recommend little or no radiologic follow-up. Recommendations for those measuring >6 mm diameter are repeat CT chest in 6–12 months and subsequent surveillance imaging every 1–2 years with a minimum of 5 years of radiologic follow-up. Those measuring >10–20 mm in diameter, those developing new solid components, and those with morphological features including bubbly fluencies, air bronchograms, spiculation, and pleural retractions warrant closer surveillance or earlier diagnostic evaluation [21]. The majority of persistent pure ground-glass nodules represent premalignant or early malignant lesions. However, exact size at which treatment is needed is not clear, with the reported frequency of invasive lung adenocarcinoma in pure ground-glass nodules >10 mm ranging from 10 to 50% [21, 53, 54].

Semisolid Nodules (Part Solid, Part Ground-Glass)

This morphology is more concerning for malignancy, particularly in the setting of a new or growing solid component within a ground-glass nodule [5, 40, 57]. The ground-glass component is often adenocarcinoma in situ, while the solid portion represents invasive adenocarcinoma. Recommendations from US societies focus on the size of the solid component to dictate follow-up and further management, recommending closer radiologic follow-up than pure ground-glass nodules. CHEST and Fleischner Society guidelines are similar, recommending CT follow-up for up to 5 years for smaller nodules with 3-month CT follow-up vs PET/CT or biopsy for larger lesions. BTS recommendations do not distinguish between pure ground-glass and semisolid nodules [49].

Pulmonary Nodule Number

Multiple pulmonary nodules are found in up to 61% of CT chest imaging studies [6]. Multiple very small (<5–6 mm) pulmonary nodules are likely benign and do not routinely require radiologic follow-up. For multiple pulmonary nodules where any nodule is >5–6 mm diameter, the recommended follow-up is dictated by the largest pulmonary nodule >6 mm in diameter (Table 4.1). Fleischner Society guidelines recommend a more aggressive radiologic follow-up for multiple pulmonary nodules where the largest nodule size is 6–8 mm in diameter [30].

Studies drawing from lung cancer screening populations suggest that multiple nodules are associated with a similar risk of malignancy as the presence of a SPN [5, 46, 47]. In the NELSON study, the largest nodule was most likely to be the malignant nodule [46]. However, it should be noted that another study evaluating pulmonary nodules in the PanCan and BCCA screening studies found that 20% of malignancies were ultimately diagnosed in a nodule other than the largest [5]. For this reason, each nodule should be considered separately as a possible malignancy, and evaluation of any enlarging pulmonary nodule or solid component of a part-solid nodule should guide subsequent evaluation. As with SPNs, the recommended duration of follow-up for multiple pulmonary nodules is 18–24 months for solid nodules and 5 years for subsolid and semisolid nodules. Computerized deep learning algorithms to discriminate subtle differences in multiple pulmonary nodules have been developed and, with further refinement and implementation, may aid in discrimination and subsequent management of benign and malignant nodules [58].

Unique Considerations for Screen-Detected Lung Nodules

LDCT along with a protocolized follow-up based on pulmonary nodule size and growth detects lung cancer at an earlier stage and reduces mortality as evidenced by two large, randomized controlled trials, together enrolling 69,246 patients [2, 36]. Several societies have endorsed lung cancer screening, including the United States Preventive Task Force (USPSTF), who give lung cancer screening a Grade B recommendation [59–64]. Revised in 2021, the USPSTF recommends screening of adults between the ages of 50 to 80 years who have a 20 pack-year cumulative smoking history, currently smoke, or have quit within the past 15 years and are willing and able to undergo yearly screening and subsequent evaluation and treatment of concerning findings [63].

Several structured reporting systems have been developed specifically for use in lung cancer screening, including Lung-RADS, International Early Lung Cancer Action Program (I-ELCAP), National Clinical Practice guidelines in Oncology (NCCN), Lung Reporting and Data System (Lu-RADS), and NODCAT/GROWCAT, among others [5, 52, 64, 65]. Of these, Lung-RADS is the most widely used in the United States [66]. Lung cancer screening is discussed in more detail in Chap. 2.

Risk Stratification Models

Several pulmonary nodule risk prediction models have been developed and validated to estimate the risk of malignancy. These are largely based on weighted incorporation of patient and imaging characteristics accepted to increase lung cancer risk. These include patient age, cigarette smoking history and duration, increased nodular diameter, and/or volume, spiculation, and upper lobe location. Commonly used risk models include the Mayo Clinic (Swensen), Herder, Veterans Administration (VA), and Brock models among others (Table 4.2). Clinical utility of these models varies based on the cancer prevalence and patient characteristics in the studied populations compared to those in the population to which it is to be applied [72]. For instance, the Brock University Model, which was developed from the Pan-Canadian Early Detection of Lung Cancer Study (PanCan), may be a better choice to estimate malignancy risk of a pulmonary nodule identified on lung cancer screening [5, 73].

While the use of specific risk calculators is recommended by some societies, several studies have shown physician intuition to be similar to published pulmonary nodule risk assessment models, particularly in those who see a large volume of pulmonary nodules in their practice [67, 74, 75].

Table 4.2 Validated pulmonary nodule risk calculators

Model	Study design	Predictors utilized	AUC (validated)	Reference
Mayo Clinic model (1997)	639 patients with newly discovered solitary nodules on CXR	Age Smoking Personal cancer history Nodule diameter Spiculation Upper lobe location	0.78–0.90	[67, 68]
Herder model (2004)	106 patients undergoing PET/CT with intermediate nodules based on Mayo Clinic model	Mayo Clinic model predictive factors plus stratification based on PET avidity	0.92	[69]
Brock University model (2013)	Two cohorts with a combined 2961 current or former smokers undergoing LDCT screening	Age Gender Family history of cancer Nodule size Part solid attenuation Upper lobe location Nodule count Spiculation Emphysema	0.90	[5]
Bayesian model (2015)	343 patients with pulmonary nodule diagnosis with biopsy or deemed stable at imaging for >2 years. All patients underwent PET/CT	Age Smoking history History of cancer Nodule size Upper lobe nodule Nodule morphology VDT Minimal focal density Enhancement PET avidity	0.89	[70]
Veterans administration (VA) model (2007)	375 VA hospital patients with new solitary nodules on CXR	Age Smoking Time since quitting (10-year intervals) Nodule diameter	0.68–0.74	[71]

AUC area under the receiver operating characteristic curve, *CXR* chest X-ray, *PET/CT* positron emission tomography/computed tomography, *LDCT* low-dose computed tomography, *VDT* volume doubling time

Diagnostic Testing

Pulmonary nodules of intermediate risk (~10–60%) often require further diagnostic evaluation. This includes noninvasive testing or invasive biopsy (percutaneous, bronchoscopic, or surgical) (Fig. 4.3). Diagnosis and staging of suspected lung cancer are discussed in more detail in Chap. 5.

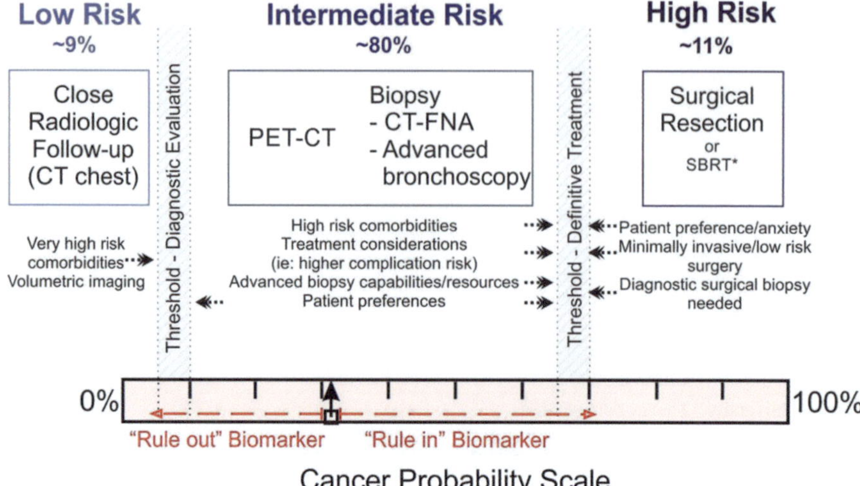

Fig. 4.3 Conceptualized impact of nodule risk assessment on diagnostic evaluation. Predicted malignancy risk, based on physician estimates, or published risk assessment tools, is used to consider aggressiveness of diagnostic evaluation. The threshold of ~5–10% malignancy risk is typically used to differentiate between low- and intermediate-risk nodules; intermediate-risk nodules require diagnostic evaluation beyond close radiologic follow-up. The threshold of ~65–70% malignancy risk is typically considered the risk above which directs surgical resection of a pulmonary nodule could be considered. These thresholds vary based on patient preferences, comorbidities, and available diagnostic and therapeutic capabilities. Underdevelopment and commercially available pulmonary nodule biomarkers can adjust the nodule posttest probability of malignancy to a value either above or below these thresholds (red). *SBRT can be considered in those unable or unwilling to have surgery. Based on the conceptual evaluation schema of Ost and Gould [76]

PET Imaging

Positron emission tomography (PET) scans, often combined with CT for better localization of radioisotope uptake, plays a large role in risk stratification of pulmonary nodules. However, it is rarely used as a first-line imaging technique for detection. PET-CT measuring fluorodeoxyglucose (FDG) uptake has good sensitivity and specificity for malignancy, with pooled data showing rates of 89% and 70%, respectively [77]. However, the utility of PET-CT decreases in those with poorly controlled diabetes, small tumors (<8–10 mm in diameter), nodules with a predominant ground-glass appearance, in tumors with a slow doubling time such as carcinoid tumors, and in lepidic-predominant, minimally invasive or mucinous adenocarcinomas, all of which are more commonly associated with false-negative PET findings [78–80]. PET is of greater utility in identifying occult mediastinal lymph node metastasis, as the sensitivity and specificity (80% and 88%) are higher than CT chest alone (55% and 81%) and can be used to identify when invasive procedures may be needed, particularly for smaller peripheral non-small cell lung cancers [81]. In select patients with nodules high/high-intermediate risk for malignancy but not fit for surgery or who are at prohibitively high risk for biopsy or have nondiagnostic biopsy attempts, increased FDG avidity in a suspicious nodule without evidence of regional or distal metastasis on PET-CT, along with other factors, may help to select those who would benefit from potentially curative stereotactic body radiation therapy (SBRT) [82].

Biopsy

Once a decision is made to biopsy a pulmonary nodule, sampling choice is determined by nodule location and characteristics, patient factors and preferences, need for concurrent tumor staging (such as concerning mediastinal adenopathy of CT or PET), required diagnostic/molecular studies, and institutional experience and availability. Biopsy may be obtained with surgical, percutaneous, or bronchoscopic techniques. Choice of technique requires complicated decision-making, and multidisciplinary tumor/nodule boards are utilized to finalize a biopsy plan.

Lymph Node Staging

Lymph node staging is recommended in instances where evaluation for locoregional disease is needed to determine optimal treatment. Lymph node staging (endobronchial ultrasound (EBUS) +/− endoscopic ultrasound (EUS) or mediastinoscopy) is recommended to evaluate enlarged or any PET-avid lymphadenopathy. Because of the increased risk of occult mediastinal upstaging (N2 or N3 lymph node involvement), systematic mediastinal lymph node staging is also recommended when PET or CT chest is concerning for ipsilateral hilar (N1) metastasis [81]. Because of the increased risk of occult thoracic lymph node metastasis, invasive thoracic lymph node staging is routinely recommended for pulmonary nodules of any size located within the proximal 1/3 of the lung and for larger (>2–3 cm) pulmonary nodules [81]. A bronchoscopic approach to pulmonary nodule diagnosis should be considered when EBUS for thoracic lymph node staging is needed to minimize the risks and costs of multiple invasive procedures. An extensive discussion of the diagnosis and staging of lung cancer is found in another chapter.

Pulmonary Biomarkers: Current and Future Directions

Although physician and nodule calculator risk assessments are useful to guide further diagnostic evaluations, fear of delayed or missed diagnosis often leads clinicians to err on the side of overly aggressive evaluations for those at low or intermediate risk of malignancy [74]. In addition to potential individual risks, one study found invasive procedures for benign disease accounted for 43% of the overall cost of lung cancer [83]. Alternatively, patients with malignant pulmonary nodules at higher risk of complications may be followed radiologically, delaying diagnoses and possibly leading to metastatic disease. This concerns intermediate-risk pulmonary nodules, which comprise the majority of nodules found on incidental and screening chest CTs. A biomarker that could identify either those intermediate nodules at low probability for malignancy ("rule-out" biomarker) or those at high probability for malignancy ("rule-in" biomarker) would be helpful to guide evaluation and management (Fig. 4.3). As scientific understanding of lung cancer continues to grow, so too does the development of biomarkers to aid in their diagnosis and management.

Biomarkers, both molecular and radiomic, have potential utility throughout the spectrum of lung cancer management, including predictive, diagnostic, prognostic, and therapeutic indications [84, 85], and molecular markers to guide personalized treatment of lung cancer are increasingly and widely incorporated into therapeutic algorithms [86–88]. Numerous biomarkers have been or are under development to aid in pulmonary nodule diagnosis, including those measuring proteins, autoantibodies, circulating tumor DNA, mRNA, miRNA, epigenetic changes, volatile chemicals, and metabolites from blood, nasal and bronchial epithelial cells, breath, sputum, and urine sources. Some of these have been analytically and clinically validated in independent, clinically appropriate cohorts, and a few biomarkers are commercially available within the United States (Table 4.3) [84, 97]. However, no randomized clinical trials have validated clinical utility, and no nodule diagnostic biomarkers have been routinely integrated into clinical practice guidelines. Several pulmonary nodule biomarkers, combined either formally with clinical risk factors or through physician pretest probability, have been studied in large, prospective studies that have retrospectively estimated their impact on patient outcomes.

Table 4.3 Commercially available (US) biomarkers for lung nodule management[a]

	Measurement	Validation cohort	Sens/Spec	Proposed use	Clinical utility study/other studies	
Nodify-CDT *Biodesix*	Blood: Autoantibody panel measured by ELISA	Patients: 1613 Cancers: 61	Sens: 37% Spec: 91%	Intermediate risk nodules Positive = aggressive management	No clinical utility trials Study of 12,208 high-risk patients (NHS Scotland, 2013–2016) randomized to screening with CT chest (biomarker +) showed increased detection of early-stage NSCLC in biomarker-led screening arm vs. usual care (no screening)	[89, 90]
Nodify-XL2 *Biodesix*	Plasma: Ratio of two proteins measured by MRM mass spectrometry +5 clinical characteristics (Mayo)	PANOPTIC: Patients: 392 (178[b]) Cancers: 29	Sens: 97% Spec: 44%	Intermediate risk nodules (pretest probability cancer <50%) Negative = CT surveillance	Utility extrapolated retrospectively from PANOPTIC with predicted utility Clinical utility trial recruiting (ALTITUDE, NCT04171492)	[91]
Percepta genomic sequence classifier (GSC) *Veracyte*	Bronchial epithelial cells: mRNA gene expression profile	AEGIS-1/ AEGIS-2 Patients: 839 Cancers: 487	Sens: 88% Spec: 47%	Intermediate risk nodules undergoing bronchoscopy Negative + nondiagnostic bronchoscopy = radiologic surveillance	Utility/change in clinical decision-making extrapolated retrospectively from large prospective observational studies No clinical utility trials	[92, 93]

(continued)

Table 4.3 (continued)

	Measurement	Validation cohort	Sens/Spec	Proposed use	Clinical utility study/other studies	
Percepta nasal swab *Veracyte*	Nasal epithelial cells: mRNA gene expression profile + clinical risk factors	AEGIS-2 Patients: 130 Cancers: 66	Sens: 91% Spec: 52%	Intermediate risk nodules Negative = radiologic surveillance	No clinical utility studies Preliminary data suggests improved sensitivity and specificity for lung cancer among those with low- and high-risk nodules, respectively	[94, 95]
REVEAL *MagArray*	Blood: mRNA by Nanostring + clinical characteristic (Mayo)	Patients: 489 Cancers: 212	10% risk threshold: Sens: 97% Spec: 36% 85% risk threshold: Sens: 27% Spec: 99%	Intermediate-risk nodule (11–84%) Low score = radiologic surveillance High score = aggressive management	No clinical utility trial	[96]

ELISA enzyme-linked immunoassay, *MRM* multiple reaction monitoring

[a] Nodule biomarker technology is changing rapidly; information is up to date at the time this chapter was written, but more information may be available soon thereafter

[b] 178 patients with low-intermediate risk nodules included in intended use group

Conclusions

Identification of pulmonary nodules on chest imaging is common and growing with the increasing use of CT chest imaging. Accurate and timely evaluation of pulmonary nodules is necessary for differentiation between benign and malignant etiologies. The goal is to choose appropriate diagnostic modalities to improve lung cancer diagnosis while minimizing the risk of unnecessary diagnostic procedures for benign disease or delays in diagnosis of malignant disease. Current guidelines for pulmonary nodule management are likely to be further improved in combination with further refinement of radiomic and molecular biomarkers to provide the best care to those diagnosed with pulmonary nodules.

COI and Funding CRS has served as a scientific/medical consultant for Bristol-Myers Squibb Company and received grant funding from Biodesix, the US Department of Veterans Affairs BLR&D (I01-BX005353) and VA CSP (#2005). The contents of this manuscript do not represent the views of the US Department of Veterans Affairs or the US Government. NTT has received grant funding from Biodesix, Nucleix, DELFI, Exact Sciences, and Eon. SV has no COI to declare.

References

1. Gould MK, Tang T, Liu I-LA, Lee J, Zheng C, Danforth K, et al. Recent trends in the identification of incidental pulmonary nodules. Am J Respir Crit Care Med. 2015;192(10):1208–14.
2. Aberle DR, Adams AM, Berg CD, Black WC, Clapp JD, Fagerstrom RM, et al. The National Lung Screening Trial Research Team. Reduced lung-cancer mortality with low-dose computed tomographic screening. N Engl J Med. 2011;265(5):395–409.
3. Kinsinger LS, Anderson C, Kim J, Larson M, Chan SH, King HA, et al. Implementation of lung cancer screening in the veterans health administration. JAMA Intern Med. 2017;177(3):399–406. https://doi.org/10.1001/jamainternmed.2016.9022.
4. Mazzone PJ, Lam L. Evaluating the patient with a pulmonary nodule: a review. JAMA. 2022;327(3):264–73. https://doi.org/10.1001/jama.2021.24287.
5. McWilliams A, Tammemagi MC, Mayo JR, Roberts H, Liu G, Soghrati K, et al. Probability of cancer in pulmonary nodules detected on first screening CT. N Engl J Med. 2013;369(10):910–9. https://doi.org/10.1056/NEJMoa1214726.
6. Verdial FC, Madtes DK, Cheng GS, Pipavath S, Kim R, Hubbard JJ, et al. Multidisciplinary team-based management of Incidentally detected lung nodules. Chest. 2020;157(4):985–93. https://doi.org/10.1016/j.chest.2019.11.032.
7. Erasmus JJ, Connolly JE, McAdams P, Roggli VL. Solitary pulmonary nodules: part I. morphologic evaluation for differentiation of benign and malignant lesions. Radiographics. 2000;20:43–58.
8. Durhan G, Ardali Duzgun S, Akpinar MG, Demirkazik F, Ariyurek OM. Imaging of congenital lung diseases presenting in the adulthood: a pictorial review. Insights Imaging. 2021;12(1):153. https://doi.org/10.1186/s13244-021-01095-2.
9. Siegel RL, Miller KD, Fuchs HE, Jemal A. Cancer statistics, 2022. CA Cancer J Clin. 2022;72(1):7–33. https://doi.org/10.3322/caac.21708.
10. The Health Consequences of Smoking - 50 Years of Progress. A report of the surgeon general. In: Services. USDoHaH ed. Atlanta: Department of Health and Human Services, Centers for

Disease Control and Prevention, National Center for Chronic Disease Prevention and Health Promotion, Office on Smoking and Health; 2014.

11. Tindle HA, Stevenson Duncan M, Greevy RA, Vasan RS, Kundu S, Massion PP, et al. Lifetime smoking history and risk of lung cancer: results from the Framingham heart study. J Natl Cancer Inst. 2018;110(11):1201–7. https://doi.org/10.1093/jnci/djy041.

12. El-Zaatari ZM, Chami HA, Zaatari GS. Health effects associated with waterpipe smoking. Tob Control. 2015;24(Suppl 1):i31–43. https://doi.org/10.1136/tobaccocontrol-2014-051908.

13. McCormack VA, Agudo A, Dahm CC, Overvad K, Olsen A, Tjonneland A, et al. Cigar and pipe smoking and cancer risk in the European prospective investigation into cancer and nutrition (EPIC). Int J Cancer. 2010;127(10):2402–11. https://doi.org/10.1002/ijc.25252.

14. Subramanian J, Govindan R. Lung cancer in 'Never-Smokers': a unique entity. Oncology. 2010;24(1):29–35.

15. Lee HW, Park SH, Weng MW, Wang HT, Huang WC, Lepor H, et al. E-cigarette smoke damages DNA and reduces repair activity in mouse lung, heart, and bladder as well as in human lung and bladder cells. Proc Natl Acad Sci U S A. 2018;115(7):E1560–E9. https://doi.org/10.1073/pnas.1718185115.

16. Tang MS, Wu XR, Lee HW, Xia Y, Deng FM, Moreira AL, et al. Electronic-cigarette smoke induces lung adenocarcinoma and bladder urothelial hyperplasia in mice. Proc Natl Acad Sci U S A. 2019;116(43):21727–31. https://doi.org/10.1073/pnas.1911321116.

17. MacRosty CR, Rivera MP. Lung cancer in women: a modern epidemic. Clin Chest Med. 2020;41(1):53–65. https://doi.org/10.1016/j.ccm.2019.10.005.

18. Sun S, Schiller JH, Gazdar AF. Lung cancer in never smokers—a different disease. Nat Rev Cancer. 2007;7(10):778–90. https://doi.org/10.1038/nrc2190.

19. Brims FJH, Kong K, Harris EJA, Sodhi-Berry N, Reid A, Murray CP, et al. Pleural plaques and the risk of lung cancer in Asbestos-exposed subjects. Am J Respir Crit Care Med. 2020;201(1):57–62. https://doi.org/10.1164/rccm.201901-0096OC.

20. Ngamwong Y, Tangamornsuksan W, Lohitnavy O, Chaiyakunapruk N, Scholfield CN, Reisfeld B, et al. Additive synergism between Asbestos and smoking in lung cancer risk: a systematic review and meta-analysis. PLoS One. 2015;10(8):e0135798. https://doi.org/10.1371/journal.pone.0135798.

21. Loverdos K, Fotiadis A, Kontogianni C, Iliopoulou M, Gaga M. Lung nodules: a comprehensive review on current approach and management. Ann Thorac Med. 2019;14(4):226–38. https://doi.org/10.4103/atm.ATM_110_19.

22. Carlos WG, Rose AS, Wheat LJ, Norris S, Sarosi GA, Knox KS, et al. Blastomycosis in Indiana: digging up more cases. Chest. 2010;138(6):1377–82. https://doi.org/10.1378/chest.10-0627.

23. Shipe ME, Deppen SA, Sullivan S, Kammer M, Starnes SL, Wilson DO, et al. Validation of histoplasmosis enzyme immunoassay to evaluate suspicious lung nodules. Ann Thorac Surg. 2021;111(2):416–20. https://doi.org/10.1016/j.athoracsur.2020.05.101.

24. Mazzone PJ, Wang XF, Lim S, Jett J, Choi H, Zhang Q, et al. Progress in the development of volatile exhaled breath signatures of lung cancer. Ann Am Thorac Soc. 2015;12(5):752–7. https://doi.org/10.1513/AnnalsATS.201411-540OC.

25. Slatore CG, Wiener RS. Pulmonary nodules: a small problem for many, severe distress for some, and how to communicate about it. Chest. 2018;153(4):1004–15. https://doi.org/10.1016/j.chest.2017.10.013.

26. Oken MM, Hocking WG, Kvale PA, Andriole GL, Buya SS, Church TR, et al. Screening by chest radiograph and lung cancer mortality: the prostate, lung, colorectal, and ovarian (PLCO) randomized trial. JAMA. 2011;306(17):E1–9.

27. Blanchon T, Brechot JM, Grenier PA, Ferretti GR, Lemarie E, Milleron B, et al. Baseline results of the Depiscan study: a French randomized pilot trial of lung cancer screening comparing low dose CT scan (LDCT) and chest X-ray (CXR). Lung Cancer. 2007;58(1):50–8. https://doi.org/10.1016/j.lungcan.2007.05.009.

28. Kaneko M, Eguchi K, Ohmatsu H, Kakinuma R, Naruke T, Suemasu K, et al. Peripheral lung cancer: screening and detection with low-dose Sprial CT versus radiography. Radiology. 1996;201:798–802.
29. Diederich S, Lenzen H. Radiation exposure associated with imaging of the chest: comparison of different radiographic and computed tomography techniques. Cancer. 2000;89(11):2457–60.
30. MacMahon H, Naidich DP, Goo JM, Lee KS, Leung ANC, Mayo JR, et al. Guidelines for management of incidental pulmonary nodules detected on CT images: from the Fleischner society 2017. Radiology. 2017;284(1):228–43. https://doi.org/10.1148/radiol.2017161659.
31. Godoy MCB, Naidich DP. Subsolid pulmonary nodules and the spectrum of peripheral adenocarcinomas of the lung: recommended interim guidelines for assessment and management. Radiology. 2009;253(3):606–22.
32. Devaraj A, van Ginneken B, Nair A, Baldwin D. Use of volumetry for lung nodule management: theory and practice. Radiology. 2017;284(3):630–44. https://doi.org/10.1148/radiol.2017151022.
33. Wormanns D, Kohl G, Klotz E, Marheine A, Beyer F, Heindel W, et al. Volumetric measurements of pulmonary nodules at multi-row detector CT: in vivo reproducibility. Eur Radiol. 2004;14(1):86–92. https://doi.org/10.1007/s00330-003-2132-0.
34. Gietema H, Schaefer-Prokop CM, Mali WPTM, Groenewegen G, Prokop M. Pulmonary nodules: interscan variabiity of Semiautomated volume measurements with multisection CT—influence of inspiration level, nodule size, and segmentation performance. Radiology. 2007;245(3):888–94.
35. Oudkerk M, Devaraj A, Vliegenthart R, Henzler T, Prosch H, Heussel CP, et al. European position statement on lung cancer screening. Lancet Oncol. 2017;18(12):e754–e66. https://doi.org/10.1016/s1470-2045(17)30861-6.
36. de Koning HJ, van der Aalst CM, de Jong PA, Scholten ET, Nackaerts K, Heuvelmans MA, et al. Reduced lung-cancer mortality with volume CT screening in a randomized trial. N Engl J Med. 2020;382:503–13. https://doi.org/10.1056/NEJMoa1911793.
37. Han D, Heuvelmans MA, Oudkerk M. Volume versus diameter assessment of small pulmonary nodules in CT lung cancer screening. Transl Lung Cancer Res. 2017;6(1):52–61. https://doi.org/10.21037/tlcr.2017.01.05.
38. Horeweg N, van der Aalst CM, Vliegenthart R, Zhao Y, Xie X, Scholten ET, et al. Volumetric computed tomography screening for lung cancer: three rounds of the NELSON trial. Eur Respir J. 2013;42(6):1659–67. https://doi.org/10.1183/09031936.00197712.
39. Thawani R, McLane M, Beig N, Ghose S, Prasanna P, Velcheti V, et al. Radiomics and radiogenomics in lung cancer: a review for the clinician. Lung Cancer. 2018;115:34–41. https://doi.org/10.1016/j.lungcan.2017.10.015.
40. Li F, Sone S, Abe H, Macmahon H, Doi K. Malignant versus benign nodules at CT screening for lung cancer: comparison of thin-section CT findings. Radiology. 2004;233(3):793-8:793. https://doi.org/10.1148/radiol.2333031018.
41. Gould MK, Donington J, Lynch WR, Mazzone PJ, Midthun DE, Naidich DP, et al. Evaluation of individuals with pulmonary nodules: when is it lung cancer? Diagnosis and management of lung cancer, 3rd ed: American College of Chest Physicians evidence-based clinical practice guidelines. Chest. 2013;143(5 Suppl):e93S–e120S. https://doi.org/10.1378/chest.12-2351.
42. Attili AK, Kazerooni EA. Imaging of the solitary pulmonary nodule. In: Medina LS, Blackmore CC, editors. Evidence-based imaging - optimizing imaging in patient care. New York, NY: Springer; 2006. p. 417–40.
43. Ravenel JG, Silvestri G. Imaging of lung cancer. In: Medina LS, Blackmore CC, editors. Evidence-based imaging—optimizing imaging in patient care. New York, NY: Springer; 2006. p. 57–78.
44. de Hoop B, van Ginneken B, Gietema H, Prokop M. Pulmonary perifissural nodules on CT scans: rapid growth is not a predictor of malignancy. Radiology. 2012;265(2):611–6. https://doi.org/10.1148/radiol.12112351.

45. Kastner J, Hossain R, Jeudy J, Dako F, Mehta V, Dalal S, et al. Lung-RADS version 1.0 versus lung-RADS version 1.1: comparison of categories using nodules from the National Lung Screening Trial. Radiology. 2021;300(1):199–206. https://doi.org/10.1148/radiol.2021203704.
46. Heuvelmans MA, Walter JE, Peters RB, Bock GH, Yousaf-Khan U, Aalst CMV, et al. Relationship between nodule count and lung cancer probability in baseline CT lung cancer screening: the NELSON study. Lung Cancer. 2017;113:45–50. https://doi.org/10.1016/j.lungcan.2017.08.023.
47. Walter JE, Heuvelmans MA, Bock GH, Yousaf-Khan U, Groen HJM, Aalst CMV, et al. Characteristics of new solid nodules detected in incidence screening rounds of low-dose CT lung cancer screening: the NELSON study. Thorax. 2018;73(8):741–7. https://doi.org/10.1136/thoraxjnl-2017-211376.
48. Henschke CI, Yankelevitz DF, Mirtcheva R, McGuinness G, McCauley D, Miettinen OS, et al. CT screening for lung cancer: frequency and significance of part-solid and nonsolid nodules. Am J Roentgenol. 2002;178:1053–7.
49. Callister ME, Baldwin DR, Akram AR, Barnard S, Cane P, Draffan J, et al. British Thoracic Society guidelines for the investigation and management of pulmonary nodules. Thorax. 2015;70 Suppl 2:ii1–ii54. https://doi.org/10.1136/thoraxjnl-2015-207168.
50. Wahidi MM, Govert JA, Goudar RK, Gould MK, McCrory DC, American College of Chest P. Evidence for the treatment of patients with pulmonary nodules: when is it lung cancer?: ACCP evidence-based clinical practice guidelines (2nd edition). Chest. 2007;132(3 Suppl):94S–107S. https://doi.org/10.1378/chest.07-1352.
51. Gould MK, Smith-Bindman R, Kelly K, Altman DE, Barjaktarevic I, Creekmur B, et al. Methods for the watch the spot trial. A pragmatic trial of more-versus less-intensive strategies for active surveillance of small pulmonary nodules. Ann Am Thorac Soc. 2019;16(12):1567–76. https://doi.org/10.1513/AnnalsATS.201903-268SD.
52. Pinsky PF, Gierada DS, Black W, Munden R, Nath H, Aberle D, et al. Performance of lung-RADS in the National Lung Screening Trial: a retrospective assessment. Ann Intern Med. 2015;162(7):485–91. https://doi.org/10.7326/M14-2086.
53. Kim HY, Shim YM, Lee KS, Han J, Yi CA, Kim YK. Persistent pulmonary nodular ground-glass opacity at thin-section CT: histopathologic comparisons. Radiology. 2007;245(1):267–75.
54. Nakata M, Sawada S, Saeki H, Takashima S, Mogami H, Teramoto N, et al. Prospective study of thoracoscopic limited resection for ground-glass opacity selected by computed tomography. Ann Thorac Surg. 2003;75(5):1601–5; discussion 5-6. https://doi.org/10.1016/s0003-4975(02)04815-4.
55. Ohtsuka T, Watanabe K, Kaji M, Naruke T, Suemasu K. A clinicopathological study of resected pulmonary nodules with focal pure ground-glass opacity. Eur J Cardiothorac Surg. 2006;30(1):160–3. https://doi.org/10.1016/j.ejcts.2006.03.058.
56. Chen K, Bai J, Reuben A, Zhao H, Kang G, Zhang C, et al. Multiomics analysis reveals distinct Immunogenomic features of lung cancer with ground-glass opacity. Am J Respir Crit Care Med. 2021;204:1180. https://doi.org/10.1164/rccm.202101-0119OC.
57. Henschke C, Yankelevitz DF, Mirtcheva R, McGuinness G, McCauley D, Miettinen OS, et al. CT screening for lung cancer: frequency and significance of part-solid and nonsolid nodules. Am J Roentgenol. 2002;178:1053–7.
58. Chen K, Nie Y, Park S, Zhang K, Zhang Y, Liu Y, et al. Development and validation of machine learning-based model for the prediction of malignancy in multiple pulmonary nodules: analysis from multicentric cohorts. Clin Cancer Res. 2021;27(8):2255–65. https://doi.org/10.1158/1078-0432.CCR-20-4007.
59. Field JK, Aberle DR, Altorki N, Baldwin DR, Dresler C, Duffy SW, et al. The international association study lung cancer (IASLC) strategic screening advisory committee (SSAC) response to the USPSTF recommendations. J Thorac Oncol. 2014;9:141–3.
60. Jacobson FL, Austin JH, Field JK, Jett JR, Keshavjee S, MacMahon H, et al. Development of the American Association for Thoracic Surgery guidelines for low-dose computed tomography scans to screen for lung cancer in North America: recommendations of the American

Association for Thoracic Surgery Task Force for lung cancer screening and surveillance. J Thorac Cardiovasc Surg. 2012;144(1):25–32. https://doi.org/10.1016/j.jtcvs.2012.05.059.

61. Mazzone PJ, Silvestri GA, Souter LH, Caverly TJ, Kanne JP, Katki HA, et al. Screening for lung cancer: CHEST guideline and expert panel report. Chest. 2021;160:e427. https://doi.org/10.1016/j.chest.2021.06.063.

62. Meza R, Jeon J, Toumazis I, Ten Haaf K, Cao P, Bastani M, et al. Evaluation of the benefits and harms of lung cancer screening with low-dose computed tomography: modeling study for the US Preventive Services Task Force. JAMA. 2021;325(10):988–97. https://doi.org/10.1001/jama.2021.1077.

63. U.S._Preventive_Services_Task_Force, Krist AH, Davidson KW, Mangione CM, Barry MJ, Cabana M, et al. Screening for lung cancer: US Preventive Services Task Force recommendation statement. JAMA. 2021;325(10):962–70. https://doi.org/10.1001/jama.2021.1117.

64. Wood DE, Kazerooni EA, Baum SL, Eapen GA, Ettinger DS, Hou L, et al. Lung cancer screening, version 3.2018, NCCN clinical practice guidelines in oncology. J Natl Compr Cancer Netw. 2018;16(4):412–41. https://doi.org/10.6004/jnccn.2018.0020.

65. Manos D, Seely JM, Taylor J, Borgaonkar J, Roberts HC, Mayo JR. The lung reporting and data system (LU-RADS): a proposal for computed tomography screening. Can Assoc Radiol J. 2014;65(2):121–34. https://doi.org/10.1016/j.carj.2014.03.004.

66. Lin Y, Fu M, Ding R, Inoue K, Jeon CY, Hsu W, et al. Patient adherence to lung-RADS recommended screening intervals in the United States: a systematic review and meta-analysis. J Thorac Oncol. 2021;17:38. https://doi.org/10.1016/j.jtho.2021.09.013.

67. Swensen SJ, Silverstein MD, Edell ES, Trastek VF, Aughenbaugh GL, Ilstrup DM, et al. Solitary pulmonary nodules: clinical prediction model versus physicians. Mayo Clin Proc. 1999;74(4):319–29. https://doi.org/10.1016/s0025-6196(11)64397-8.

68. Swensen SJ, Silverstein MD, Ilstrup DM, Schleck CD, Edell ES. The probability of malignancy in solitary pulmonary nodules. Arch Intern Med. 1997;157:849–55.

69. Herder GJ, van Tinteren H, Golding RP, Kostense PJ, Comans EF, Smit EF, et al. Clinical prediction model to characterize pulmonary nodules: validation and added value of 18F-Fluorodeoxyglucose positron emission tomography. Chest J. 2005;128(4):2490–6.

70. Soardi GA, Perandini S, Motton M, Montemezzi S. Assessing probability of malignancy in solid solitary pulmonary nodules with a new Bayesian calculator: improving diagnostic accuracy by means of expanded and updated features. Eur Radiol. 2015;25(1):155–62. https://doi.org/10.1007/s00330-014-3396-2.

71. Gould MK, Ananth L, Barnett PG, Veterans Affairs SCSG. A clinical model to estimate the pretest probability of lung cancer in patients with solitary pulmonary nodules. Chest. 2007;131(2):383–8. https://doi.org/10.1378/chest.06-1261.

72. Schultz EM, Sanders GD, Trotter PR, Patz EF Jr, Silvestri GA, Owens DK, et al. Validation of two models to estimate the probability of malignancy in patients with solitary pulmonary nodules. Thorax. 2008;63(4):335–41. https://doi.org/10.1136/thx.2007.084731.

73. Sundaram V, Gould MK, Nair VS. A comparison of the PanCan model and lung-RADS to assess cancer probability among people with screening-detected, solid lung nodules. Chest. 2021;159(3):1273–82. https://doi.org/10.1016/j.chest.2020.10.040.

74. Tanner NT, Porter A, Gould MK, Li XJ, Vachani A, Silvestri GA. Physician assessment of pretest probability of malignancy and adherence with guidelines for pulmonary nodule evaluation. Chest. 2017;152(2):263–70. https://doi.org/10.1016/j.chest.2017.01.018.

75. Baldwin DR, Eaton T, Kolbe J, Christmas T, Milne D, Mercer J, et al. Management of solitary pulmonary nodules: how do thoracic computed tomography and guided fine needle biopsy influence clinical decisions? Thorax. 2002;57:817–22.

76. Ost DE, Gould MK. Decision making in patients with pulmonary nodules. Am J Respir Crit Care Med. 2012;185(4):363–72. https://doi.org/10.1164/rccm.201104-0679CI.

77. Li ZZ, Huang YL, Song HJ, Wang YJ, Huang Y. The value of 18F-FDG-PET/CT in the diagnosis of solitary pulmonary nodules: a meta-analysis. Medicine (Baltimore). 2018;97(12):e0130. https://doi.org/10.1097/MD.0000000000010130.

78. Khalaf M, Abdel-Nabi H, Baker J, Shao Y, Lamonica D, Gona J. Relation between nodule size and 18F-FDG-PET SUV for malignant and benign pulmonary nodules. J Hematol Oncol. 2008;1:13. https://doi.org/10.1186/1756-8722-1-13.

79. Berger KL, Nicholson SA, Dehdashti F, Siegel BA. FDG PET evaluation of mucinous neoplasms: correlation of FDG uptake with histopathologic features. Am J Roentgenol. 2000;174:1005–8.

80. Ambrosini V, Nicolini S, Caroli P, Nanni C, Massaro A, Marzola MC, et al. PET/CT imaging in different types of lung cancer: an overview. Eur J Radiol. 2011;81:988. https://doi.org/10.1016/j.ejrad.2011.03.020.

81. Silvestri GA, Gonzalez AV, Jantz MA, Margolis ML, Gould MK, Tanoue LT, et al. Methods for staging non-small cell lung cancer: diagnosis and management of lung cancer, 3rd ed: American College of Chest Physicians evidence-based clinical practice guidelines. Chest. 2013;143(5 Suppl):e211S–e50S. https://doi.org/10.1378/chest.12-2355.

82. Schneider BJ, Daly ME, Kennedy EB, Antonoff MB, Broderick S, Feldman J, et al. Stereotactic body radiotherapy for early-stage non-small-cell lung cancer: American Society of Clinical Oncology endorsement of the American Society for Radiation Oncology evidence-based guideline. J Clin Oncol. 2018;36(7):710–9. https://doi.org/10.1200/JCO.2017.74.9671.

83. Lokhandwala T, Bittoni MA, Dann RA, D'Souza AO, Johnson M, Nagy RJ, et al. Costs of diagnostic assessment for lung cancer: a medicare claims analysis. Clin Lung Cancer. 2017;18(1):e27–34. https://doi.org/10.1016/j.cllc.2016.07.006.

84. Sears CR, Mazzone PJ. Biomarkers in lung cancer. Clin Chest Med. 2020;41(1):115–27. https://doi.org/10.1016/j.ccm.2019.10.004.

85. Mazzone PJ, Sears CR, Arenberg DA, Gaga M, Gould MK, Massion PP, et al. Evaluating molecular biomarkers for the early detection of lung cancer: when is a biomarker ready for clinical use? An official American Thoracic Society policy statement. Am J Respir Crit Care Med. 2017;196(7):e15–29. https://doi.org/10.1164/rccm.201708-1678ST.

86. Singh N, Temin S, Baker S Jr, Blanchard E, Brahmer JR, Celano P, et al. Therapy for stage IV non-small-cell lung cancer with driver alterations: ASCO living guideline. J Clin Oncol. 2022;40:JCO2200824. https://doi.org/10.1200/JCO.22.00824.

87. Lindeman NI, Cagle PT, Aisner DL, Arcila ME, Beasley MB, Bernicker E, et al. Updated molecular testing guideline for the selection of lung cancer patients for treatment with targeted tyrosine kinase inhibitors. J Thorac Oncol. 2018;13:323. https://doi.org/10.1016/j.jtho.2017.12.001.

88. National_Comprehensive_Cancer_Network. Non-small cell lung cancer (Version 6.2021). https://www.nccn.org/professionals/physician_gls/pdf/nscl.pdf. Accessed 16 July 2022.

89. Jett JR, Peek LJ, Fredericks L, Jewell W, Pingleton WW, Robertson JF. Audit of the autoantibody test, EarlyCDT(R)-lung, in 1600 patients: an evaluation of its performance in routine clinical practice. Lung Cancer. 2014;83(1):51–5. https://doi.org/10.1016/j.lungcan.2013.10.008.

90. Sullivan FM, Mair FS, Anderson W, Armory P, Briggs A, Chew C, et al. Earlier diagnosis of lung cancer in a randomised trial of an autoantibody blood test followed by imaging. Eur Respir J. 2021;57(1):2000670. https://doi.org/10.1183/13993003.00670-2020.

91. Silvestri GA, Tanner NT, Kearney P, Vachani A, Massion PP, Porter A, et al. Assessment of plasma proteomics biomarker's ability to distinguish benign from malignant lung nodules: results of the PANOPTIC (pulmonary nodule plasma proteomic classifier) trial. Chest. 2018;154:491. https://doi.org/10.1016/j.chest.2018.02.012.

92. Silvestri GA, Vachani A, Whitney D, Elashoff M, Porta Smith K, Ferguson JS, et al. A bronchial genomic classifier for the diagnostic evaluation of lung cancer. N Engl J Med. 2015;373(3):243–51. https://doi.org/10.1056/NEJMoa1504601.

93. Lee HJ, Mazzone P, Feller-Kopman D, Yarmus L, Hogarth K, Lofaro LR, et al. Impact of the Percepta genomic classifier on clinical management decisions in a multicenter prospective study. Chest. 2021;159(1):401–12. https://doi.org/10.1016/j.chest.2020.07.067.

94. Perez-Rogers JF, Gerrein J, Anderlind C, Liu G, Zhang S, Alekseyev Y, et al. Shared gene expression alterations in nasal and bronchial epithelium for lung cancer detection. J Natl Cancer Inst. 2017;109(7):djw327. https://doi.org/10.1093/jnci/djw327.
95. Mazzone PJ, Lamb C, Rieger-Christ KM, Reddy CB, Qu J, Wu S, et al. Early candidate nasal swab classifiers developed using machine learning and whole transcriptome sequencing may improve early lung cancer detection. J Clin Oncol. 2021;39(15_suppl):8551. https://doi.org/10.1200/JCO.2021.39.15_suppl.8551.
96. Vachani A, Lam S, Massion PP, Brown JK, Beggs M, Fish AL, et al. Development and validation of a risk assessment model for pulmonary nodules using plasma proteins and clinical factors. Chest. 2022;163:966. https://doi.org/10.1016/j.chest.2022.10.038.
97. Seijo LM, Peled N, Ajona D, Boeri M, Field JK, Sozzi G, et al. Biomarkers in lung cancer screening: achievements, promises, and challenges. J Thorac Oncol. 2019;14(3):343–57. https://doi.org/10.1016/j.jtho.2018.11.023.

Chapter 5
Staging and Diagnosis of Lung Cancer

Ghosh Sohini, Marshall Tanya, and Baltaji Stephanie

Significance of Staging

In the United States, lung cancer incidence is 35 per 100,000 people and causes more deaths than colon, breast, and prostate cancer combined [1, 2]. The approach to treatment is driven by the size of the primary tumor, extent of lymph node involvement, and the presence or absence of extrathoracic metastases. Accurate lung cancer staging is essential to achieve the most favorable outcomes in patients. On a larger scale, appropriate staging and nomenclature also facilitate the exchange of information between providers and healthcare centers using a common language, allowing for enrollment of patients into clinical trials nationwide [3].

Staging Overview

Lung cancer is categorized as either small cell or non-small cell lung cancer (NSCLC). NSCLC is staged using the tumor, nodes, and metastases (TNM) classification. The first TNM staging for lung cancer was developed by Mountain et al. in 1974. The letter T represents the size of the primary tumor with subscripts to indicate degree of direct extension. The letter N represents lymph node involvement, and the letter M represents the presence or absence of distant metastatic disease. Using data from 2155 cases of bronchogenic carcinoma (including squamous cell,

G. Sohini (✉) · M. Tanya
Department of Pulmonary and Critical Care, Allegheny Health Network, Pittsburgh, PA, USA
e-mail: Sohini.Ghosh@AHN.ORG; Tanya.Marshall@AHN.ORG

B. Stephanie
Department of Pulmonary Disease and Critical Care, Virginia Commonwealth University, Richmond, VA, USA

C. MacRosty, M. P. Rivera (eds.), *Lung Cancer*, Respiratory Medicine,
https://doi.org/10.1007/978-3-031-38412-7_5

adenocarcinoma, undifferentiated large cell, small cell, and undifferentiated cell type), they plotted the survival of patients with T1 to T3, N0 to N3 disease, and then stage I to stage III [4].

Small cell can be staged using TNM or dichotomously as "limited" versus "extensive" disease as defined by the size of the radiation field. TNM stages I–III are considered limited stage, excluding those tumors with multiple nodules or those nodules/nodes that are too large to be safely included in the radiation plan. Extensive stage encompasses all T4 and some T3 lesions. Clinically, the dichotomous classification, developed by the Veteran's Administration (VA), is more commonly utilized. TNM staging is most useful for early-stage small cell lung cancer, which may be eligible for surgical resection or radiation [5].

The TNM classification system has undergone multiple iterations, most recently the eighth edition released by the International Association for the Study of Lung Cancer (IASLC) in 2018. The TNM classification groups patients with similar survival outcomes and assists with prognostication. It does not consider all variables contributing to lung cancer outcomes and, thus, is not designed to predict an individual's survival [6].

The IASLC eighth TNM edition guidelines are derived from a database with 94,708 patients from 16 countries diagnosed with lung cancer between 1999 and 2010. These guidelines are endorsed by the Union Internationale Contre le Cancer (UICC) and the American Joint Committee on Cancer (AJCC) [7, 8].

Clinical Versus Pathological Staging Prefixes

When considering lung cancer staging, it is important to differentiate between clinical (c) and pathologic (p) stage.

Clinical staging, cTNM, is based on pretreatment data from imaging studies, lab work, and staging procedures, including bronchoscopy, endoscopy, mediastinoscopy, thoracentesis, and thoracoscopy. Pathological staging, pTNM, is assigned after the analysis of surgical resections and is used to guide adjuvant therapy [9]. There are additional prefix classifiers that can be added to TNM staging. These include "R," "y," "r," and "a." The "R" identifier indicates a postsurgical specimen which is discussed later in this chapter. The "y" identifier denotes a patient who received neoadjuvant therapy before surgical resection. The "r" identifier denotes disease recurrence, and "a" denotes staging performed at autopsy [3].

Among both clinical and pathological staging, the 5-year survival rates are lower the higher the stage. The most recent IASLC database included lung cancers staged both clinically and pathologically and found similar survival rates. For example, 5-year survival rates for clinical stage IA1 versus IIIC were 92% versus 13%, respectively. Among pathological stages, 5-year survival rates for IA1 versus IIIC were 90% versus 12% [8].

TNM

T Component

The T (tumor) component, or tumor size, is the most important prognostic factor in the TNM staging system [10]. The updated T categories are split into 1 cm intervals. Each 1 cm T designation has its own statistically separate survival curve ($p < 0.001$), illustrating the prognostic importance of tumor size [3, 6]. For solid tumors, size should be measured during full inspiration, and the T designation is assigned using the largest diameter in any projection. The clinical T staging is assigned for subsolid nodules by measuring the solid or invasive component, often done after surgical resection [10]. Further details on T staging are described in the Pathologic Staging section and outlined in Table 5.1.

Table 5.1 Definitions for T descriptor *(adapted with permission from Detterbeck* et al. *The Eight Edition Lung Cancer Stage Classification. Chest 2017; 151: 193–203)*

T: Tumor		Description
T0		
	Tis	Carcinoma in situ (adenocarcinoma or squamous cell)
T1		
	T1a(mi)	Minimally invasive adenocarcinoma (MIA)
	T1a	Superficial spreading tumor confined to tracheal or bronchial wall
	T1a	≤ 1 cm
	T1b	>1 to ≤2 cm
	T1c	>2 to ≤3 cm
T2		Tumor >3 cm and ≤ 5 cm or
		Involving the visceral pleura or main bronchus (not carina) or
		Causing lobar atelectasis
	T2a	>3 to <4 cm or
		Invasion of visceral pleura or
		Involving the main bronchus not involving the carina or
		Causing lobar atelectasis
	T2b	>4 to <5 cm or
		Involving the main bronchus <2 cm from the carina without carinal involvement
T3		Tumor >5 to ≤7 cm or
		Separate nodule(s) in same lobe or
		Invasion of chest wall, pericardium, phrenic nerve
T4		Tumor >7 cm or
		Invasion of mediastinum, diaphragm, heart, great vessels, recurrent laryngeal nerve, carina, trachea, esophagus, spine, or
		Tumor nodule(s) in a different ipsilateral lobe

N Component

In 1929, Rouvière first described lymph node drainage within the thorax [11]. Since then, multiple corroborative studies have indicated that, in general, right upper lobe tumors first metastasize to the right paratracheal area [12, 13]. Left upper lobe tumors metastasize to para- and subaortic lymph nodes. Middle and lower lobe tumors metastasize to subcarinal and right paratracheal lymph nodes [12]. The establishment of this drainage pattern led to the classification of nodal disease.

The N (nodal) component is assigned N0-N3, with a higher N classification indicating more advanced stage and worse prognosis. A summary of N descriptors is outlined in Table 5.2. Nodal status is classified as N0 when there is no evidence of thoracic lymph node metastases. N1 is characterized by ipsilateral hilar, peribronchial, and/or intrapulmonary node involvement. N2 refers to the involvement of subcarinal, para-aortic, subaortic, and/or ipsilateral mediastinal lymph nodes. N3 involves contralateral mediastinal, hilar, and/or supraclavicular nodes [14]. Outcomes are the most favorable when no evidence of lymph node metastasis exists. Single-station N1 disease has a worse prognosis than N0 disease. This is followed by multi-station N1 involvement, which has a similar prognosis to single-station N2 disease without N1 metastases (i.e., skip metastases). Skip metastases bypass the hilar lymph nodes and metastasize directly to mediastinal lymph nodes at rates ranging from 7 to 26% [11]. This is more common in adenocarcinomas and upper lobe tumors [11, 12]. Single-station N2 disease with N1 disease, followed by multi-station N2 lymph node metastases, has the worst prognosis—involvement of N1 node stages a tumor as at least a stage IIB. N2 nodal involvement denotes at least a stage IIIA, while N3 nodal involvement denotes at least a stage IIIB.

The lymph node map has remained constant since the seventh edition of IASLC staging guidelines and has been adopted by multiple international organizations. This map provides distinct borders for lymph nodes (see Fig. 5.1). Notable borders include the subcarinal station [7], which extends to the origin of the left lower lobe and right middle lobe. The right lower paratracheal station (4R) lateral border is located at the left lateral border of the trachea and encompasses both the right and anterior tracheal walls [9, 11]. Station 4R's upper border is the inferior margin of the innominate vein, and its lower border is the distal border of the azygos vein, with 10R starting just beyond the azygos vein.

Table 5.2 Definitions for N descriptor *(adapted with permission from Detterbeck* et al. *The Eight Edition Lung Cancer Stage Classification. Chest 2017; 151: 193–203)*

N: regional lymph nodes	Description
N0	No regional lymph node metastases
N1	Ipsilateral hilar or pulmonary nodes
N2	Subcarinal and/or ipsilateral mediastinal nodes
N3	Contralateral mediastinal and/or hilar nodes and/or supraclavicular nodes

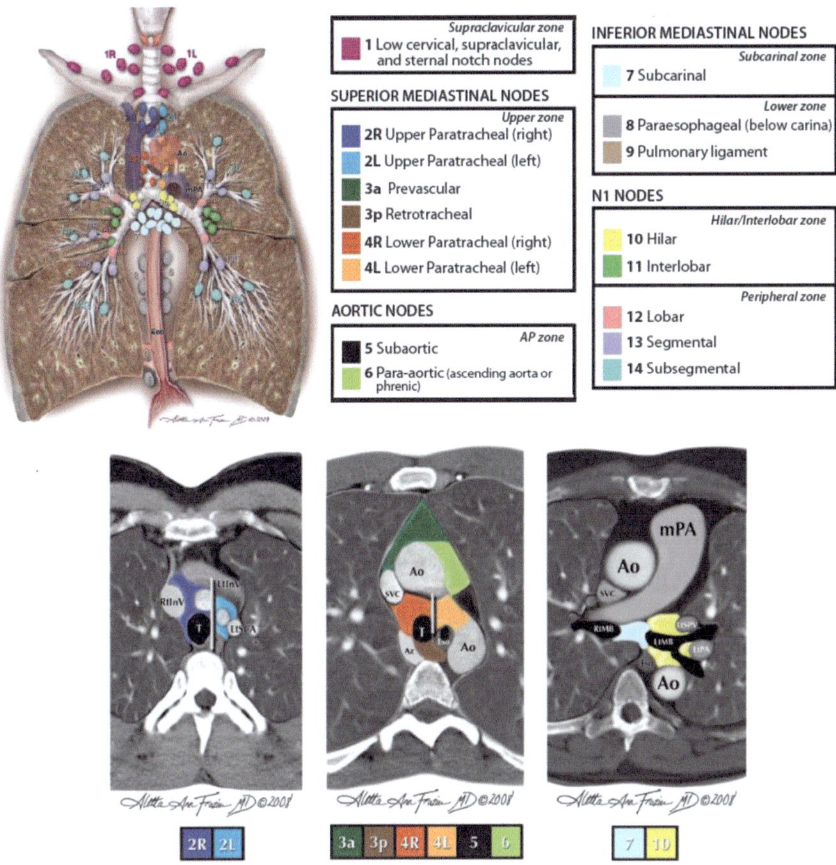

Fig. 5.1 Lymph node station. IASLC lymph node map with delineated borders *(reproduced with permission from Rusch VW, et al. The IASLC lung cancer staging project: a proposal for a new international lymph node map in the forthcoming seventh edition of the TNM classification for lung cancer. J Thorac Oncol 2009; 4: 568–577)*

M Component and Stage Grouping

The IASLC database demonstrated that the number of metastatic foci was a better prognostic indicator than metastatic location. This led to the subclassification of metastases (M) with a, b, and c, as outlined in Table 5.3. Intrathoracic metastases (M1a) have the same prognosis as a single extrathoracic metastasis (M1b). Multiple extrathoracic metastases (M1c) have the worst prognosis [6]. Using TNM, up to 64 combinations can occur, subsequently grouped into 1 of 11 stages as outlined in Fig. 5.2. Each TNM combination within a stage (as illustrated in Table 5.4) shares similar survival outcomes, while 5-year overall survival decreases with more advanced stages (Table 5.5).

Table 5.3 Definitions for M descriptor *(adapted with permission from Detterbeck* et al. *The Eight Edition Lung Cancer Stage Classification. Chest 2017; 151: 193–203)*

M: distant metastases	Description
M0	No distant metastases
M1a	Malignant pleural or pericardial effusion and/or nodules or tumor in contralateral lung
M1b	Single extrathoracic lymph node or metastases
M1c	Multiple extrathoracic metastases

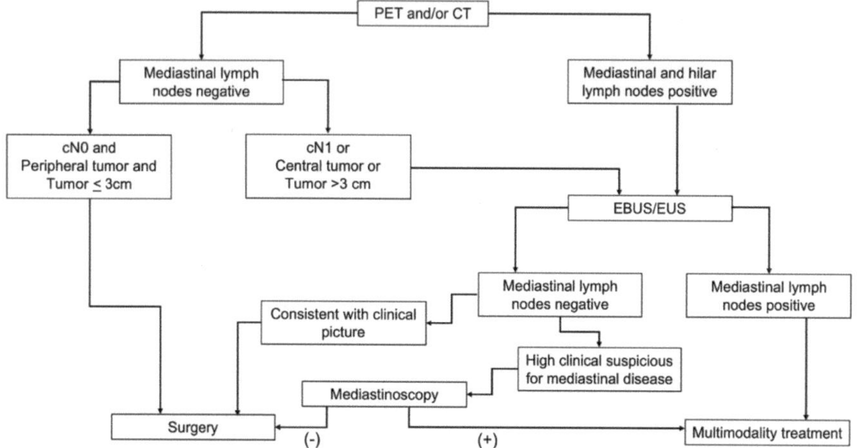

Fig. 5.2 Proposed approach to staging

Lung Cancers with Multiple Lesions

In patients with two or more pulmonary lesions, it is important to determine whether these lesions represent synchronous primary lung cancers or metastatic disease.

Synchronous primaries may have different histologies; however, it is possible to see the same histology. The following parameters can help distinguish second primary tumor versus metastasis:

- Differing rates of growth.
- Varying degrees of metabolic uptake.
- Lack of nodal metastases.
- Differing biomarkers/genetic profiles.

When two or more primary tumors are present, i.e., synchronous primary lung cancers, each tumor should be classified separately using TNM staging [3, 6]. If the pulmonary tumors exhibit the same histology and do not meet the above criteria, they are considered intrapulmonary metastases. Lesions located in the same lobe are classified as T3 disease; if an intrapulmonary metastasis is in a different lobe but in

Table 5.4 Lung cancer stage grouping (reproduced with permission from Detterbeck et al. The Eight Edition Lung Cancer Stage Classification. Chest 2017; 151: 193–203)

T/M	Label	N0	N1	N2	N3
T1	T1a ≤*1*	IA1	IIB	IIIA	IIIB
	T1b >*1-2*	IA2	IIB	IIIA	IIIB
	T1c >*2-3*	IA3	IIB	IIIA	IIIB
T2	T2a *cent*, Visc Pl	IB	IIB	IIIA	IIIB
	T2a >*3-4*	IB	IIB	IIIA	IIIB
	T2b >*4-5*	IIA	IIB	IIIB	IIIB
T3	T3 >*5-7*	IIB	IIIA	IIIB	IIIC
	T3 *Inv*	IIB	IIIA	IIIB	IIIC
	T3 *Satell*	IIB	IIIA	IIIB	IIIC
T4	T4 >*7*	IIIA	IIIA	IIIB	IIIC
	T4 *Inv*	IIIA	IIIA	IIIB	IIIC
	T4 *Ipsi Nod*	IIIA	IIIA	IIIB	IIIC
M1	M1a *Contr Nod*	IVA	IVA	IVA	IVA
	M1a Pl *Dissem*	IVA	IVA	IVA	IVA
	M1b *Single*	IVA	IVA	IVA	IVA
	M1c *Multi*	IVB	IVB	IVB	IVB

Cent=central, Visc = Visceral, Inv = Invasion, Satell=Satellite nodule, Ispi Nod = Ipsilateral nodule, Contr Nod = Contralateral Nodule, Pl Dissem = Pleural disseminated,

Table 5.5 Five-year survival percentages. Average overall survival in IASLC of patients diagnosed between 1999 and 2010 *(reproduced with permission from Detterbeck* et al. *The Eight Edition Lung Cancer Stage Classification. Chest 2017; 151: 193–203)*

Type	IA1	IA2	IA3	IB	IIA	IIB	IIIA	IIIB	IIIC	IVA	IVB
Clinical	92	83	77	68	60	53	36	26	13	10	0
Pathologic	90	85	80	73	65	56	41	24	12	-	-

the ipsilateral lung, it is classified as T4 disease. Lesions located in the contralateral lung are classified as M1a.

Multifocal adenocarcinoma has multiple lesions but a different entity than synchronous primaries or metastatic lung cancer. These lesions are staged using the nodule with the largest T classification as measured by the solid component (c) or invasive component (p). This designation is then followed by the number of lesions in parenthesis. For innumerable lesions, the prefix (m) for multiple is appropriate. N and M classifications are then given according to the nodules as one group [6].

Noninvasive Staging

Initial evaluation of a patient with suspected lung cancer should begin with a history and physical examination. For patients with systemic symptoms such as weight loss or neurologic symptoms like a new headache, the likelihood of metastatic disease is higher, and the workup should be tailored as such [15]. Other new diagnoses and symptoms unrelated to the lung may indicate a para-neoplastic syndrome, frequently seen in small cell lung cancer. These syndromes include syndrome of inappropriate antidiuretic hormone secretions (SIADH), hypercalcemia, Cushing's syndrome, Lambert-Eaton syndrome, limbic encephalitis, encephalomyelitis, and paraneoplastic cerebellar degeneration syndrome [16]. Diagnostic evaluation should begin with lab testing tailored toward explaining systemic symptoms (i.e., unintentional weight loss) and chest imaging. Chest X-ray is limited in identifying lymphadenopathy or early-stage lung cancer but can identify large tumors and pleural or pericardial effusions indicative of advanced-stage disease. Computed tomographic (CT) chest imaging is the first-line modality for evaluating lung nodules and allows for the best assessment of the mediastinum and lung parenchyma. The use of contrast-enhanced CT is typically not necessary but does allow for better visualization of the hila, and the assessment of potential vascular invasion in preoperative patients [15, 17].

On chest CT, pathologic lymphadenopathy is defined as any lymph node measuring greater than 1 cm in the short axis on a transverse cut. However, lymphadenopathy does not necessarily translate to metastatic disease [15]. CT imaging alone has a 55% sensitivity and 81% specificity for detecting mediastinal metastatic disease [9]. In one study of 256 patients, up to 77% of patients without nodal involvement had lymph nodes on CT measuring 1 cm or more, while up to 12% of patients with N1 and/or N2 disease did not have any lymphadenopathy on CT [18]. At the time of surgery, 5–15% of patients with clinical T1N0 are still found to have positive lymph nodes with resection [9]. If findings on CT are suspicious for lung cancer, assessment for metastatic spread can be further evaluated with positron emission tomography (PET).

PET is recommended for patients with a CT concerning metastatic disease and patients with a reassuring CT but an abnormal clinical evaluation suspicious for metastatic disease. These symptoms include unexplained weight loss, morning headaches, bone/back pain, and/or recent fracture concerning for pathological fracture. PET can also be done before curative treatment in patients without evidence of metastatic disease but is not required [9]. Compared to CT alone, PET is more accurate at identifying mediastinal metastases with a sensitivity and specificity of 80% and 88%, respectively [9]. In a population with a median lung cancer prevalence of 28%, the positive predictive value was 75%, and the negative predictive value was 91% [9]. Approximately 4% of patients with clinical stage I disease by PET still have unexpected mediastinal disease at the time of surgery. In patients with adrenal metastases, PET has high sensitivity and specificity of 97% and 91%, respectively [19]. Given the nearly 10% false-positive rate of benign adrenal lesions, isolated foci of FDG avidity should be sampled to confirm metastatic disease [10, 18]. In addition to identifying metastases, PET can be useful for prognostication; one meta-analysis showed that greater uptake was an independent risk factor for shorter survival in stage I–III NSCLC [20]. In centers where PET is unavailable, bone scanning and abdominal CT should be completed to look for metastatic disease [9].

One limitation of PET is that it is not specific to cancer. Both infection and sterile inflammation, such as granulomas, can cause an increase in fluorodeoxyglucose (FDG) uptake similar to that seen with malignancy [9]. Limited spatial resolution and decreased sensitivity for nodes and nodules measuring less than 7–10 mm also limit the utility of PET. The sensitivity for lymph nodes equal to or greater than 10 mm is relatively high at 85% but drops to 32% for lymph nodes measuring less than 10 mm [21]. PET/CT hybrid imaging may help identify the specific anatomic location of a metabolic focus; however, the sensitivity and specificity are similar to PET alone at 62% and 90%, respectively. Assessing pure ground-glass opacities (GGOs) and GGOs with a solid component less than 10 mm via PET is unreliable and is not recommended [6, 9].

Magnetic resonance imaging (MRI) of the chest is limited in lung cancer staging. It is most useful in preoperative planning for superior sulcus (or Pancoast) tumors to better evaluate chest wall invasion [6, 10]. MRI of the brain with and without gadolinium is recommended for all patients with stage III or IV disease [9]. In patients unable to have MRIs, contrast-enhanced brain CT is recommended. One meta-analysis of 19 studies evaluated the diagnostic utility of MRI in evaluating nodal metastases by comparing diffusion MRI to PET [22]. The sensitivity was statistically equal in both groups (75% and 72%, respectively), but MRI did have a higher specificity of 95% compared to 89% in PET. Further studies have yet to reproduce this difference [23, 24].

While noninvasive radiologic staging can help determine TNM staging, adequate tissue sampling is required to confirm the histology and perform molecular characterization [14]. Over the past two decades, significant advancements have been made in genomic profiling of NSCLC, leading to the discovery of driver oncogenes activated by mutations [25], fusion, and translocations [26]. Detection of molecular markers and tumor protein expression (i.e., programmed death-ligand 1 or PDL1) is critical to make decisions about therapy and requires tissue for analysis. While noninvasive staging is an important part of the workup, invasive sampling with adequate material is crucial for histological workup and molecular testing [27].

Invasive Staging

Invasive staging with tissue biopsy is frequently needed before a patient can receive definitive treatment. In patients without a confirmed tissue diagnosis, a thoughtful and thorough evaluation should provide a diagnosis and staging while minimizing the number of procedures a patient experiences. If extrathoracic lesions such as axillary, abdominal, or pelvic lymphadenopathy, skin lesions, adrenal nodules or masses, liver lesions, or pleural effusions are identified on imaging, the most advanced stage should be sampled first to allow for simultaneous staging and diagnosis [15, 28]. A multidisciplinary approach is frequently required between medical oncology, surgery, pulmonology, interventional radiology, and pathology. Lymph node sampling establishes nodal involvement for patients without evidence of extrathoracic disease. No single invasive technique can provide access to all mediastinal and hilar lymph nodes. Table 5.2 diagrams which lymph nodes can be accessed using which method.

The American College of Chest Physicians (ACCP) [9], European Society of Thoracic Surgeons (ESTS) [29], National Comprehensive Cancer Network (NCCN) [28], and European Society for Medical Oncology (ESMO) [30] have all published recommendation on how to stage a patient appropriately. A summary of these recommendations with a proposed approach is seen in Fig. 5.2.

Who Requires Invasive Staging

Invasive mediastinal staging, in addition to imaging, is recommended in the following scenarios [9, 29, 31]:

- Patients without evidence of distant metastasis with evidence of mediastinal and/or hilar node enlargement ($\geq$1 cm), regardless of FDG uptake on PET.
- Patients without distant metastases with normal-sized mediastinal and/or hilar lymph nodes (<1 cm) on CT *with* FDG avidity on PET.
- Patients with central tumor.
- Patients with tumor size greater than 3 cm.

For these patients, a needle technique with endobronchial ultrasound (EBUS), endoscopic ultrasound (EUS), or combined EBUS/EUS is recommended, given the intermediate to high suspicion for N2 or N3 disease [9, 29, 31]. If the results from a needle aspiration technique show lymphocytes without tumor or a sample insufficient for examination, video-assisted mediastinoscopy (VAM) can be pursued before definitive treatment if clinical suspicion for nodal metastatic disease remains high.

Conventional TBNA

Conventional transbronchial needle aspiration (TBNA) of lymph nodes has existed since 1978 using a Wang™ needle [32]. The Wang needle, developed by Dr. Ko Pen Wang, is a retractable needle with a smooth hub to allow for safe passage through the bronchoscope's working channel. It contains a locking mechanism to provide stability with sampling. Conventional TBNA was done before the visualization of lymph nodes by EBUS. It is a blind technique mainly used for sampling the lymph nodes in the subcarinal or lower paratracheal regions (stations 7, 4 L, 4R). This procedure is safe and can be done outpatient, without significant morbidity. However, this technique has a low sensitivity of only 78% in patients with clinical N2 disease and fell out of favor with the introduction of EBUS [33, 34].

EBUS/TBNA

EBUS-TBNA was initially introduced in 2002 and is now the recommended first-line approach in diagnosing and staging lung cancer. EBUS allows for needle aspiration of mediastinal, hilar, and central lung lesions under direct ultrasound visualization. Since its development, multiple publications, including meta-analyses and systematic reviews, have proven the safety and efficacy of EBUS in staging [35, 36].

The EBUS scope is a flexible bronchoscope combined with a convex transducer that allows scanning the mediastinum parallel to the scope. Ultrasound images are obtained by direct contact of the probe with the airway wall or with the help of a balloon inflated with saline to minimize air artifact (Fig. 5.3). A needle (19 g–25 g) is inserted into the working channel of the EBUS scope and deployed into the lymph under continuous visualization by ultrasound. Lymph nodes that are accessible with the EBUS scope include paratracheal (stations 2R/L, 4R/L), subcarinal (station 7), hilar (station 10R/L), interlobar (station 11R/L), and interlobar (stations 12R/L).

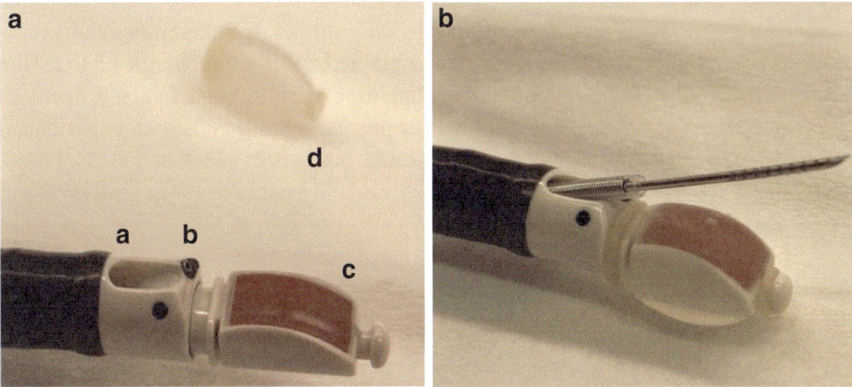

Fig. 5.3 Endobronchial ultrasound scope. (**a**) The distal tip of the EBUS bronchoscope. A. Working channel. B. Light and camera. C. Linear ultrasound. D. Latex balloon. (**b**) Flexible EBUS scope with a 21-gauge needle deployed parallel to the ultrasound. Latex balloon applied and filled with saline to minimize air artifact

When invasive staging is required, a systematic approach is implemented to optimize yield and minimize contamination. Assessment and sampling of the lymph nodes by EBUS should start with an evaluation of nodes contralateral to the lesion, i.e., N3 stations. This is followed by sampling of N2 stations, including the subcarinal lymph node and ipsilateral mediastinal lymph nodes. Sampling of ipsilateral hilar lymph nodes, i.e., N1 stations, should occur last. This sequential method prevents possible contamination of the needle with cells from a positive lower lymph node station (i.e., N1 node) with a higher, more distal, negative station (i.e., N2/N3 node) [37]. While all lymph node stations are assessed, only those greater than 5 mm in the short axis require sampling. A minimum of three samples from each lymph node is recommended to ensure adequacy. A study by Lee et al. demonstrated that after the third sample, adequacy was 100% with a sensitivity of 95.3% and NPV of 97.6% [38]. No guidelines currently exist for the optimal number of passes required for molecular analysis; however, studies suggest four to five passes are sufficient [36, 37, 39, 40]. Other biopsy tools, such as mini-forceps, have been utilized to increase tissue acquisition for molecular characterization, however this is yet to be rigorously analyzed [41]. PET FDG avid lymph nodes measuring less than 5 mm should also be sampled. However, the yield for lymph nodes measuring less than 5 mm is low [42].

EBUS-TBNA is safe and well-tolerated, with a mortality rate of 0.01%. Incidence of complication is 1–2% and includes bleeding, infection, and pneumothorax. EBUS bronchoscopy is generally an outpatient procedure performed under general anesthesia (GA) or moderate sedation with a topical anesthetic. Initial studies showed that the diagnostic yield and the number of lymph nodes visualized and sampled were higher when the procedure was performed under GA [43]. More recent comparison studies have demonstrated that the diagnostic yield, rates of complications, and patient comfort were similar between moderate sedation and GA [44, 45, 46].

*R*apid *O*n-*S*ite cytologic *E*valuation (ROSE) allows for the immediate intraprocedural examination of the specimens obtained. While the benefit of ROSE is not universal, many studies have shown it can improve sampling adequacy, decrease procedure time, and decrease the number of passes [47–49]. When an experienced cytologist performs ROSE, it can increase the diagnostic yield of EBUS-TBNA [50]. The sensitivity of TBNA utilizing ROSE in malignancy is between 85.7% and 96.1% [51, 52].

Endoscopic Ultrasound

Endoscopic ultrasound (EUS) fine needle aspiration is a well-established technique used in diagnosing and staging gastrointestinal and pancreatobiliary malignancy. EUS has also been utilized in the staging of lung cancer as it allows for the sampling of some mediastinal lymph nodes accessible by EBUS (stations 2 L, 4 L, 7, 3p) as well as some which are not accessible via EBUS (stations 8, 9). The right paratracheal lymph nodes (stations 2R, 4R) have limited visualization with EUS as the trachea lies between the lymph nodes and the esophagus. Structures below the diaphragm can also be sampled using EUS, including lesions in the left liver lobe, adrenal glands, and spleen. New techniques to sample the aortopulmonary and para-aortic lymph nodes (stations 5 and 6) using EUS are under development [53, 54]. EUS has been shown in multiple studies to safely upstage patients, avoiding inappropriate resections or the need for surgical staging [55–60].

Combined EUS/EBUS

A combination of EUS and EBUS allows access to most mediastinal lymph nodes (excluding para-aortic and aortopulmonary window) and is more sensitive than either technique alone [61–64]. A prospective single-center study in Montreal enrolled 166 patients with suspected resectable lung cancer who met the criteria for surgical mediastinal staging. Under general anesthesia, all patients were staged with EBUS, followed by EUS staging and surgical mediastinal staging. When compared to surgical staging, combined EUS/EBUS had a sensitivity and NPV of 91% and 96% compared to EBUS alone at 72% and 88%, respectively. Of 166 patients, five (3%) had negative ultrasound assessments and were ultimately found to have N2 disease on surgical staging. Conversely, 14% of patients with negative surgical stage had N2 disease detected via EUS/EBUS [61]. One meta-analysis reported a pooled sensitivity of 83–94% with combined EUS/EBUS. Given this data, the ESTS recommends the combination of EBUS/EUS over either technique alone for mediastinal staging in patients with NSCLC [29].

Endobronchial Ultrasound Using the EBUS Scope (EUS-B)

Although EUS allows access to more mediastinal lymph nodes, gastroenterologists traditionally do it via an esophagogastroduodenoscopy (EGD) scope. The gain in diagnostic yield in staging with EUS/EBUS is still observed when the EUS portion is done using the EBUS scope, i.e., EUS-B [65]. Among 150 patients with NSCLC, Herth et al. performed EBUS and EUS consecutively using the same linear EBUS scope [66]. The combined sensitivity remained higher at 95% compared to EBUS or EUS alone at 92 and 89%, respectively. This strategy allows for a quicker and more cost-effective approach for mediastinal staging when done by an experienced practitioner. A patient-centered approach should be adopted depending on the target location, physician expertise, and available resources.

Sampling of Metastatic Disease

If there is a concern for metastatic disease on imaging, tissue sampling for confirmation should be performed. Much of this can be done in a minimally invasive manner with CT-guided or ultrasound (US)-guided techniques.

Transthoracic needle aspiration (TTNA) of lung nodules is most frequently done under CT guidance and has reported accuracy rates of up to 90% [10]. When staging a patient, TTNA is most helpful in sampling contralateral nodules concerning for metastases. CT guidance is also necessary for sampling adrenal nodules, and either CT or US can be utilized for liver lesions.

Malignant pleural effusions (MPEs) automatically upstage a patient to M1a disease; therefore, any pleural effusion should be sampled by a US-guided thoracentesis [10, 27]. Diagnostic rates range from 14 to 82% and depend on the cell type. The overall yield for diagnosing MPE via pleural fluid analysis remains less than 60% after the second thoracentesis and does not increase with further pleural fluid sampling [67, 68]. Additionally, analysis of volumes greater than 75 mL does not improve yield [68, 69]. If there is clinical suspicion for a MPE in a recurrent exudative effusion with negative cytology, more invasive pleural sampling should be done with pleuroscopy or video-assisted thoracoscopy (VATS) [10].

Surgical Staging

Mediastinoscopy

Standard cervical mediastinoscopy uses a video mediastinoscope (VAM) under general anesthesia via a cervical incision just above the sternal notch [70, 71]. VAM allows for sampling of superior and inferior bilateral paratracheal nodes (stations 2R/L, 4R/L), subcarinal (station 7), and bilateral hilar nodes (station 10R/L) [10]. VAM does not allow sampling of the aortopulmonary window, anterior mediastinal (stations 5 and 6), or inferior mediastinal (stations 8 and 9) lymph nodes [10]. Compared to EBUS, VAM is more invasive as lymph nodes are accessed via a skin incision. Specificity is 100%, with sensitivity ranging from 78 to 97% [10]. Complication rates of cervical mediastinoscopy are low, with a mortality rate of 0.05%. The most common complication is left recurrent laryngeal nerve palsy occurring at a rate of 2% [10, 72]. The median negative predictive value (NPV) of cervical mediastinoscopy is 91%, and about one-half of the false negatives are due to the inability to access stations [9]. Mediastinoscopy is most useful when EBUS is inconclusive and/or clinical suspicion remains high despite negative EBUS/EUS.

Anterior mediastinoscopy, also known as the Chamberlain procedure, is done via a left parasternal incision at the level of the second or third intercostal space to access the aortopulmonary window and para-aortic lymph nodes (stations 5 and 6). The median sensitivity among 238 patients with left upper lobe tumors was approximately 71%, with a NPV of 91% [9]. Many surgeons use VATS Chamberlain procedure as a minimally invasive alternative to traditional mediastinoscopy.

Extended cervical mediastinoscopy starts with VAM to assess the paratracheal lymph nodes and is then directed laterally to the aortic arch. The sensitivity and NPV of extended cervical mediastinoscopy are similar to those of the Chamberlain procedure at 71% and 91%, respectively [10, 70, 71, 73–75].

Transcervical Lymphadenectomies

While mediastinoscopy only allows for lymph node sampling, video-assisted mediastinoscopic lymphadenectomy (VAMLA) and transcervical extended mediastinal lymphadenectomy (TEMLA) allow for complete lymph node excision. VAMLA is an endoscopic technique utilizing VAM, and TEMLA is an open procedure assisted by VAM or video thoracoscopy (VAT). Both procedures are well tolerated, with recurrent laryngeal nerve palsy being the most common complication occurring at similar rates to cervical mediastinoscopy [10]. These may be useful procedures prior to performing an extended resection as the NPV is nearly 100%.

Endosonography Versus Mediastinoscopy

Since the implementation of EBUS, multiple studies have been done comparing endosonography to mediastinoscopy staging [42, 76, 77]. The ACCP and ESTS guidelines recommend combined mediastinoscopy plus EBUS over mediastinoscopy alone due to its higher sensitivity of 94% versus 79%, respectively ($p = 0.02$) [56]. When comparing surgical staging to endosonography, studies have shown no significant differences in NPV, sensitivity, or diagnostic accuracy [42, 78]. Despite being more invasive and allowing for more tissue acquisition, mediastinoscopy has limited access to nodal stations and may contribute less information than EBUS/EUS. A study of 418 patients found 14% nodal disease at the time of resection despite a negative EBUS and a negative confirmatory mediastinoscopy [79]. This data has contributed to the shifting trend of only performing mediastinoscopy after negative EBUS/EUS when clinical suspicion remains high [80].

VATS

VATS has a limited role in the staging paradigm as it only allows for the assessment of ipsilateral lymph nodes. The sensitivity varies from 58 to 100% with 100% specificity and a false-negative rate of 4% [10]. Left-sided VATS does allow for sampling of the aortopulmonary and para-aortic (stations 5 and 6), which are most likely to be involved in left upper lobe tumors [9, 10]. The left paratracheal nodes (station 2 L and 4 L) are not accessible by VATS without transecting the ligamentum arteriosum and mobilizing the aorta. VATs is useful for biopsying levels 5 and 6 lymph nodes as an alternative to the Chamberlain procedure.

Table 5.6 outlines which procedural approaches can access which lymph node stations.

Prediction Models

While invasive staging is recommended in patients with larger tumors or lymphadenopathy, hospital capabilities or individual patient factors, such as functional status and co-morbidities, may limit the feasibility of invasive staging. Prediction models can help assess the risk of forgoing invasive mediastinal staging in these scenarios [81, 82].

The *H*elp with the assessment of *A*denopathy in *L*ung cancer (HAL) prediction model is a multivariable logistic regression model to predict the likelihood of N2/N3 disease. It incorporates patient age, the location and histology of the primary cancer, and the N stage by CT and PET imaging. The model was first derived from data from the AQuIRE (American College of Chest Physicians Quality Improvement Registry, Evaluation, And Education) registry and was validated using data from 722 patients from 3 other hospitals. It is designed to provide a likelihood of N2/N3 disease in a particular patient, which can then be utilized to weigh the risks of invasive staging versus going directly to surgical resection [82].

Table 5.6 Lymph nodes accessibility via different modalities

Station	Lymph nodes	EBUS	EUS	VATS	CM
2	Upper paratracheal	✓	✓[a]	✓[b]	✓
3	Pre-vascular retro tracheal	✓	✓	✓	
4	Lower paratracheal	✓	✓[a]	✓[b]	✓
5	Aortopulmonary window		✓[c]	✓	
6	Para-aortic		✓[c]	✓	
7	Subcarinal	✓	✓	✓	✓
8	Paraesophageal		✓	✓	
9	Pulmonary ligament		✓	✓	
10	Hilar	✓		✓[b]	✓
11	Interlobar	✓		✓[b]	
12	Lobar	✓		✓[b]	

EBUS endobronchial ultrasound, *EUS* endoscopic ultrasound, *CM* cervical mediastinoscopy, *VATS* video-assisted thoracoscopic surgery
[a]Right sided only
[b]Ipsilateral only
[c]Limited data

ESTS recommends that surgical candidates with a 10% or less predicted chance of N2 disease may proceed directly to surgery without invasive mediastinal staging [10]. Mediastinal lymph node staging is performed in these patients during surgery. This approach aims to minimize complications, procedure costs, and treatment delays associated with unnecessary testing and procedures. Per ESTS guidelines, however, patients with >10% risk of N2 disease should undergo invasive mediastinal staging before surgery. Without invasive staging, these patients would go straight to surgery and be more likely to find N2 disease, therefore having had unnecessary surgery [10].

The HAL prediction model is not designed to predict N1 disease. N1 involvement would not alter surgical plans but would extend the radiation field in a patient undergoing SBRT. The *H*elp with *O*ncologic *M*ediastinal *E*valuation for *R*adiation (HOMER) prediction model was designed to predict N1 disease in a patient before radiation therapy [81]. HOMER is an ordinal logistical regression model that uses patient age, location, and histology of the primary cancer and N stage by CT and PET. It is designed to compare the likelihood of nodal metastases in a nonsurgical candidate against the sensitivity of EBUS, the possibility of procedural complications, and the harm of treating possible N0 disease.

However, HOMER and HAL have only been studied in patients with NSCLC, and their applicability in small cell lung cancer is yet to be determined.

Pathologic Staging

At the time of surgery, the primary tumor and any adjacent or invaded structures should be resected en bloc to avoid contamination of the field with cancer cells. The pathological staging of nodal disease requires a complete lobe-specific nodal dissection starting from mediastinum to hilum to intrapulmonary lymph nodes. A complete resection requires a minimum of six stations. Regardless of the lobe resected, appropriate resection includes the subcarinal station, two mediastinal nodes, and three hilar or intrapulmonary nodes. Lower lobe tumors require removal of stations 8 and 9, and left upper lobe tumors require resection of stations 5 and 6; these are all stations not accessible via bronchoscopy. If a minimum of six stations are not resected, the resection is classified as pN0 or pNo(un), depending on the classification system used [6, 10, 83]. If macroscopic or microscopic tumor is left within the chest, the resection is considered incomplete and is associated with worse survival [84].

For tumors near the pleura, elastin stains evaluate for tumor invasion beyond the elastic layer of the pleura and establish PL classification, which may affect T staging [6, 9]. The greater the degree of pleural invasion, the worse the prognosis. When there is no invasion of the elastic layer, the tumor is PL0, and T staging is unaffected. Any invasion of the visceral pleural classifies a tumor as PL1 or PL2, which is at least a T2 tumor. If there is involvement of the parietal pleural (i.e., PL3) that increases the tumor staging to a T3 [10] and if the pathological specimen shows the invasion of the inner pericardial surface or great vessels (pulmonary artery, pulmonary vein, vena cava, or aorta), the tumor is staged T4 [9]. Thoracic nerve root involvement classifies a tumor as T3, while higher nerve root (C8 or higher) or spine involvement is classified as T4. Based on imaging alone, these classifications are difficult to determine and are not part of the clinical staging paradigm.

After resection, surgical specimens can be further classified beyond TNM using the "R" identifier [3]:

- R0 denotes a specimen with negative margins.
- R1 denotes a specimen with microscopic positive margins.
- R2 demotes a specimen with grossly positive margins.

The ACCP guidelines still recommend the p prefix when extensive biopsy samples were taken during an attempted resection [83].

Pathologic Staging of Adenocarcinoma

Tumor in situ, or Tis category, includes squamous cell carcinoma (SCIS) and adenocarcinoma in situ (AIS). On pathological specimens, AIS is less than 3 cm in size, and the neoplastic growth lacks any invasion and is limited to alveolar structures. This is also known as lepidic growth. The pathological specimen in AIS lacks any evidence of spread through the air spaces (STAS) beyond the edge of the tumor. Most AIS lesions are non-mucinous and, on imaging, appear to be pure GGOs. This diagnosis cannot be made on a biopsy specimen and requires complete surgical excision [6, 10].

Due to its low prevalence, there is minimal data on lepidic tumors measuring greater than 3 cm. These are classified as lepidic predominant adenocarcinomas (LPA) and assigned to a pathological T1a category. Lack of invasion should still be commented on in the final pathology report as the outcomes of such tumors are not yet well understood [10].

Tumors are invasive if they have any of the following [10]:

- Lymphatic, vasculature, alveolar space, or pleural involvement.
- Tumor necrosis.
- STAS.

Minimally invasive adenocarcinomas (MIA) are lepidic predominant, measuring up to 3 cm, but contain an invasive component measuring no more than 0.5 cm in its largest dimension [6, 10, 85]. In cases where the invasive components are not contiguous, a percentage of the invasive tumor with respect to total tumor size can be calculated. For example, a 2 cm tumor with a 20% invasive component would be 0.4 cm and therefore be classified as MIA [10]. Any invasive component larger than 0.5 cm would be classified as an adenocarcinoma, not MIA.

Non-mucinous adenocarcinomas are classified as either lepidic or invasive; invasive tumors are further classified as having acinar, papillary, solid, or micropapillary patterns. Subsolid nodules contain both lepidic and invasive components. Similar to the clinical staging of subsolid nodules, the T staging is categorized based on the invasive component, as this component is a better predictor of survival than overall nodule size [6, 86].

Patients Without Nodal Metastases

After a patient has been appropriately staged, those without evidence of nodal metastases still require further evaluation to diagnose the lung lesion. If a patient with a high pretest probability of malignancy is deemed a surgical candidate, diagnosis and treatment can be done simultaneously with surgical resection [27] (see Chap. 6). If a patient is not a surgical candidate, diagnosis can be achieved with either transthoracic needle (TTNA) biopsy or navigational bronchoscopy [28].

For peripheral nodules, navigational bronchoscopy, with or without radial ultrasound and fluoroscopic guidance, is recommended given the higher false-negative rate and higher complication risk with TTNA [27]. However, the appropriate diagnostic procedure will depend on the location of the lesion, the patient's comorbidities, and the center's capabilities and expertise. Electromagnetic navigation (EMN) bronchoscopy has historically been the most available form of peripheral bronchoscopy. EMN relies on creation of an electromagnetic field around the patient's body, and using a tracked sensor within biopsy tools (needle or forceps), the patient's airways are mapped and matched to a 3D reconstruction of the patient's anatomy from CT imaging. This technique creates a virtual 3D map of the lung and a suggested bronchoscopic pathway to the suspicious lesion. The bronchoscopist can then navigate the bronchoscope and tracked biopsy tools through the airways to the target lesion [87]. The use of multiple tools, thin and ultrathin bronchoscopy, and the use of radial EBUS have helped improve ability to navigate and sample peripheral pulmonary nodules; however, diagnostic yield remains between 40% and 60%, depending on the study cited [88–91]. Challenges with EMN-guided bronchoscopy include difficulty navigating to peripheral lesions due to small size of peripheral airways and difficulty reaching lesions that are not adjacent to or surrounding an airway. These limitations decrease diagnostic certainty [92].

In 2019, robotic systems were introduced, allowing for more peripheral reach and stability during biopsy. Pilot study demonstrated safety and feasibility of robotic bronchoscopy [92], while retrospective and prospective studies have demonstrated promising results for diagnostic yields for peripheral pulmonary nodules with complication rates similar to conventional ENB and radial EBUS-guided bronchoscopy [92–94]. Diagnostic yield may be increased with the presence of an airway into the nodule (bronchus sign), increased size of the nodule. Newer technologies such as cone beam CT, digital tomosynthesis augmentation, and others may be added to existing platforms to enhance visualization; however, further study is needed to determine their effect on diagnostic yield. A multidisciplinary discussion can help elucidate the best diagnostic approach while minimizing the number of procedures a patient requires.

Conclusion

While not all patients require invasive staging, tissue confirmation is frequently required as PET scans, and CT scans have limited sensitivity and specificity for lung cancer staging. The TNM guidelines provide a framework that allows for clear and consistent communication between providers and helps to dictate the course of treatment for patients.

References

1. O'Neil ME, Henley SJ, Rohan EA, Ellington TD, Gallaway MS. Lung cancer incidence in nonmetropolitan and metropolitan counties—United States, 2007-2016. MMWR Morb Mortal Wkly Rep. 2019;68(44):993–8.
2. Toumazis I, Bastani M, Han SS, Plevritis SK. Risk-based lung cancer screening: a systematic review. Lung cancer. 2020;147:154–86.
3. Tanoue LT. Lung cancer staging. Clin Chest Med. 2020;41(2):161–74.
4. Mountain CF, Carr DT, Anderson WA. A system for the clinical staging of lung cancer. Am J Roentgenol. 1974;120(1):130–8.
5. Ganti AKP, Loo BW, Bassetti M, Blakely C, Chiang A, D'Amico TA, et al. Small cell lung cancer, version 2.2022, NCCN clinical practice guidelines in oncology. J Natl Compr Cancer Netw. 2021;19(12):1441–64.
6. Amin M. Part VII Thorax. AJCC Cancer Staging Manual (8th ed.). American College of Surgeons. (2017). https://www.r2library.com/Resource/Title/3319406175/pt0007.
7. Rami-Porta R, Bolejack V, Giroux DJ, Chansky K, Crowley J, Asamura H, et al. The IASLC lung cancer staging project: the new database to inform the eighth edition of the TNM classification of lung cancer. J Thorac Oncol. 2014;9(11):1618–24.
8. Detterbeck FC, Boffa DJ, Kim AW, Tanoue LT. The eighth edition lung cancer stage classification. Chest. 2017;151(1):193–203.
9. Silvestri GA, Gonzalez AV, Jantz MA, Margolis ML, Gould MK, Tanoue LT, et al. Methods for staging non-small cell lung cancer: diagnosis and management of lung cancer, 3rd ed: American College of Chest Physicians evidence-based clinical practice guidelines. Chest. 2013;143(5 Suppl):e211S–e50S.
10. Rami-Porta R, Call S, Dooms C, Obiols C, Sanchez M, Travis WD, et al. Lung cancer staging: a concise update. Eur Respir J. 2018;51(5):1800190.
11. Rusch VW, Asamura H, Watanabe H, Giroux DJ, Rami-Porta R, Goldstraw P, et al. The IASLC lung cancer staging project: a proposal for a new international lymph node map in the forthcoming seventh edition of the TNM classification for lung cancer. J Thorac Oncol. 2009;4(5):568–77.
12. Libshitz HI, McKenna RJ Jr, Mountain CF. Patterns of mediastinal metastases in bronchogenic carcinoma. Chest. 1986;90(2):229–32.
13. Watanabe Y, Shimizu J, Tsubota M, Iwa T. Mediastinal spread of metastatic lymph nodes in bronchogenic carcinoma. Mediastinal nodal metastases in lung cancer. Chest. 1990;97(5):1059–65.

14. Feng SH, Yang ST. The new 8th TNM staging system of lung cancer and its potential imaging interpretation pitfalls and limitations with CT image demonstrations. Diagn Interv Radiol. 2019;25(4):270–9.
15. Almeida FA, Uzbeck M, Ost D. Initial evaluation of the nonsmall cell lung cancer patient: diagnosis and staging. Curr Opin Pulm Med. 2010;16(4):307–14.
16. van Meerbeeck JP, Fennell DA, De Ruysscher DK. Small-cell lung cancer. Lancet. 2011;378(9804):1741–55. https://doi.org/10.1016/S0140-6736(11)60165-7.
17. Marshall T, Kalanjeri S, Almeida FA. Lung cancer staging, the established role of bronchoscopy. Curr Opin Pulm Med. 2022;28(1):17–30.
18. Prenzel KL, Monig SP, Sinning JM, Baldus SE, Brochhagen HG, Schneider PM, et al. Lymph node size and metastatic infiltration in non-small cell lung cancer. Chest. 2003;123(2):463–7.
19. Boland GW, Dwamena BA, Jagtiani Sangwaiya M, Goehler AG, Blake MA, Hahn PF, et al. Characterization of adrenal masses by using FDG PET: a systematic review and meta-analysis of diagnostic test performance. Radiology. 2011;259(1):117–26.
20. Paesmans M, Garcia C, Wong CY, Patz EF Jr, Komaki R, Eschmann S, et al. Primary tumour standardised uptake value is prognostic in nonsmall cell lung cancer: a multivariate pooled analysis of individual data. Eur Respir J. 2015;46(6):1751–61.
21. Lv YL, Yuan DM, Wang K, Miao XH, Qian Q, Wei SZ, et al. Diagnostic performance of integrated positron emission tomography/computed tomography for mediastinal lymph node staging in non-small cell lung cancer: a bivariate systematic review and meta-analysis. J Thorac Oncol. 2011;6(8):1350–8.
22. Wu LM, Xu JR, Gu HY, Hua J, Chen J, Zhang W, et al. Preoperative mediastinal and hilar nodal staging with diffusion-weighted magnetic resonance imaging and fluorodeoxyglucose positron emission tomography/computed tomography in patients with non-small-cell lung cancer: which is better? J Surg Res. 2012;178(1):304–14.
23. Sommer G, Wiese M, Winter L, Lenz C, Klarhofer M, Forrer F, et al. Preoperative staging of non-small-cell lung cancer: comparison of whole-body diffusion-weighted magnetic resonance imaging and 18F-fluorodeoxyglucose-positron emission tomography/computed tomography. Eur Radiol. 2012;22(12):2859–67.
24. Pauls S, Schmidt SA, Juchems MS, Klass O, Luster M, Reske SN, et al. Diffusion-weighted MR imaging in comparison to integrated [(1)(8)F]-FDG PET/CT for N-staging in patients with lung cancer. Eur J Radiol. 2012;81(1):178–82.
25. Lynch TJ, Bell DW, Sordella R, et al. Activating mutations in the epidermal growth factor receptor underlying responsiveness of non-small-cell lung cancer to gefitinib. N Engl J Med. 2004;350:2129–39.
26. Shaw AT, Kim DW, Nakagawa K, et al. Crizotinib versus chemotherapy in advanced ALK-positive lung cancer. N Engl J Med. 2013;368:2285–394.
27. Rivera MP, Mehta AC, Wahidi MM. Establishing the diagnosis of lung cancer: diagnosis and management of lung cancer, 3rd ed: American College of Chest Physicians evidence-based clinical practice guidelines. Chest. 2013;143(5 Suppl):e142S–65S.
28. (NCCN) NCCN. NCCN Practice Guide- lines in Oncology. Non Small Cell Lung Cancer Version 5.2021. https://www.Nccn.Org/Professionals/Physician_gls/Pdf/Nscl.Pdf. Accessed 30 Aug 2022.
29. De Leyn P, Dooms C, Kuzdzal J, Lardinois D, Passlick B, Rami-Porta R, et al. Revised ESTS guidelines for preoperative mediastinal lymph node staging for non-small-cell lung cancer. Eur J Cardiothorac Surg. 2014;45(5):787–98.
30. Vansteenkiste J, Crino L, Dooms C, Douillard JY, Faivre-Finn C, Lim E, et al. 2nd ESMO consensus conference on lung cancer: early-stage non-small-cell lung cancer consensus on diagnosis, treatment and follow-up. Ann Oncol. 2014;25(8):1462–74.
31. Detterbeck FC, Lewis SZ, Diekemper R, Addrizzo-Harris D, Alberts WM. Executive summary: diagnosis and management of lung cancer, 3rd ed: American College of Chest Physicians evidence-based clinical practice guidelines. Chest. 2013;143(5 Suppl):7S–37S.

32. Wang KP, Terry P, Marsh B. Bronchoscopic needle aspiration biopsy of paratracheal tumors. Am Rev Respir Dis. 1978;118(1):17–21.
33. Holty JE, Kuschner WG, Gould MK. Accuracy of transbronchial needle aspiration for mediastinal staging of non-small cell lung cancer: a meta-analysis. Thorax. 2005;60(11):949–55.
34. Detterbeck FC, Jantz MA, Wallace M, Vansteenkiste J, Silvestri GA, American College of Chest P. Invasive mediastinal staging of lung cancer: ACCP evidence-based clinical practice guidelines (2nd edition). Chest. 2007;132(3 Suppl):202S–20S.
35. Adams K, Shah PL, Edmonds L, Lim E. Test performance of endobronchial ultrasound and transbronchial needle aspiration biopsy for mediastinal staging in patients with lung cancer: systematic review and meta-analysis. Thorax. 2009;64(9):757–62.
36. Gu P, Zhao YZ, Jiang LY, Zhang W, Xin Y, Han BH. Endobronchial ultrasound-guided transbronchial needle aspiration for staging of lung cancer: a systematic review and meta-analysis. Eur J Cancer. 2009;45(8):1389–96.
37. Block MI. Endobronchial ultrasound for lung cancer staging: how many stations should be sampled? Ann Thorac Surg. 2010;89(5):1582–7.
38. Lee HS, Lee GK, Lee HS, Kim MS, Lee JM, Kim HY, et al. Real-time endobronchial ultrasound-guided transbronchial needle aspiration in mediastinal staging of non-small cell lung cancer: how many aspirations per target lymph node station? Chest. 2008;134(2):368–74.
39. Yarmus L, Akulian J, Gilbert C, Feller-Kopman D, Lee HJ, Zarogoulidis P, et al. Optimizing endobronchial ultrasound for molecular analysis. How many passes are needed? Ann Am Thorac Soc. 2013;10(6):636–43.
40. Labarca G, Folch E, Jantz M, Mehta HJ, Majid A, Fernandez-Bussy S. Adequacy of samples obtained by endobronchial ultrasound with transbronchial needle aspiration for molecular analysis in patients with non-small cell lung cancer. Systematic review and meta-analysis. Ann Am Thorac Soc. 2018;15(10):1205–16.
41. Cheng G, Mahajan A, Oh S, Benzaquen S, Chen A. Endobronchial ultrasound-guided intranodal forceps biopsy (EBUS-IFB)-technical review. J Thorac Dis. 2019;11(9):4049–58.
42. Yasufuku K, Pierre A, Darling G, de Perrot M, Waddell T, Johnston M, et al. A prospective controlled trial of endobronchial ultrasound-guided transbronchial needle aspiration compared with mediastinoscopy for mediastinal lymph node staging of lung cancer. J Thorac Cardiovasc Surg. 2011;142(6):1393–400.e1.
43. Yarmus LB, Akulian JA, Gilbert C, Mathai SC, Sathiyamoorthy S, Sahetya S, et al. Comparison of moderate versus deep sedation for endobronchial ultrasound transbronchial needle aspiration. Ann Am Thorac Soc. 2013;10(2):121–6.
44. Cornelissen CG, Dapper J, Dreher M, Muller T. Endobronchial ultrasound-guided transbronchial needle aspiration under general anesthesia versus bronchoscopist-directed deep sedation: a retrospective analysis. Endosc Ultrasound. 2019;8(3):204–8.
45. Casal RF, Lazarus DR, Kuhl K, Nogueras-Gonzalez G, Perusich S, Green LK, et al. Randomized trial of endobronchial ultrasound-guided transbronchial needle aspiration under general anesthesia versus moderate sedation. Am J Respir Crit Care Med. 2015;191(7):796–803.
46. Fernandes MGO, Santos VF, Martins N, Sucena MC, Passos MM, Marques MM, et al. Endobronchial ultrasound under moderate sedation versus general anesthesia. J Clin Med. 2018;7(11):421.
47. Chandra S, Chandra H, Sindhwani G. Role of rapid on-site evaluation with cyto-histopathological correlation in diagnosis of lung lesion. J Cytol. 2014;31(4):189–93.
48. Madan K, Dhungana A, Mohan A, Hadda V, Jain D, Arava S, et al. Conventional transbronchial needle aspiration versus endobronchial ultrasound-guided transbronchial needle aspiration, with or without rapid on-site evaluation, for the diagnosis of sarcoidosis: a randomized controlled trial. J Bronchology Interv Pulmonol. 2017;24(1):48–58.
49. Schacht MJ, Toustrup CB, Madsen LB, Martiny MS, Larsen BB, Simonsen JT. Endobronchial ultrasound-guided transbronchial needle aspiration: performance of biomedical scientists on rapid on-site evaluation and preliminary diagnosis. Cytopathology. 2016;27(5):344–50.

50. Li C, Sun W-W, Feng J, Cao J, Zhang P. Utilization of rapid on-site evaluation (ROSE) in transbronchial needle aspiration (TBNA), it is not a simple statistical issue. Int J Clin Exp Med. 2016;9:13298.
51. Simon M, Pop B, Toma IL, Vallasek AK, Simon I. The use of EBUS-TBNA and ROSE in the diagnosis of lung cancer. Romanian J Morphol Embryol. 2017;58(1):79–87.
52. Caupena C, Esteban L, Jaen A, Barreiro B, Albero R, Perez-Ochoa F, et al. Concordance between rapid on-site evaluation and final cytologic diagnosis in patients undergoing endobronchial ultrasound-guided transbronchial needle aspiration for non-small cell lung cancer staging. Am J Clin Pathol. 2020;153(2):190–7.
53. Liberman M, Duranceau A, Grunenwald E, Martin J, Thiffault V, Khereba M, et al. New technique performed by using EUS access for biopsy of para-aortic (station 6) mediastinal lymph nodes without traversing the aorta (with video). Gastrointest Endosc. 2011;73(5):1048–51.
54. Liberman M, Duranceau A, Grunenwald E, Thiffault V, Khereba M, Ferraro P. Initial experience with a new technique of endoscopic and ultrasonographic access for biopsy of para-aortic (station 6) mediastinal lymph nodes without traversing the aorta. J Thorac Cardiovasc Surg. 2012;144(4):787–92; discussion 92–3.
55. Singh P, Camazine B, Jadhav Y, Gupta R, Mukhopadhyay P, Khan A, et al. Endoscopic ultrasound as a first test for diagnosis and staging of lung cancer: a prospective study. Am J Respir Crit Care Med. 2007;175(4):345–54.
56. Annema JT, Versteegh MI, Veselic M, Voigt P, Rabe KF. Endoscopic ultrasound-guided fine-needle aspiration in the diagnosis and staging of lung cancer and its impact on surgical staging. J Clin Oncol Off J Am Soc Clin Oncol. 2005;23(33):8357–61.
57. Herth FJ, Rabe KF, Gasparini S, Annema JT. Transbronchial and transoesophageal (ultrasound-guided) needle aspirations for the analysis of mediastinal lesions. Eur Respir J. 2006;28(6):1264–75.
58. Tournoy KG, Praet MM, Van Maele G, Van Meerbeeck JP. Esophageal endoscopic ultrasound with fine-needle aspiration with an on-site cytopathologist: high accuracy for the diagnosis of mediastinal lymphadenopathy. Chest. 2005;128(4):3004–9.
59. Eloubeidi MA, Cerfolio RJ, Chen VK, Desmond R, Syed S, Ojha B. Endoscopic ultrasound-guided fine needle aspiration of mediastinal lymph node in patients with suspected lung cancer after positron emission tomography and computed tomography scans. Ann Thorac Surg. 2005;79(1):263–8.
60. Micames CG, McCrory DC, Pavey DA, Jowell PS, Gress FG. Endoscopic ultrasound-guided fine-needle aspiration for non-small cell lung cancer staging: a systematic review and meta-analysis. Chest. 2007;131(2):539–48.
61. Liberman M, Sampalis J, Duranceau A, Thiffault V, Hadjeres R, Ferraro P. Endosonographic mediastinal lymph node staging of lung cancer. Chest. 2014;146(2):389–97.
62. Wallace MB, Pascual JM, Raimondo M, Woodward TA, McComb BL, Crook JE, et al. Minimally invasive endoscopic staging of suspected lung cancer. JAMA. 2008;299(5):540–6.
63. Korevaar DA, Crombag LM, Cohen JF, Spijker R, Bossuyt PM, Annema JT. Added value of combined endobronchial and oesophageal endosonography for mediastinal nodal staging in lung cancer: a systematic review and meta-analysis. Lancet Respir Med. 2016;4(12):960–8.
64. Zhang R, Ying K, Shi L, Zhang L, Zhou L. Combined endobronchial and endoscopic ultrasound-guided fine needle aspiration for mediastinal lymph node staging of lung cancer: a meta-analysis. Eur J Cancer. 2013;49(8):1860–7.
65. Oki M, Saka H, Ando M, Kitagawa C, Kogure Y, Seki Y. Endoscopic ultrasound-guided fine needle aspiration and endobronchial ultrasound-guided transbronchial needle aspiration: are two better than one in mediastinal staging of non-small cell lung cancer? J Thorac Cardiovasc Surg. 2014;148(4):1169–77.
66. Herth FJ, Krasnik M, Kahn N, Eberhardt R, Ernst A. Combined endoscopic-endobronchial ultrasound-guided fine-needle aspiration of mediastinal lymph nodes through a single bronchoscope in 150 patients with suspected lung cancer. Chest. 2010;138(4):790–4.

67. Porcel JM, Esquerda A, Vives M, Bielsa S. Etiology of pleural effusions: analysis of more than 3,000 consecutive thoracenteses. Arch Bronconeumol. 2014;50(5):161–5.
68. Kaul V, McCracken DJ, Rahman NM, Epelbaum O. Contemporary approach to the diagnosis of malignant pleural effusion. Ann Am Thorac Soc. 2019;16(9):1099–106.
69. Rooper LM, Ali SZ, Olson MT. A minimum fluid volume of 75 mL is needed to ensure adequacy in a pleural effusion: a retrospective analysis of 2540 cases. Cancer Cytopathol. 2014;122(9):657–65.
70. Obiols C, Call S, Rami-Porta R, Iglesias M, Saumench R, Serra-Mitjans M, et al. Extended cervical mediastinoscopy: mature results of a clinical protocol for staging bronchogenic carcinoma of the left lung. Eur J Cardiothorac Surg. 2012;41(5):1043–6.
71. Witte B, Wolf M, Hillebrand H, Kriegel E, Huertgen M. Extended cervical mediastinoscopy revisited. Eur J Cardiothorac Surg. 2014;45(1):114–9.
72. Lemaire A, Nikolic I, Petersen T, Haney JC, Toloza EM, Harpole DH Jr, et al. Nine-year single center experience with cervical mediastinoscopy: complications and false negative rate. Ann Thorac Surg. 2006;82(4):1185–9; discussion 9–90.
73. Ginsberg RJ, Rice TW, Goldberg M, Waters PF, Schmocker BJ. Extended cervical mediastinoscopy. A single staging procedure for bronchogenic carcinoma of the left upper lobe. J Thorac Cardiovasc Surg. 1987;94(5):673–8.
74. Metin M, Citak N, Sayar A, Pekcolaklar A, Melek H, Kok A, et al. The role of extended cervical mediastinoscopy in staging of non-small cell lung cancer of the left lung and a comparison with integrated positron emission tomography and computed tomography: does integrated positron emission tomography and computed tomography reduce the need for invasive procedures? J Thorac Oncol. 2011;6(10):1713–9.
75. Freixinet Gilart J, Garcia PG, de Castro FR, Suarez PR, Rodriguez NS, de Ugarte AV. Extended cervical mediastinoscopy in the staging of bronchogenic carcinoma. Ann Thorac Surg. 2000;70(5):1641–3.
76. Ernst A, Anantham D, Eberhardt R, Krasnik M, Herth FJ. Diagnosis of mediastinal adenopathy-real-time endobronchial ultrasound guided needle aspiration versus mediastinoscopy. J Thorac Oncol. 2008;3(6):577–82.
77. Um SW, Kim HK, Jung SH, Han J, Lee KJ, Park HY, et al. Endobronchial ultrasound versus mediastinoscopy for mediastinal nodal staging of non-small-cell lung cancer. J Thorac Oncol. 2015;10(2):331–7.
78. Figueiredo VR, Cardoso PFG, Jacomelli M, Santos LM, Minata M, Terra RM. EBUS-TBNA versus surgical mediastinoscopy for mediastinal lymph node staging in potentially operable non-small cell lung cancer: a systematic review and meta-analysis. J Bras Pneumol. 2020;46(6):e20190221.
79. Visser MPJ, van Grimbergen I, Holters J, Barendregt WB, Vermeer LC, Vreuls W, et al. Performance insights of endobronchial ultrasonography (EBUS) and mediastinoscopy for mediastinal lymph node staging in lung cancer. Lung Cancer. 2021;156:122–8.
80. Sanz-Santos J, Almagro P, Malik K, Martinez-Camblor P, Caro C, Rami-Porta R. Confirmatory mediastinoscopy after negative endobronchial ultrasound-guided transbronchial needle aspiration for mediastinal staging of lung cancer: systematic review and meta-analysis. Ann Am Thorac Soc. 2022;19(9):1581–90.
81. Martinez-Zayas G, Almeida FA, Simoff MJ, Yarmus L, Molina S, Young B, et al. A prediction model to help with oncologic mediastinal evaluation for radiation: HOMER. Am J Respir Crit Care Med. 2020;201(2):212–23.
82. O'Connell OJ, Almeida FA, Simoff MJ, Yarmus L, Lazarus R, Young B, et al. A prediction model to help with the assessment of adenopathy in lung cancer: HAL. Am J Respir Crit Care Med. 2017;195(12):1651–60.
83. Detterbeck FC, Postmus PE, Tanoue LT. The stage classification of lung cancer: diagnosis and management of lung cancer, 3rd ed: American College of Chest Physicians evidence-based clinical practice guidelines. Chest. 2013;143(5 Suppl):e191S–210S.

84. Gagliasso M, Migliaretti G, Ardissone F. Assessing the prognostic impact of the International Association for the Study of Lung Cancer proposed definitions of complete, uncertain, and incomplete resection in non-small cell lung cancer surgery. Lung Cancer. 2017;111:124–30.
85. Travis WD, Asamura H, Bankier AA, Beasley MB, Detterbeck F, Flieder DB, et al. The IASLC lung cancer staging project: proposals for coding T categories for subsolid nodules and assessment of tumor size in part-solid tumors in the forthcoming eighth edition of the TNM classification of lung cancer. J Thorac Oncol. 2016;11(8):1204–23.
86. Maeyashiki T, Suzuki K, Hattori A, Matsunaga T, Takamochi K, Oh S. The size of consolidation on thin-section computed tomography is a better predictor of survival than the maximum tumour dimension in resectable lung cancer. Eur J Cardiothorac Surg. 2013;43(5):915–8.
87. Cicenia J, Avasarala SK, Gildea TR. Navigational bronchoscopy: a guide through history, current use, and developing technology. J Thorac Dis. 2020;12(6):3263–71.
88. Tanner NT, Yarmus L, Chen A. Standard bronchoscopy with fluoroscopy vs thin bronchoscopy and radial endobronchial ultrasound for biopsy of pulmonary lesions: a multicenter, prospective, randomized trial. Chest. 2018;154(5):1035–43.
89. Eberhardt R, Anantham D, Ernst A. Multimodality bronchoscopic diagnosis of peripheral lung lesions: a randomized controlled trial. Am J Respir Crit Care Med. 2007;176(1):36–41.
90. Oki M, Saka H, Ando M. Ultrathin bronchoscopy with multimodal devices for peripheral pulmonary lesions: a randomized trial. Am J Respir Crit Care Med. 2015;192(4):468–76.
91. Folch EE, Pritchett MA, Nead MA, et al. Electromagnetic navigation bronchoscopy for peripheral pulmonary lesions: one-year results of the prospective, multicenter NAVIGATE study. J Thorac Oncol. 2019;14(3):445–58.
92. Chen et al. Chest. 2021;159(2):845–52. https://doi.org/10.1016/j.chest.2020.08.2047. Epub 2020 Aug 19.
93. Chaddha U, Kovacs SP, Manley C, et al. Robot-assisted bronchoscopy for pulmonary lesion diagnosis: results from the initial multicenter experience. BMC Pulm Med. 2019;19(1):243.
94. Kalchiem-Dekel O, Connolly JG, Lin IH, et al. Shape-sensing robotic-assisted bronchoscopy in the diagnosis of pulmonary parenchymal lesions. Chest. 2022;161(2):572–82.

Chapter 6
Treatment of Early-Stage (Stage I and II) Non-Small Cell Lung Cancer

Panagiotis Tasoudis, Ashley A. Weiner, and Gita N. Mody

Introduction

Lung cancer is the second commonest malignancy in the United States and the number one cause of cancer-related mortality, with approximately 240,000 new cases and 130,000 deaths annually nationally per year [1]. Most lung cancers are non-small cell lung cancers (NSCLC), representing 80–85% of cases, of which adenocarcinoma and squamous cell carcinoma are the most common histologies [1]. Disease-specific recurrence and survival rates are impacted primarily by presenting stage and histology. Treatments for early-stage disease include surgery (e.g., pulmonary lobectomy) or radiotherapy followed by adjuvant chemotherapy (for stage II disease) with emerging roles for adjuvant chemoimmunotherapy and neo-adjuvant chemoimmunotherapy.

Advances in public health including smoking cessation and screening programs have resulted in lung cancer downstaging, with 30% of the patients newly diagnosed with non-small cell lung cancer presenting with early-stage disease [2]. This chapter briefly describes the current diagnostic and staging approaches and provides a detailed discussion of the treatment for early-stage NSCLC. Treatment for limited stage small cell cancer is addressed in Chap. 9.

P. Tasoudis · G. N. Mody (✉)
Division of Cardiothoracic Surgery, Department of Surgery, University of North Carolina at Chapel Hill, Chapel Hill, NC, USA
e-mail: tasoudis@email.unc.edu; gita_mody@med.unc.edu

A. A. Weiner
Department of Radiation Oncology, University of North Carolina at Chapel Hill, Chapel Hill, NC, USA
e-mail: ashley_weiner@med.unc.edu

C. MacRosty, M. P. Rivera (eds.), *Lung Cancer*, Respiratory Medicine, https://doi.org/10.1007/978-3-031-38412-7_6

Presentation

Early-stage lung cancer most commonly presents without symptoms and is often found incidentally or on screening chest computed tomography (CT) scans. Endobronchial tumors may present with respiratory symptoms (dyspnea, cough, hemoptysis, sputum production). Regardless of the presentation at the time of diagnosis, a patient with chest imaging concerning for primary lung cancer will undergo further assessment to define the clinical stage of the disease.

Staging Schema

Disease staging is the foundation for cancer treatment planning. We will briefly review the eighth edition of the American Joint Committee on Cancer (AJCC) staging system for early-stage NSCLC, as lung cancer staging is covered in more detail in Chap. 5. Early-stage lung cancer includes tumors that are classified as stage IA (T1miN0M0 or T1N0M0), IB (T2aN0M0), IIA (T2bN0M0), and IIB (T1-2N1M0 or T3N0M0). Briefly, T1mi classification includes tumors with a primarily lepidic pattern, an invasive component <=0.5 cm, and overall nodule size of <= 3 cm. T1 classification involves tumors ranging from 1 to 3 cm, T2 classification refers tumors that range from 3 to 5 cm, and finally T3 refers to tumors ranging from 5 to 7 cm. The N classifications of the AJCC eighth edition staging system refer to the location of regional lymph node metastases. N0 disease refers to cancers that have not metastasized to any neighboring or distant lymph nodes. N1 disease includes cancers that have spread in ipsilateral peribronchial, intrapulmonary, or hilar lymph node(s) [3, 4].

Despite advancements in imaging including chest CT and positron emission tomography (PET) scans, clinical staging may underestimate tumor extent, and many patients are reclassified pathologically following surgery [5]. This is especially important for patients with N2 disease that were initially misclassified as having early-stage disease due to the presence of radiographically occult lymph nodes; current guidelines recommend different treatment plans for early-stage versus advanced stage NSCLC [6]. As studies emerge on the role of neoadjuvant chemoimmunotherapy for tumor downstaging prior to resection, limitations of imaging will become increasingly relevant, leading to increased roles for thoracic surgeons and pulmonologists for obtaining tissue samples.

Treatment Options for Early-Stage Lung Cancer

Advancements in minimally invasive surgical techniques, refinements in radiotherapy, and a burgeoning of new systemic therapies targeting molecular and immune pathways have broadened the therapeutic options available for treatment of lung cancer. For patients with early-stage NSCLC deemed eligible for surgery, pulmonary resections remain the cornerstone of treatment [6], with roles for neoadjuvant and adjuvant therapies in select cases. For nonoperable patients or patients who prefer nonoperative management, stereotactic body radiotherapy (SBRT, also known as stereotactic ablative radiotherapy [SABR]) is the first-line recommendation.

Adjuvant Chemotherapy in Resected Early-Stage NSCLC

The use of adjuvant chemotherapy in resected lung cancer patients is historically a topic of debate. According to the National Commission on Cancer Network (NCCN) guidelines, adjuvant chemotherapy should be offered for stage II NSCLC as defined by large tumors (>4 cm) and/or N1 involvement [6]. Outside of this, the benefit of adjuvant therapy in early-stage NSCLC is unclear, with studies providing support for either adjuvant chemotherapy or observation in stage I disease [7–9]. A landmark meta-analysis on this topic incorporating approximately 350 patients with stage IA NSCLC resected with negative margins reported that adjuvant chemotherapy was associated with worse outcomes compared to no therapy [9]. Conversely, preliminary reports on high-risk stage IA patients (cancers with visceral or lymphatic or vascular invasion) showed adjuvant chemotherapy might improve overall survival [7, 8]. The use of adjuvant chemotherapy is an equally controversial topic in patients with stage IB disease, and this is reflected in the discrepancy between the American Society of Clinical Oncology (ASCO) Cancer Care Ontario guidelines, in which adjuvant chemotherapy is not recommended [10], and the NCCN guidelines in which adjuvant chemotherapy is considered a potential option for stage IB [6]. Finally, regarding patients with stage II disease, studies on adjuvant chemotherapy after complete resections have demonstrated improved survival and therefore are recommended in the NCCN guidelines [6]. Data from contemporary clinical trials [10–14] conclude that platinum-based regimens are useful for patients with completely resected stage II NSCLC. Overall survival (OS) among patients with stage II NSCLC was found to be 41 months in patients who did not receive chemotherapy and 80 months in the patients that received chemotherapy (hazard ratio [HR]: 0.59; 95 percent confidence interval [CI], 0.42–0.85; $P = 0.004$) [11]. To summarize, the role of adjuvant chemotherapy in resected stage IA NSCLC has not been found to be beneficial; is limited in resected IB NSCLC and has yet to be defined; and in resected stage II, NSCLC has shown to be beneficial. Emerging trial evidence may ultimately support the use of adjuvant chemoimmunotherapy, immune monotherapy in resected early-stage lung cancer patients [15], or targeted therapy for patients with molecular mutations [16].

Radiotherapy in Resected Early-Stage NSCLC

The role of radiotherapy after resection of lung cancer has been controversial. Local adjuvant radiation for stage I NSCLC after complete resection of the tumor has not been shown to have benefit [17]. Postoperative radiotherapy was historically considered in patients who underwent surgical resection for presumed early-stage disease and were incidentally found to have positive mediastinal (N2) lymph nodes based on an unplanned secondary analysis of a trial evaluating postoperative chemotherapy [18]. The recently published Lung ART study, which randomized patients with resected lung cancer with N2 nodal involvement to postoperative radiotherapy versus observation, showed no significant increase in progression-free survival with postoperative radiotherapy, and radiation was associated with an increase in cardiopulmonary deaths [19]. As such, postoperative radiotherapy for resected early-stage NSCLC is often considered only on a case-by-case basis, primarily in the case of positive surgical margins or incomplete resection.

Radiotherapy in Unresected Early-Stage NSCLC

For patients with early-stage NSCLC who are medically inoperable or prefer a non-invasive approach, SBRT is an alternative definitive treatment option [20]. SBRT delivers high (ablative)-dose, hypofractionated radiation with curative intent in early-stage lung cancer. The advantages of SBRT are the precision and the accuracy with which high-intensity radiation doses can be delivered to small-volume targets minimizing post-radiation tissue injury to the healthy lung parenchyma. The major difference with conventionally fractionated radiotherapy is that instead of ensuring tissue safety by leveraging principles of radiobiology (small dose each day, for many weeks), SBRT precisely localizes the target using image guidance and motion management technology with larger doses of radiation given over fewer treatments (typically five or fewer sessions). The role of radiation to early-stage NSCLC will be discussed in more detail in the "Radiation" section below. Clinical outcomes of patients who have undergone SBRT for treatment of early-stage lung cancer can be challenging to compare to surgical outcomes, as patients undergoing SBRT have been historically medically inoperable and have a poorer general prognosis than the patients undergoing surgical management; nevertheless, local control following SBRT is ~97% at 3 years [21].

In selected patients with endobronchial tumors that are not invasive beyond the mucosa, bronchoscopic techniques including thermal ablative, mechanical, and ultrasound-guided techniques could be utilized to mechanically debride the tumor [22].

Other less common treatment options for patients who are deemed inoperable after diagnosis include a variety of image-guided ablative techniques such as thermal ablation, laser ablation, and cryoablation, all of which are considered alternative treatment options for NSCLC in inoperable patients [23–25].

Determination of Operability

Surgery is the cornerstone of the treatment plan for early-stage NSCLC; however, patients must be reasonably fit in order to undergo surgery, determined primarily by cardiopulmonary reserve and secondarily by age and comorbidities. The selection of patients eligible for pulmonary resections is based on a guidelines from various professional societies, including the American College of Chest Physicians (ACCP) [26], the European Respiratory Society and the European Society of Thoracic Surgeons (ERS/ESTS) [27], and the British Thoracic Society [28]. Both ACCP and ERS/ESTS guidelines are similar with differences in the timing and indications of cardiopulmonary exercise testing (CPET). Preoperative evaluation and physiologic assessment are discussed in detail in Chap. 13.

Evaluating a patient's eligibility for a lung resection requires a functional capacity assessment and pulmonary function tests (PFTs) [26]. In practice, functional capacity is typically done by surgeon assessment, which allows for physical exam and estimation of physical activity levels quantified as metabolic equivalents (METs). The PFTs typically include the forced expiratory volume in 1 s (FEV1) and carbon monoxide diffusing capacity (DLCO), though for FEV1 > 1.5 L, DLCO may be deferred [28]. These tests allow estimation of the tolerance of one lung ventilation and prediction of postoperative morbidity and mortality. The PPO lung function should be calculated using preoperative values for FEV1 and DLCO and the amount of lung tissue to be resected [26, 28, 29]. Patients with a PPO FEV1 and DLCO that are both ≥40% of the predicted values are considered average risk patients, and further testing is usually deferred [28]. On the other hand, patients with a PPO FEV1 and DLCO that are <40% of the predicted values should undergo quantitative lung scintigraphy ("perfusion" scan) to verify the segment count calculation and further risk stratification through physiologic testing with cardiopulmonary exercise testing (CPET) [26, 27, 29].

Determination of Extent of Resection

The extent of lung resection indicated for early-stage lung cancer is determined by the location and size of the tumor. The guiding principles are to provide an adequate margin (at least twice the size of the tumor) and perform an adequate lymph node dissection. In general, for those with acceptable pulmonary and physical functioning, lobectomy has been traditionally considered the gold standard due to the resulting thorough evaluation of the hilar lymph nodes. However, recent studies (Cancer and Leukemia Group B (CALGB) 140503 [31, 32] and Japanese Cooperative Oncology Group 0802 [33]) have supported the equivalency of sublobar resection (nonanatomic wedge resection with an adequate margin for peripheral tumors) or segmentectomy for small (< 2 cm) invasive lung cancers. This approach may be particularly useful for patients with limited functional reserve or multifocal disease, though special attention should be given to margins and lymph node clearance, which must still be done adequately to maintain equivalent locoregional recurrence rate and allow complete pathologic staging.

For centrally located tumors in which a lobectomy cannot achieve radical removal of the mass, sleeve lobectomy (e.g., removal of an upper lobe with reimplantation of the distal airway for endobronchial tumors) or bilobectomy (e.g., right middle and lower lobectomy for a tumor crossing the fissure and/or invading the pulmonary artery) may be required. Pneumonectomy (e.g., for main stem airway involvement) also can be considered. Less commonly, a more centrally located early-stage tumor or associated lymph node involving the vascular hilum may require pneumonectomy. Parenchymal sparing operations such as sleeve lobectomy have lower morbidity and mortality than pneumonectomy with 5-year OS of 52.4% in the sleeve lobectomy group and 48.7% in the pneumonectomy group; quality of life (QoL) also was found to be significantly better in the sleeve lobectomy group [34].

For cases in which the tumor has invaded the chest wall, the pericardium or the diaphragm (T3), extended pulmonary resection would be done. The term extended means that the lung parenchyma resection is accompanied with excision of the invaded structures followed by reconstruction with mesh as needed and can be done with good results in carefully selected patients [35, 36].

Preoperative Workup

A comprehensive history and physical examination are critical for every patient presenting with suspected lung cancer, primarily to identify other systemic diseases that may contraindicate biopsy or resection. Paying close attention to any extrapulmonary symptoms, signs, or laboratory findings that might indicate metastases (e.g., focal neurological signs or elevated GGT) or related conditions is important to ensure more workup is not required.

In the case of a screen or incidentally detected indeterminate pulmonary nodule, biopsy (image-guided transthoracic [37] or transbronchial [38, 39]) may be indicated prior to deciding on treatment, especially for those nodules with intermediate pretest probability of being a lung cancer. Bronchoscopy can facilitate both staging and diagnosis using techniques such as endobronchial ultrasound (EBUS), transbronchial biopsy, brushings, washings, bronchoalveolar lavage, and transbronchial needle aspiration (TBNA) with complication rates less than 1% [38–40]. CT-guided transthoracic fine needle aspiration (FNA) is also a safe approach to diagnose lung cancer especially for peripheral lesions [30, 41]. For peripheral nodules, excisional biopsy (wedge) with frozen section preceding tentatively planned resection may be preferred for highly suspicious nodules in fit patients [42] or in the case that needle biopsy is not feasible due to the mass location or yields an inconclusive diagnosis [43]. Approach to pulmonary nodules is discussed in detail in Chap. 4.

After a suspected diagnosis sof lung cancer, establishing the clinical stage of the disease is the next priority as it will define treatment recommendations. Noncontrast chest CT scan (protocoled to evaluate through the upper abdomen) is usually adequate for operative planning and preliminary/clinical staging of hilar and mediastinal lymph nodes (clinically positive for size >1 cm), adrenal glands, and liver [44, 45]. For hilar tumors, contrast-enhanced CT scan should be done to assess the relationship of the mass with adjacent structures (pulmonary artery, pulmonary veins, atrium, great vessels, etc.) [45]. For tumors abutting the chest wall or superior sulcus, MRI may be considered.

Following axial imaging, whole-body positron emission tomography (PET)/CT using 18F-flurodeoxyglucose (FDG) is routinely obtained given its high sensitivity 85% and specificity 90% for further disease staging [46–48]. Brain metastases are uncommon (0% to 10%) in patients who are neurologically asymptomatic at the time of lung cancer diagnosis [49]. Therefore, MRI scans are not recommended in asymptomatic patients with early-stage lung cancer unless tumor size is >4 cm, and N1 nodes are involved in PET scan and/or biopsy or for those patients with new onset of neurological symptoms including headaches, diplopia, or ataxia [49].

It is important to note that PET scan findings of involved lymph nodes should be confirmed with a pathologic staging modality including mediastinoscopy (cervical or anterior) or EBUS [50–52]. If EBUS is nondiagnostic, cervical mediastinoscopy for paratracheal notes or anterior mediastinoscopy (Chamberlin procedure, which allows access to the aortopulmonary window area through dissection of the left second costosternal cartilage). If the results of the frozen section analysis during the mediastinoscopy fail to demonstrate malignant infiltration to the mediastinal lymph nodes, a pulmonary resection can be performed under the same setting, making workflow for diagnosis, staging, and resection more streamlined [50–52].

Surgical Approach

Minimally invasive approaches to pulmonary resection are increasingly routine. Video-assisted thoracoscopic surgery (VATS) and robotic-assisted thoracic surgery (RATS) are two contemporary surgical approaches that have gained popularity. These minimally invasive approaches emerged with the aim to eliminate the need for an open thoracotomy that leads to rib spreading, large incisions, long recovery periods, and increased postoperative pain. Indeed, the utilization and the indications of these approaches for thoracic diseases are steadily increasing [53], and the outcomes reported in the current literature of VATS and RATS are very encouraging [54–57]. Further, VATS lobectomy leads to faster recovery rates and better QoL and health services utilization postoperatively [58–60], including improved pain levels, decreased utilization of pain medications, shorter length of hospitalization, fewer postoperative complications, shorter overall recovery period, and fewer readmissions without worsening in adverse event rates or oncologic outcomes compared to thoracotomy [61].

RATS for pulmonary resection was introduced in 2001 and is increasingly considered an alternative to VATS; however, there is still scarcity of reports comparing RATS to VATS in patients with early-stage diseases [62, 63]. In general, RATS has several potential advantages compared with VATS, including enhanced vision with three-dimensional views, greater agility, and precision in movement which can offer reduced intraoperative tissue trauma and reduced postoperative pain [64]. On the other hand, RATS is associated with high operative costs, steeper learning curves, and potentially higher risk for cardiovascular complications compared to VATS [65, 66]. A recent study using the National Cancer Database to compare RATS and VATS outlined the superiority of VATS in terms of 1-year survival outcomes compared to RATS in patients with tumors larger than 2 cm (HR, 1.58; 95% CI, 1.06–2.36) but not in patients with tumors <2 cm [62]. Another contemporary report comparing RATS with both VATS and open thoracotomy in patients with stage I disease noted that all three approaches are comparable in terms of long-term survival rates [63]. Nevertheless, VATS and RATS were associated with shorter hospitalizations, and RATS in particular was linked with higher numbers of lymph nodes assessed [63].

Another minimally invasive approach that can facilitate pulmonary resections is the uniportal VATS. VATS is typically performed though three or four incisions. By definition, uniportal VATS requires only one incision through which a single port is inserted in the chest cavity, and with the use of this port, the surgeon performs the whole operation [67–69]. Although there are only few studies examining the role of uniportal VATS, recent data from single institutional reports indicate that this approach is safe, feasible, and offers comparable results to the traditional VATS [67–69]. For early-stage NSCLC patients, uniportal VATS seems to offer similar oncologic results to traditional VATS [68, 69]. The major advantage of the uniportal VATS is the low levels of postoperative pain that comes along with the single incision required to perform the whole operation [68].

Even though all the aforementioned minimally invasive techniques are constantly gaining popularity, there are many patients with early-stage NSCLC with postinfectious, postradiation, posttraumatic, and anatomic variations that render them unable to undergo VATS or RATS. Emerging experience with resection after neoadjuvant chemoimmunotherapy has led to reports of a dense fibrosis (particularly in patients with high levels of immune checkpoint expression and ultimately pathologic complete response) that may limit the feasibility of minimally invasive surgery [70]. In these cases, a posterolateral thoracotomy is typically used as the incision for the lung resection because it gives the surgeon excellent exposure and mobility. Other approaches include muscle-sparing lateral or axillary thoracotomies, median sternotomies, and anterolateral thoracotomies.

Surgical Techniques

Lobectomy

Anatomic and Positioning Considerations

Most individuals have five distinct pulmonary lobes with named bronchial, venous, and arterial supply. While venous and bronchial anatomy are fairly consistent, the pulmonary artery has some important variations that largely follow the segmental anatomy and are well described [71]. For example, the truncus anterior (TA) branch of the right pulmonary artery is the first branch to the right upper lobe and has one to two branches to the apical and anterior segments and sometimes a third branch to the posterior segment. A variable in size more distal posterior ascending artery branches to the posterior segment. Regardless of the lobe to be resected, patient positioning is typically in full lateral decubitus, as a posterior lateral approach leads to efficient exposure of the hilum. An alternative is supine position, and this may be used in a substernal uniportal approach.

Operative Flow

The sequence of steps of lobectomy will depend on the approach (i.e., open, thoracoscopic, robotic), though there are variations within these approaches. In modern practice in high-resource settings, endoscopic staplers are used for all approaches (including open). The general flow of the operation involves opening the pleura and dissecting individually the vein, artery, and bronchus of the lobe to be resected. The lymph nodes are individually dissected as well. After dissection, the hilar structures may be divided in variable order depending on their actual relationships. For right upper lobectomy, as depicted in Fig. 6.1, the pulmonary artery branches may be divided first to prevent congestion of the lobe. Sequentially, division of the vein and the right upper bronchus are performed. The fissure between the adjacent lobe(s) may be divided before or after the hilar structures.

During a right middle lobectomy, the middle pulmonary artery is identified within the major fissure and is divided. Following that the middle lobe vein is dissected and divided, the middle bronchus is stapled, and finally the parenchyma between the upper lobe and lower lobe is removed again with the use of the stapler.

A right lower lobectomy is considered the least technically challenging of the lobectomies. Often the inferior pulmonary ligament is divided first, leading to the inferior pulmonary vein. The lower lobe artery is approached through the fisure.

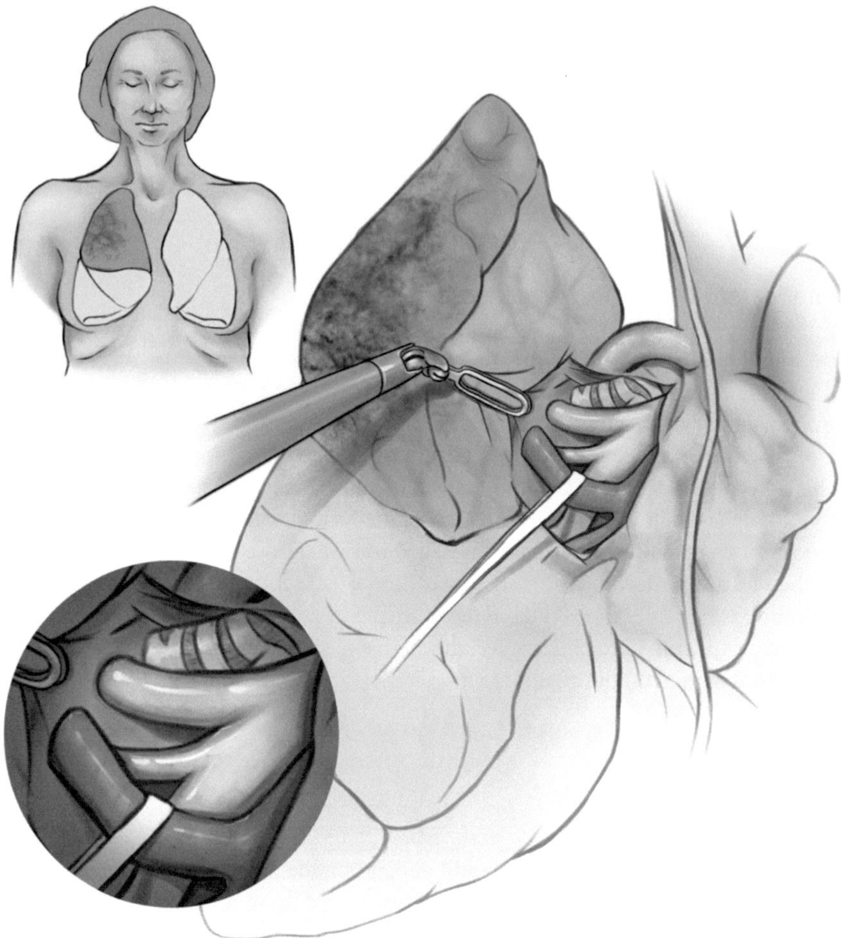

Fig. 6.1 Right upper lobectomy: hilar exposure with retraction of the upper lobe division of the superior pulmonary vein

Next, the fissure is divided, and this only leaves the bronchus, which must be cut at an angle to preserve the middle lobe bronchus.

The left upper lobectomy is unique due to the highly variable pulmonary artery branching pattern (three to five divisions) and proximity to the aorta and recurrent laryngeal nerve. In general, the superior vein is mobilized away from the artery and is divided first followed by the arterial vessels, the lung parenchyma, and the bronchus.

Lastly, it is worth noting that the sequence in which a left lower lobectomy is performed depends on the integrity of the fissure. If the fissure is complete, the parenchyma is divided first followed by the arterial vessels and the vein with the inferior ligament. On the other hand, if the fissure is incomplete, the vascular structures may be divided first, followed by the bronchus and finally the parenchyma if any remains.

Segmentectomy

Segmentectomy refers to an anatomical resection of one or more of the lung segments (Fig. 6.2). Each segment has a pyramidal shape, with the hilum serving as the apex and the surface of the lung as the base. It is supplied by the following

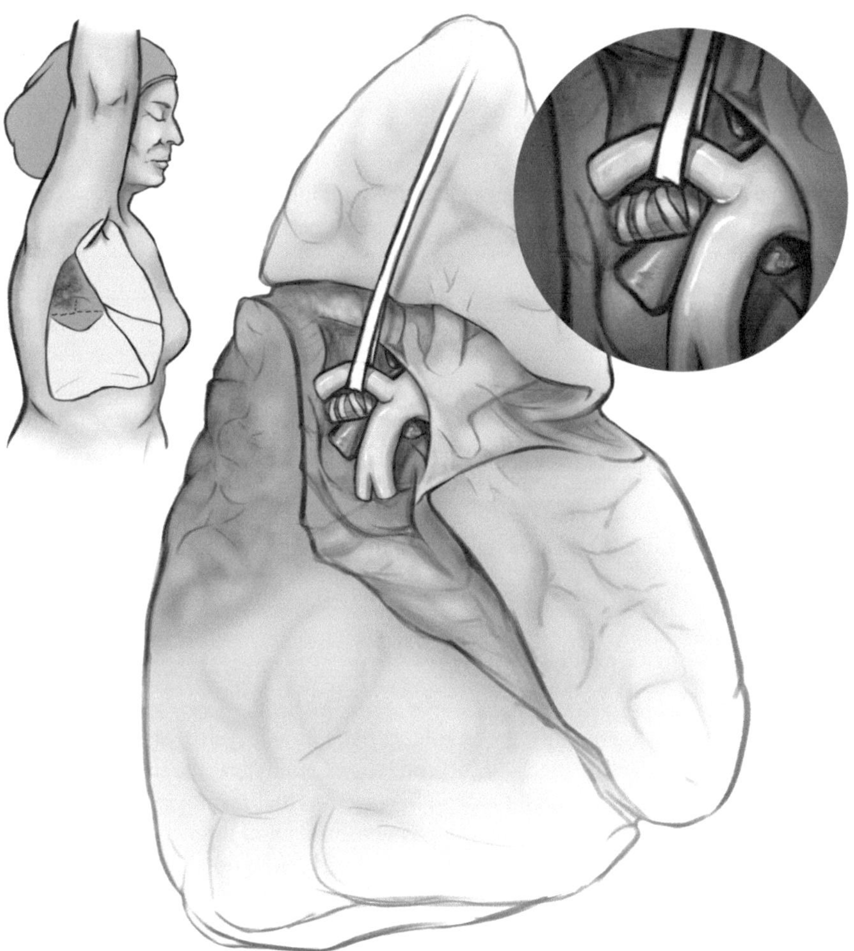

Fig. 6.2 Right lower lobe superior segment (S6) segmentectomy: exposure of the right lower lobe pulmonary artery and segmental branch in the fissure

structures, with few collateral connections between segments: (1) a tertiary branch of the bronchial tree; (2) a segmental branch of the pulmonary artery (along with the bronchial artery); and (3) a segmental branch of the pulmonary vein along with lymphatics. Accounting for the anatomic structure of each segment, removal of a segment does not affect the functionality of the remaining lung. In segmentectomies the order of dividing the individual bronchovascular structures varies according to the individual segment. An additional challenge includes identification of the appropriate planes for lung parenchyma removal, which may be accomplished using several techniques. These include clamping the segmental bronchus before (or after) full inflation to better delineate the targeted segment or using fluorescent dye such as Indocyanine Green (ICG) to delineate the nonperfused area after division of vascular structures. The segmental bronchus is usually divided using a stapler followed by the parenchyma.

Wedge Resection

Wedge resections can be performed in patients with tumors located in the periphery. A U-type resection is preferable than a V-type resection for wedge resections, to ensure adequate margins around the lesion. This resection could be facilitated with the use of stapling manufacturing devices or with electrocautery. The major advantages of wedge resections are decreased postoperative morbidity and mortality that accompany the procedure. A study using the Society of Thoracic Surgeons database reported that the morbidity and mortality of wedge resections were decreased when compared to anatomic lung resections (lobectomy and segmentectomy) [72]. However, wedge resections have been associated with increased risk of locoregional recurrence when compared with segmentectomies [73]. In addition, segmentectomies allow larger parenchyma margins and better accuracy in disease staging due to the possibility of hilar node retrieval compared to wedge resections [74, 75].

Pneumonectomy and Sleeve Lobectomy

Sleeve resections are generally preferable in patients with early-stage NSCLC as they can facilitate avoiding the need for a pneumonectomy and the morbidity of this procedure. Pneumonectomy is an anatomic resection that results in removal of the entire lung. The operation is usually done via posterolateral thoracotomy or median sternotomy in cases of left lung cancer with carinal invasion, though minimally invasive pneumonectomy also is described. In all appraoches, the mediastinal pleura is resected, and the hilar structures are dissected away from the lung. The arterial supply is divided first followed by the veins and the bronchus. The procedure is completed with mediastinal lymph node dissections. In comparison to other standard anatomic lung resections, pneumonectomy is the only lung resection that leaves an empty pleural space; hence perioperative management calls for additional special considerations. It is worth noting that the mortality following a pneumonectomy ranges from 0 to 26% depending on the patient's baseline characteristics and the operating center [76].

A sleeve lobectomy is an alternative to pneumonectomy for early-stage lung cancer and consists of the removal of a portion of main bronchus in conjunction with the involved lobar bronchus and associated lung tissue followed by direct reimplantation of the lobe(s) to be preserved. Similarly, a vascular sleeve lobectomy involves clamping and partial resection of the involved pulmonary artery. A sleeve lobectomy is usually performed via a posterolateral thoracotomy though may also be done robotically. A variation on sleeve resection may involve a bronchoplastic technique, defined as partial resection of a lobar bronchial orifice and closure without removing a segment of main bronchus. Although sleeve lobectomies are technically more challenging procedures than pneumonectomies, they have been associated with better morbidity and mortality and therefore are recommended in patients who are deemed eligible for this type of surgery [77].

Mediastinal Lymph Sampling Versus Dissection

The standard approach to mediastinal lymph nodes assessment (complete dissection versus sampling) at time of pulmonary resection for NSCLC has been debated for several decades. The American College of Surgery Oncology Group conducted the Z0030 Trial aiming to elucidate the role of mediastinal lymph node dissection in patients with early-stage NSCLC undergoing resection [78]. The Z0030 trial concluded that systematic lymph node dissection did not improve the survival of patients with early-stage NSCLC nor decrease the incidence of local or regional recurrence [78]. On the other hand, a meta-analysis on this topic reported that systematic mediastinal nodal dissection is linked with improved accuracy of staging which translated to better survival outcomes compared to lymph node sampling alone [79]. In practice, the surgical approach and surgeon preference may dictate the degree of lymph node dissection intraoperatively.

Surgical Outcomes

A population-level analysis of the overall survival (OS) for patients with early-stage NSCLC has been reported from the Surveillance, Epidemiology, and End Results (SEER) database to validate the 8th edition TNM (Tumor, Node, and Metastasis) staging system [80]. According to this report, the 2-year OS of patients with clinical stage IA1, IA2, and IA3 was 97%, 94%, and 90%, respectively. Patients with stage IB, IIA, and IIB were reported to have a 2-year OS of 87%, 79%, and

72%, respectively. Patients with clinical stage IA, IB, IIA, and IIB had a 5-year OS of 77–92%, 68%, 60%, and 53%, respectively [80].

Incidence of local recurrence following surgery for early-stage NSCLC ranges from 6 to 55% in different studies [81–83]. A comprehensive institutional series examining 975 patients with early-stage NSCLC reported a 5-year local and/or distant recurrence rate of 36% [84]. The majority of the recurrences were noted in local sites [84]. Another study conducted by the American College of Surgeons reported that the 5-year disease-free survival (DFS) for stage T1 and T2 was approximately 60% and 75%, respectively [85].

Quality of Life

Health-related quality of life (HRQOL) following treatment for lung cancer is gaining increased attention. Although there are no reports assessing the HRQOL specifically for patients with early-stage NSCLC, one study examining the effect of lung resections on HRQOL longitudinally demonstrated that lobectomy had a transient impact on physical functioning of the patients, but the magnitude of this influence decreased over time [86]. Pneumonectomies, however, were found to have a large impact on both physical and emotional domains of HRQOL, and interestingly, this impact persisted over time [86]. Of note, patients with NSCLC awaiting surgical treatment were found to have impaired HRQOL in most assessed domains compared to healthy individuals [87]. Finally, it is worth noting that the HRQOL of patients who undergo VATS is significantly better both in the early postoperative period and during the 6-month follow-up compared to open thorocotomies [61, 88].

Disparities

Unfortunately, disparities still exist in lung cancer treatment. These disparities are multifaceted and may be attributed to social determinants of health. A study using the National Cancer Database noted that non-Hispanic Black patients and elderly patients were less likely to receive predefined, stage-specific, guideline-concordant treatments [89]. Specifically for early-stage NSCLC, several studies found that Black patients are less likely to receive curative-intent surgery [90–92]. These disparities were reflected on the OS outcomes of Black patients, which for the past two decades, have been worse than White patients. Increased awareness of this issue has led to further work to reduce disparities in modern healthcare systems. For example, a pragmatic trial conducted in five cancer centers of a system-based intervention showed that this approach reduced the racial disparities in lung cancer care [93]. Further action is needed to achieve a significant reduction in racial and other health disparities gaps and improve the health outcomes for all patients.

Radiotherapy Techniques

SBRT is an alternative curative intent treatment for early-stage NSCLC in patients who are not operative candidates or who elect to undergo nonoperative management. SBRT is highly conformal radiation with large fraction size (10–30 Gy) delivered in one to five treatments over 1–2 weeks. The SBRT treatment planning process begins with a CT simulation. During CT image acquisition, the patient is immobilized using a stereotactic body frame or a vacuum-locked body cast to provide reproducible alignment during imaging and treatment.

To account for respiratory motion, a 4D CT scan is acquired. During this scan, each axial slice is imaged multiple times throughout the breathing cycle, and the images are recombined to create a library of CT images to allow accurate delineation of tumor motion.

After CT simulation, the radiation oncologist contours, or draws, the tumor target on the CT dataset. The gross tumor volume (GTV) is drawn on either the free-breathing CT or on the average of the 4D-CT dataset. For gated treatment, radiation is delivered only when the tumor is within a specified region of the breathing cycle. When gating is not used, an internal target volume (ITV) is generated as expansion of the GTV to account for respiratory motion using the phases of the 4D-CT. A planning target volume (PTV) is then created as a geometric expansion of the GTV (with gating) or the ITV (without gating) to account for uncertainty in daily positioning or setup. The desired dose is prescribed to cover the PTV. Organs at risk (heart, normal lung parenchyma, esophagus, great vessels, spinal cord, and chest wall) are also delineated as avoidance structures.

The radiation treatment plan is then optimized by dosimetrists and medical physicists by selecting beam arrangements to deliver the prescribed dose to the PTV, while sparing the organs at risk. SBRT is typically planned with significant dose heterogeneity, such that the center of the tumor often receives over 120% of the prescription dose. Once the plan is finalized, there are multiple quality assurance checks to ensure that the plan is physically deliverable and that dosimetry is appropriate. For treatment, the patient is positioned on the treatment table in the same immobilization devices that are used at simulation. Imaging (typically X-ray or CT) is obtained on the treatment table to ensure proper patient alignment and to verify respiratory motion. When localization is verified, the prescribed radiation dose is delivered.

Outcomes After SBRT

A number of important dose-escalation trials were performed at Indiana University and have guided the standard lung SBRT dose/fractionation schemes used today. An initial phase I dose escalation trial found the maximum tolerated dose to be 60 Gy/3 fractions [94]. There were local recurrences in six patients in this study, all of whom received less than 54Gy in three fractions. A subsequent phase II trial confirmed excellent 2-year local control rate of 95% but identified a high rate of severe toxicity for central tumors located within 2 cm of the proximal bronchial tree [21]. A subsequent cooperative group study (RTOG 0236) was a phase II multi-institution trial of medically inoperable patients with peripheral stage I–II NSCLC (< 5 cm) [21]. Patients were prescribed 60Gy in three fractions (roughly equivalent to 54 Gy in three fractions when accounting for heterogeneity of lung parenchyma). Long-term results demonstrated 5-year local control of 93%, lobar control 80%, distant failure rate of 31%, and overall survival 40% [95]. Of note, the low overall survival following SBRT for lung cancer in medically inoperable patients is often driven by deaths from intercurrent disease and not cancer-related deaths.

Since the landmark Hammersmith study in the 1950s showing that early-stage NSCLC patients had improved overall survival with pneumonectomy or lobectomy compared with conventionally fractionated radiation, surgery has been the standard of care for this patient population [96]. Indeed, in comparison to SBRT, surgical approaches have the benefit of staging the mediastinum, although positron emission tomography with CT (PET-CT) scans are fairly sensitive and specific in detecting mediastinal adenopathy [97] and invasive mediastinal staging (via mediastinoscopy or endobronchial ultrasound-guided lymph node aspiration (EBUS-TBNA)) can be performed if there are concerning or questionable lymph nodes on chest CT or PET-CT. Given the excellent local control and favorable toxicity profile of SBRT, recently, a number of groups have become interested in evaluating SBRT for operable patients with early-stage NSCLC, though it is not the current standard of care.

RTOG 0618 evaluated operable patients with peripheral T1N0 NSCLC (<5 cm) treated with SBRT (54 Gy/3 fx) [98]. With a median follow-up in 4 years, local control rate was 96%, regional failure 12%, and distant metastases 12%. Four patients had grade 3 toxicity, and no grade 4–5 toxicities were reported. Two randomized phase III trials (STARS and ROSEL) were being conducted in the USA and Europe. There were differences in study design; however, both trials randomized operable patients with stage I NSCLC to lobectomy versus SBRT. Unfortunately, both trials closed early due to poor accrual. A combined analysis of patients accrued to both studies (58 patients) demonstrated no difference in recurrence-free survival (86% for SBRT and 80% for surgery, $p = 0.54$) [99]. With a median follow-up of approximately 3 years, overall survival was found to be higher in the SBRT group (95%) versus 79% in the surgery group. Toxicity was also worse in the surgery group—rates of any grade 3–4 toxicity were 10% for SBRT patients and 44% for surgical patients. Dyspnea and chest/chest wall pain were the most common grade 3 toxicities overall. A number of ongoing randomized trials (VALOR, Stablemates, SAbRtooth and POSTILV) aim to answer this important question of whether lobectomy or SBRT has superior tumor control and/or toxicity profile for early-stage operable NSCLC. At the present time, SBRT can be considered a reasonable alternative to lobectomy in patients who are high operative risk or decline surgery.

Two randomized trials have evaluated the efficacy and safety of SBRT versus conventionally fractionated radiation therapy. The SPACE trial was a phase II trial that randomized medically inoperable patients with stage I NSCLC to SBRT

(66Gy/3 fractions) or 3D conformal radiation (70 Gy/35 fractions) [99]. Progression-free survival (~54%) and overall survival (~70%) were similar between the two arms; however, higher rates of pneumonitis and esophagitis and worse patient reported quality of life were reported in the patients receiving conventionally fractionated radiation. CHISEL was a randomized phase III trial that randomized patients with stage I NSCLC who were either medically inoperable or refused surgery to receive SBRT (54 Gy/3 fractions or 48 Gy/4 fractions if the tumor was <2 cm from the chest wall) versus conventionally fractionated radiotherapy (66 Gy/33 fractions or 50 Gy/20 fractions, depending on institutional preference) [100]. The primary endpoint was time to local treatment failure, which occurred at 2.1 years in the standard radiotherapy or 2.6 years in the SBRT arm. Furthermore, median survival was 5 years in the SBRT arm versus 3 years in the conventional radiation arm. Thus, the CHISEL trial provides prospective evidence supporting the use of SBRT for definitive radiotherapy for early-stage NSCLC [100].

Conclusion

Early-stage lung cancer care is increasingly multidisciplinary in the diagnostic and treatment approaches. Coordinated programmatic and system-based approaches will be needed to ensure high-quality and equitable care delivery and ultimately improved survival and patient-centered outcomes.

References

1. Lung Cancer Statistics|How Common is Lung Cancer?. Accessed 8 Oct 2022. https://www.cancer.org/cancer/lung-cancer/about/key-statistics.html.
2. Siegel RL, Miller KD, Jemal A. Cancer statistics, 2018. CA Cancer J Clin. 2018;68(1):7–30. https://doi.org/10.3322/CAAC.21442.
3. Thomas KW, Gould MK. Tumor, node, metastasis (TNM) staging system for lung cancer—UpToDate. Accessed 2 Oct 2022. https://www.uptodate.com/contents/tumor-node-metastasis-tnm-staging-system-for-lung-cancer.
4. Non-small Cell Lung Cancer Staging|Stages of Lung Cancer. Accessed 2 Oct 2022. https://www.cancer.org/cancer/lung-cancer/detection-diagnosis-staging/staging-nsclc.html.
5. Dyas AR, King RW, Ghanim AF, Cerfolio RJ. Clinical misstagings and risk factors of occult nodal disease in non-small cell lung cancer. Ann Thorac Surg. 2018;106(5):1492–8. https://doi.org/10.1016/J.ATHORACSUR.2018.05.045.
6. NCCN Clinical practice guidelines in oncology. Non-Small Cell Lung Cancer Version 1.2023. Accessed 12 Sep 2022. https://www.nccn.org/guidelines/recently-published-guidelines.
7. Pathak R, Hoag JR, Goldberg SB, Monsalve AF, Resio B, Boffa DJ. Refining the role of adjuvant chemotherapy in stage IB and IIA NSCLC. J Clin Oncol. 2019;37(15_suppl):8519. https://doi.org/10.1200/JCO.2019.37.15_SUPPL.8519.
8. Tsutani Y, Imai K, Ito H, et al. Adjuvant chemotherapy for pathological stage I non-small cell lung cancer with high-risk factors for recurrence: a multicenter study. J Clin Oncol. 2019;37(15_suppl):8500. https://doi.org/10.1200/JCO.2019.37.15_SUPPL.8500.

9. Pignon JP, Tribodet H, Scagliotti GV, et al. Lung adjuvant cisplatin evaluation: a pooled analysis by the LACE collaborative group. J Clin Oncol. 2008;26(21):3552–9. https://doi.org/10.1200/JCO.2007.13.9030.

10. Kris MG, Gaspar LE, Chaft JE, et al. Adjuvant systemic therapy and adjuvant radiation therapy for stage I to IIIA completely resected non-small-cell lung cancers: American society of clinical oncology/cancer care Ontario clinical practice guideline update. J Clin Oncol. 2017;35(25):2960–74. https://doi.org/10.1200/JCO.2017.72.4401.

11. Winton T, Livingston R, Johnson D, et al. Vinorelbine plus cisplatin vs. observation in resected non-small-cell lung cancer. N Engl J Med. 2005;352(25):2589–97. https://doi.org/10.1056/NEJMOA043623.

12. Douillard JY, Rosell R, de Lena M, et al. Adjuvant vinorelbine plus cisplatin versus observation in patients with completely resected stage IB-IIIA non-small-cell lung cancer (Adjuvant Navelbine International Trialist Association [ANITA]): a randomised controlled trial. Lancet Oncol. 2006;7(9):719–27. https://doi.org/10.1016/S1470-2045(06)70804-X.

13. Scagliotti GV, Fossati R, Torri V, et al. Randomized study of adjuvant chemotherapy for completely resected stage I, II, or IIIA non-small-cell lung cancer. J Natl Cancer Inst. 2003;95(19):1453–61. https://doi.org/10.1093/JNCI/DJG059.

14. Arriagada R, Bergman B, Dunant A, Le Chevalier T, Pignon JP, Vansteenkiste J, International Adjuvant Lung Cancer Trial Collaborative Group. Cisplatin-based adjuvant chemotherapy in patients with completely resected non-small-cell lung cancer. N Engl J Med. 2004;350(4):351–60. https://doi.org/10.1056/NEJMOA031644.

15. Horn L, Mansfield AS, Szczęsna A, et al. First-line atezolizumab plus chemotherapy in extensive-stage small-cell lung cancer. N Engl J Med. 2018;379(23):2220–9. https://doi.org/10.1056/NEJMOA1809064/SUPPL_FILE/NEJMOA1809064_DATA-SHARING.PDF.

16. Wu YL, Tsuboi M, He J, et al. Osimertinib in resected EGFR -mutated non–small-cell lung cancer. N Engl J Med. 2020;383(18):1711–23. https://doi.org/10.1056/NEJMOA2027071/SUPPL_FILE/NEJMOA2027071_DATA-SHARING.PDF.

17. Stewart LA, Burdett S, Parmar MKB, et al. Postoperative radiotherapy in non-small-cell lung cancer: systematic review and meta-analysis of individual patient data from nine randomised controlled trials. Lancet. 1998;352(9124):257–63. https://doi.org/10.1016/S0140-6736(98)06341-7.

18. Douillard JY, Rosell R, Delena M, Legroumellec A, Torres A, Carpagnano F. ANITA: Phase III adjuvant vinorelbine (N) and cisplatin (P) versus observation (OBS) in completely resected (stage I-III) non-small-cell lung cancer (NSCLC) patients (pts): Final results after 70-month median follow-up. On behalf of the Adjuvant Navelbine International Trialist Association. J Clin Oncol. 2005;23(16_suppl):7013. https://doi.org/10.1200/JCO.2005.23.16_SUPPL.7013.

19. le Pechoux C, Pourel N, Barlesi F, et al. Postoperative radiotherapy versus no postoperative radiotherapy in patients with completely resected non-small-cell lung cancer and proven mediastinal N2 involvement (lung ART): an open-label, randomised, phase 3 trial. Lancet Oncol. 2022;23(1):104–14. https://doi.org/10.1016/S1470-2045(21)00606-9.

20. Prezzano KM, Ma SJ, Hermann GM, Rivers CI, Gomez-Suescun JA, Singh AK. Stereotactic body radiation therapy for non-small cell lung cancer: a review. World J Clin Oncol. 2019;10(1):14. https://doi.org/10.5306/WJCO.V10.I1.14.

21. Timmerman R, Paulus R, Galvin J, et al. Stereotactic body radiation therapy for inoperable early stage lung cancer. JAMA. 2010;303(11):1070–6. https://doi.org/10.1001/JAMA.2010.261.

22. Herth F, Becker HD, LoCicero J, Ernst A. Endobronchial ultrasound in therapeutic bronchoscopy. Eur Respir J. 2002;20(1):118–21. https://doi.org/10.1183/09031936.02.01642001.

23. Moore W, Talati R, Bhattacharji P, Bilfinger T. Five-year survival after cryoablation of stage I non-small cell lung cancer in medically inoperable patients. J Vasc Interv Radiol. 2015;26(3):312–9. https://doi.org/10.1016/J.JVIR.2014.12.006.

24. Uhlig J, Ludwig JM, Goldberg SB, Chiang A, Blasberg JD, Kim HS. Survival rates after thermal ablation versus stereotactic radiation therapy for stage 1 non-small cell lung cancer: A National Cancer Database Study. Radiology. 2018;289(3):862–70. https://doi.org/10.1148/RADIOL.2018180979.
25. Liao Z, Lee JJ, Komaki R, et al. Bayesian adaptive randomization trial of passive scattering proton therapy and intensity-modulated photon radiotherapy for locally advanced non-small-cell lung cancer. J Clin Oncol. 2018;36(18):1813–22. https://doi.org/10.1200/JCO.2017.74.0720.
26. Brunelli A, Kim AW, Berger KI, Addrizzo-Harris DJ. Physiologic evaluation of the patient with lung cancer being considered for resectional surgery: diagnosis and management of lung cancer, 3rd ed: American College of Chest Physicians evidence-based clinical practice guidelines. Chest. 2013;143(5 Suppl):e166S. https://doi.org/10.1378/CHEST.12-2395.
27. Brunelli A, Charloux A, Bolliger CT, et al. ERS/ESTS clinical guidelines on fitness for radical therapy in lung cancer patients (surgery and chemo-radiotherapy). Eur Respir J. 2009;34(1):17–41. https://doi.org/10.1183/09031936.00184308.
28. Armstrong P, Congleton J, Fountain SW, et al. BTS guidelines: guidelines on the selection of patients with lung cancer for surgery. Thorax. 2001;56(2):89–108. https://doi.org/10.1136/THORAX.56.2.89.
29. Datta D, Lahiri B. Preoperative evaluation of patients undergoing lung resection surgery. Chest. 2003;123(6):2096–103. https://doi.org/10.1378/CHEST.123.6.2096.
30. Gould MK, Donington J, Lynch WR, et al. Evaluation of individuals with pulmonary nodules: when is it lung cancer? Diagnosis and management of lung cancer, 3rd ed: American college of chest physicians evidence-based clinical practice guidelines. Chest. 2013;143(5 SUPPL):e93S–e120S. https://doi.org/10.1378/CHEST.12-2351/ATTACHMENT/62CD9F06-7D2E-4FCF-A041-2B5F781CEFFE/MMC4.XLS.
31. Altorki NK, Kamel MK, Narula N, et al. Anatomical segmentectomy and wedge resections are associated with comparable outcomes for patients with small cT1N0 non-small cell lung cancer. J Thorac Oncol. 2016;11(11):1984–92. https://doi.org/10.1016/J.JTHO.2016.06.031.
32. Altorki NK, Wang X, Wigle D, et al. Perioperative mortality and morbidity after sublobar versus lobar resection for early-stage non-small-cell lung cancer: post-hoc analysis of an international, randomised, phase 3 trial (CALGB/Alliance 140503). Lancet Respir Med. 2018;6(12):915–24. https://doi.org/10.1016/S2213-2600(18)30411-9.
33. Saji H, Okada M, Tsuboi M, et al. Segmentectomy versus lobectomy in small-sized peripheral non-small-cell lung cancer (JCOG0802/WJOG4607L): a multicentre, open-label, phase 3, randomised, controlled, non-inferiority trial. Lancet. 2022;399(10335):1607–17. https://doi.org/10.1016/S0140-6736(21)02333-3.
34. Ferguson MK, Lehman AG. Sleeve lobectomy or pneumonectomy: optimal management strategy using decision analysis techniques. Ann Thorac Surg. 2003;76(6):1782–8. https://doi.org/10.1016/S0003-4975(03)01243-8.
35. Oka S, Matsumiya H, Shinohara S, et al. Total or partial vertebrectomy for lung cancer invading the spine. Ann Med Surg. 2016;12:1. https://doi.org/10.1016/J.AMSU.2016.10.002.
36. Borri A, Leo F, Veronesi G, et al. Extended pneumonectomy for non-small cell lung cancer: morbidity, mortality, and long-term results. J Thorac Cardiovasc Surg. 2007;134(5):1266–72. https://doi.org/10.1016/J.JTCVS.2007.01.021.
37. Steinfort DP, Vincent J, Heinze S, Antippa P, Irving LB. Comparative effectiveness of radial probe endobronchial ultrasound versus CT-guided needle biopsy for evaluation of peripheral pulmonary lesions: a randomized pragmatic trial. Respir Med. 2011;105(11):1704–11. https://doi.org/10.1016/J.RMED.2011.08.008.
38. El-Bayoumi E, Silvestri GA. Bronchoscopy for the diagnosis and staging of lung cancer. Semin Respir Crit Care Med. 2008;29(3):261–70. https://doi.org/10.1055/S-2008-1076746.
39. Dooms C, Seijo L, Gasparini S, Trisolini R, Ninane V, Tournoy KG. Diagnostic bronchoscopy: state of the art. Eur Respir Rev. 2010;19(117):229–36. https://doi.org/10.1183/09059180.00005710.

40. Maldonado F, Edell ES, Barron PJ, et al. Novel bronchoscopic strategies for the diagnosis of peripheral lung lesions: present techniques and future directions. Respirology. 2014;19(5):636–44. https://doi.org/10.1111/RESP.12301.

41. Wiener RS, Schwartz LM, Woloshin S, Gilbert WH. Population-based risk for complications after transthoracic needle lung biopsy of a pulmonary nodule: an analysis of discharge records. Ann Intern Med. 2011;155(3):137–44. https://doi.org/10.7326/0003-4819-155-3-201108020-00003.

42. Howington JA. The role of VATS for staging and diagnosis in patients with non-small cell lung cancer. Semin Thorac Cardiovasc Surg. 2007;19(3):212–6. https://doi.org/10.1053/J.SEMTCVS.2007.07.007.

43. Giroux DJ, Rami-Porta R, Chansky K, et al. The IASLC lung cancer staging project data elements for the prospective project. J Thorac Oncol. 2009;4(6):679–83. https://doi.org/10.1097/JTO.0b013e3181a52370.

44. Purandare NC, Rangarajan V. Imaging of lung cancer: implications on staging and management. Indian J Radiol Imaging. 2015;25(2):109. https://doi.org/10.4103/0971-3026.155831.

45. Verschakelen JA, Bogaert J, de Wever W. Computed tomography in staging for lung cancer. Eur Respir J. 2002;19(35 suppl):40S–8s. https://doi.org/10.1183/09031936.02.00270802.

46. de Wever W, Vankan Y, Stroobants S, Verschakelen J. Detection of extrapulmonary lesions with integrated PET/CT in the staging of lung cancer. Eur Respir J. 2007;29(5):995–1002. https://doi.org/10.1183/09031936.00119106.

47. Wever W, Ceyssens S, Mortelmans L, et al. Additional value of PET-CT in the staging of lung cancer: comparison with CT alone, PET alone and visual correlation of PET and CT. Eur Radiol. 2007;17(1):23–32. https://doi.org/10.1007/S00330-006-0284-4.

48. Gould MK, Kuschner WG, Rydzak CE, et al. Test performance of positron emission tomography and computed tomography for mediastinal staging in patients with non-small-cell lung cancer: a meta-analysis. Ann Intern Med. 2003;139(11):879. https://doi.org/10.7326/0003-4819-139-11-200311180-00013.

49. Silvestri GA, Gonzalez AV, Jantz MA, et al. Methods for staging non-small cell lung cancer: diagnosis and management of lung cancer, 3rd ed: American college of chest physicians evidence-based clinical practice guidelines. Chest. 2013;143(5 SUPPL):e211S–50S. https://doi.org/10.1378/CHEST.12-2355/ATTACHMENT/19E9A976-6185-4CE8-AAEE-B4A713FEACCA/MMC1.DOCX.

50. Mentzer SJ. Mediastinoscopy, thoracoscopy, and video-assisted thoracic surgery in the diagnosis and staging of lung cancer. Hematol Oncol Clin North Am. 1997;11(3):435–47. https://doi.org/10.1016/S0889-8588(05)70442-1.

51. Detterbeck FC, Boffa DJ, Tanoue LT. The new lung cancer staging system. Chest. 2009;136(1):260–71. https://doi.org/10.1378/CHEST.08-0978.

52. Detterbeck F, Puchalski J, Rubinowitz A, Cheng D. Classification of the thoroughness of mediastinal staging of lung cancer. Chest. 2010;137(2):436–42. https://doi.org/10.1378/CHEST.09-1378.

53. Dezube AR, Hirji S, Shah R, et al. Pre-COVID-19 national mortality trends in open and video-assisted lobectomy for non-small cell lung cancer. J Surg Res. 2022;274:213–23. https://doi.org/10.1016/J.JSS.2021.12.047.

54. Villamizar NR, Darrabie MD, Burfeind WR, et al. Thoracoscopic lobectomy is associated with lower morbidity compared with thoracotomy. J Thorac Cardiovasc Surg. 2009;138(2):419–25. https://doi.org/10.1016/J.JTCVS.2009.04.026.

55. Paul S, Altorki NK, Sheng S, et al. Thoracoscopic lobectomy is associated with lower morbidity than open lobectomy: a propensity-matched analysis from the STS database. J Thorac Cardiovasc Surg. 2010;139(2):366–78. https://doi.org/10.1016/J.JTCVS.2009.08.026.

56. Fernandez FG, Kosinski AS, Burfeind W, et al. The society of thoracic surgeons lung cancer resection risk model: higher quality data and superior outcomes. Ann Thorac Surg. 2016;102(2):370–7. https://doi.org/10.1016/J.ATHORACSUR.2016.02.098.

57. Ceppa DP, Kosinski AS, Berry MF, et al. Thoracoscopic lobectomy has increasing benefit in patients with poor pulmonary function: a Society of Thoracic Surgeons database analysis. Ann Surg. 2012;256(3):487–93. https://doi.org/10.1097/SLA.0B013E318265819C.
58. Zhang L, Gao S. Robot-assisted thoracic surgery versus open thoracic surgery for lung cancer: a system review and meta-analysis. Int J Clin Exp Med. 2015;8(10):17804; /pmc/articles/PMC4694272/. Accessed 2 Oct 2022.
59. Bendixen M, Jørgensen OD, Kronborg C, Andersen C, Licht PB. Postoperative pain and quality of life after lobectomy via video-assisted thoracoscopic surgery or anterolateral thoracotomy for early stage lung cancer: a randomised controlled trial. Lancet Oncol. 2016;17(6):836–44. https://doi.org/10.1016/S1470-2045(16)00173-X.
60. Yang CFJ, Kumar A, Klapper JA, et al. A national analysis of long-term survival following thoracoscopic versus open lobectomy for stage I non-small-cell lung cancer. Ann Surg. 2019;269(1):163–71. https://doi.org/10.1097/SLA.0000000000002342.
61. Lim EKS, Batchelor TJP, Dunning J, et al. Video-assisted thoracoscopic versus open lobectomy in patients with early-stage lung cancer: one-year results from a randomized controlled trial (VIOLET). J Clin Oncol. 2021;39(15_suppl):8504. https://doi.org/10.1200/JCO.2021.39.15_SUPPL.8504.
62. Cui Y, Grogan EL, Deppen SA, et al. Mortality for robotic- vs video-assisted lobectomy-treated stage I non-small cell lung cancer patients. JNCI Cancer Spectr. 2020;4(5):pkaa028. https://doi.org/10.1093/JNCICS/PKAA028.
63. Yang HX, Woo KM, Sima CS, et al. Long-term survival based on the surgical approach to lobectomy for clinical stage I nonsmall cell lung cancer: comparison of robotic, video-assisted thoracic surgery, and thoracotomy lobectomy. Ann Surg. 2017;265(2):431–7. https://doi.org/10.1097/SLA.0000000000001708.
64. Ma J, Li X, Zhao S, Wang J, Zhang W, Sun G. Robot-assisted thoracic surgery versus video-assisted thoracic surgery for lung lobectomy or segmentectomy in patients with non-small cell lung cancer: a meta-analysis. BMC Cancer. 2021;21(1):1–16. https://doi.org/10.1186/S12885-021-08241-5/FIGURES/8.
65. Paul S, Jalbert J, Isaacs AJ, Altorki NK, Isom OW, Sedrakyan A. Comparative effectiveness of robotic-assisted vs thoracoscopic lobectomy. Chest. 2014;146(6):1505–12. https://doi.org/10.1378/CHEST.13-3032.
66. Swanson SJ, Miller DL, McKenna RJ, et al. Comparing robot-assisted thoracic surgical lobectomy with conventional video-assisted thoracic surgical lobectomy and wedge resection: results from a multihospital database (premier). J Thorac Cardiovasc Surg. 2014;147(3):929–37. https://doi.org/10.1016/J.JTCVS.2013.09.046.
67. Gonzalez-Rivas D, Paradela M, Fernandez R, et al. Uniportal video-assisted thoracoscopic lobectomy: two years of experience. Ann Thorac Surg. 2013;95(2):426–32. https://doi.org/10.1016/J.ATHORACSUR.2012.10.070.
68. Ng CSH, Kim HK, Wong RHL, Yim APC, Mok TSK, Choi YH. Single-port video-assisted thoracoscopic major lung resections: experience with 150 consecutive cases. Thorac Cardiovasc Surg. 2016;64(4):348–53. https://doi.org/10.1055/S-0034-1396789.
69. Rocco G, Martucci N, la Manna C, et al. Ten-year experience on 644 patients undergoing single-port (uniportal) video-assisted thoracoscopic surgery. Ann Thorac Surg. 2013;96(2):434–8. https://doi.org/10.1016/J.ATHORACSUR.2013.04.044.
70. Forde PM, Spicer J, Lu S, et al. Neoadjuvant nivolumab plus chemotherapy in resectable lung cancer. N Engl J Med. 2022;386(21):1973–85. https://doi.org/10.1056/NEJMOA2202170/SUPPL_FILE/NEJMOA2202170_DATA-SHARING.PDF.
71. Kandathil A, Chamarthy M. Pulmonary vascular anatomy & anatomical variants. Cardiovasc Diagn Ther. 2018;8(3):201. https://doi.org/10.21037/CDT.2018.01.04.
72. Linden PA, D'Amico TA, Perry Y, et al. Quantifying the safety benefits of wedge resection: a society of thoracic surgery database propensity-matched analysis. Ann Thorac Surg. 2014;98(5):1705–12. https://doi.org/10.1016/J.ATHORACSUR.2014.06.017.

73. Schuchert MJ, Abbas G, Pennathur A, et al. Sublobar resection for early-stage lung cancer. Semin Thorac Cardiovasc Surg. 2010;22(1):22–31. https://doi.org/10.1053/J. SEMTCVS.2010.04.004.

74. Kent M, Landreneau R, Mandrekar S, et al. Segmentectomy versus wedge resection for non-small cell lung cancer in high-risk operable patients. Ann Thorac Surg. 2013;96(5):1747–55. https://doi.org/10.1016/J.ATHORACSUR.2013.05.104.

75. El-Sherif A, Fernando HC, Santos R, et al. Margin and local recurrence after sublobar resection of non-small cell lung cancer. Ann Surg Oncol. 2007;14(8):2400–5. https://doi. org/10.1245/S10434-007-9421-9.

76. Gudbjartsson T, Gyllstedt E, Pikwer A, Jönsson P. Early surgical results after pneumonectomy for non-small cell lung cancer are not affected by preoperative radiotherapy and chemotherapy. Ann Thorac Surg. 2008;86(2):376–82. https://doi.org/10.1016/j.athoracsur.2008.04.013.

77. Shi W, Zhang W, Sun H, Shao Y. Sleeve lobectomy versus pneumonectomy for non-small cell lung cancer: a meta-analysis. World J Surg Oncol. 2012;10:265. https://doi.org/10.118 6/1477-7819-10-265.

78. Darling GE, Allen MS, Decker PA, et al. Randomized trial of mediastinal lymph node sampling versus complete lymphadenectomy during pulmonary resection in the patient with N0 or N1 (less than hilar) non-small cell carcinoma: results of the American college of surgery oncology group Z0030 trial. J Thorac Cardiovasc Surg. 2011;141(3):662–70. https://doi. org/10.1016/J.JTCVS.2010.11.008.

79. Manser R, Wright G, Hart D, et al. Surgery for early stage non-small cell lung cancer. Cochrane Database Syst Rev. 2005;2005(1):CD004699. https://doi.org/10.1002/14651858. CD004699.PUB2.

80. Goldstraw P, Chansky K, Crowley J, et al. The IASLC lung cancer staging project: proposals for revision of the TNM stage groupings in the forthcoming (eighth) edition of the TNM classification for lung cancer. J Thorac Oncol. 2016;11(1):39–51. https://doi.org/10.1016/j. jtho.2015.09.009.

81. Pisters KMW, le Chevalier T. Adjuvant chemotherapy in completely resected non-small-cell lung cancer. J Clin Oncol. 2005;23(14):3270–8. https://doi.org/10.1200/JCO.2005.11.478.

82. Saynak M, Veeramachaneni NK, Hubbs JL, et al. Local failure after complete resection of N0-1 non-small cell lung cancer. Lung Cancer. 2011;71(2):156–65. https://doi.org/10.1016/J. LUNGCAN.2010.06.001.

83. Choi MS, Park JS, Kim HK, et al. Analysis of 1,067 cases of video-assisted thoracic surgery lobectomy. Korean J Thorac Cardiovasc Surg. 2011;44(2):169–77. https://doi.org/10.5090/ KJTCS.2011.44.2.169.

84. Kelsey CR, Marks LB, Hollis D, et al. Local recurrence after surgery for early stage lung cancer: an 11-year experience with 975 patients. Cancer. 2009;115(22):5218–27. https://doi. org/10.1002/CNCR.24625.

85. Su S, Scott WJ, Allen MS, et al. Patterns of survival and recurrence after surgical treatment of early stage non–small cell lung carcinoma in the ACOSOG Z0030 (ALLIANCE) trial. J Thorac Cardiovasc Surg. 2014;147(2):747–53. https://doi.org/10.1016/J.JTCVS.2013.10.001.

86. Brunelli A, Pompili C, Koller M. Changes in quality of life after pulmonary resection. Thorac Surg Clin. 2012;22(4):471–85. https://doi.org/10.1016/J.THORSURG.2012.07.006.

87. Handy JR, Asaph JW, Skokan L, et al. What happens to patients undergoing lung cancer surgery? Outcomes and quality of life before and after surgery. Chest. 2002;122(1):21–30. https://doi.org/10.1378/CHEST.122.1.21.

88. Handy JR, Asaph JW, Douville EC, Ott GY, Grunkemeier GL, Wu YX. Does video-assisted thoracoscopic lobectomy for lung cancer provide improved functional outcomes compared with open lobectomy? Eur J Cardiothorac Surg. 2010;37(2):451–5. https://doi.org/10.1016/J. EJCTS.2009.07.037.

89. Blom EF, ten Haaf K, Arenberg DA, de Koning HJ. Disparities in receiving guideline-concordant treatment for lung cancer in the United States. Ann Am Thorac Soc. 2020;17(2):186–94. https://doi.org/10.1513/ANNALSATS.201901-094OC.

90. Coughlin SS, Matthews-Juarez P, Juarez PD, Melton CE, King M. Opportunities to address lung cancer disparities among African Americans. Cancer Med. 2014;3(6):1467–76. https://doi.org/10.1002/CAM4.348.
91. Lathan CS. Lung cancer care: the impact of facilities and area measures. Transl Lung Cancer Res. 2015;4(4):385–91. https://doi.org/10.3978/J.ISSN.2218-6751.2015.07.23.
92. Check DK, Albers KB, Uppal KM, et al. Examining the role of access to care: racial/ethnic differences in receipt of resection for early-stage non-small cell lung cancer among integrated system members and non-members. Lung Cancer. 2018;125:51–6. https://doi.org/10.1016/J.LUNGCAN.2018.09.006.
93. Cykert S, Eng E, Walker P, et al. A system-based intervention to reduce black-white disparities in the treatment of early stage lung cancer: a pragmatic trial at five cancer centers. Cancer Med. 2019;8(3):1095–102. https://doi.org/10.1002/CAM4.2005.
94. Timmerman R, Papiez L, McGarry R, et al. Extracranial stereotactic radioablation: results of a phase I study in medically inoperable stage I non-small cell lung cancer. Chest. 2003;124(5):1946–55. https://doi.org/10.1378/CHEST.124.5.1946.
95. Timmerman RD, Hu C, Michalski JM, et al. Long-term results of stereotactic body radiation therapy in medically inoperable stage I non-small cell lung cancer. JAMA Oncol. 2018;4(9):1287–8. https://doi.org/10.1001/JAMAONCOL.2018.1258.
96. Morrison R, Deeley TJ, Cleland WP. The treatment of carcinoma of the bronchus: a clinical trial to compare surgery and supervoltage radiotherapy. Lancet. 1963;281(7283):683–4. https://doi.org/10.1016/s0140-6736(63)91444-2.
97. Darling GE, Maziak DE, Inculet RI, et al. Positron emission tomography-computed tomography compared with invasive mediastinal staging in non-small cell lung cancer: results of mediastinal staging in the early lung positron emission tomography trial. J Thorac Oncol. 2011;6(8):1367–72. https://doi.org/10.1097/JTO.0B013E318220C912.
98. Timmerman RD, Paulus R, Pass HI, et al. Stereotactic body radiation therapy for operable early-stage lung cancer: findings from the NRG oncology RTOG 0618 trial. JAMA Oncol. 2018;4(9):1263. https://doi.org/10.1001/JAMAONCOL.2018.1251.
99. Chang JY, Senan S, Paul MA, et al. Stereotactic ablative radiotherapy versus lobectomy for operable stage I non-small-cell lung cancer: a pooled analysis of two randomised trials. Lancet Oncol. 2015;16(6):630–7. https://doi.org/10.1016/S1470-2045(15)70168-3.
100. Ball D, Mai GT, Vinod S, et al. Stereotactic ablative radiotherapy versus standard radiotherapy in stage 1 non-small-cell lung cancer (TROG 09.02 CHISEL): a phase 3, open-label, randomised controlled trial. Lancet Oncol. 2019;20(4):494–503. https://doi.org/10.1016/S1470-2045(18)30896-9.

Chapter 7
Treatment of Stage III Non-small Cell Lung Cancer

Shinsuke Kitazawa, Alexander Gregor, and Kazuhiro Yasufuku

Introduction

Stage III non-small cell lung cancer (NSCLC), commonly referred to as "locally advanced lung cancer," encompasses a group of heterogeneous clinical presentations ranging from bulky primary tumors to small-sized lesions with extensive lymph node involvement. The anatomic extent of cancer is described by the American Joint Committee on Cancer (AJCC) tumor, node, and metastasis (TNM) staging system (Table 7.1). According to the eighth edition of the AJCC staging system, stage III NSCLC is subclassified into stages IIIA, IIIB, and IIIC [2]. Stage IIIA includes locally invasive tumors (T3 or T4) with ipsilateral hilar lymph node (N1) involvement, T4 tumors without nodal involvement, and smaller (T1-2) tumors with mediastinal lymph node (N2) involvement. Stage IIIB includes T1-2 tumors with spread to contralateral mediastinal or supraclavicular (N3) nodes and T3-4 tumors with N2 involvement. Stage IIIC encompasses patients with T3-4 and N3 disease. Approximately 20% of lung cancer patients present with stage III NSCLC; clinical outcomes, unfortunately, remain dismal, with 5-year overall survival (OS) at 36%/41% for clinical/pathological stage IIIA disease, 26%/24% for stage IIIB disease, and 13%/12% for stage IIIC disease [3–5]. These poor outcomes likely reflect that many with stage III disease represent micrometastatic stage IV disease undetectable by modern imaging. Therefore, therapeutic approaches to stage III disease must invariably address local and distant disease control. This complexity has encouraged coordinated care provided by a multidisciplinary team (MDT) to optimize the entire diagnostic and therapeutic process. MDTs are fundamental to

S. Kitazawa · A. Gregor · K. Yasufuku (✉)
Division of Thoracic Surgery, Department of Surgery, Toronto General Hospital, University Health Network, Toronto, ON, Canada
e-mail: skitazawa@md.tsukuba.ac.jp; Alexander.Gregor@uhn.ca; kazuhiro.yasufuku@uhn.ca

© The Author(s), under exclusive license to Springer Nature Switzerland AG 2023
C. MacRosty, M. P. Rivera (eds.), *Lung Cancer*, Respiratory Medicine,
https://doi.org/10.1007/978-3-031-38412-7_7

Table 7.1 Lung cancer stage grouping (eighth edition) [1]

T/M	Label	N0	N1	N2	N3
T1	T1a (≤1 cm)	IA1	IIB	IIIA	IIIB
	T1b (>1–2 cm)	IA2	IIB	IIIA	IIIB
	T1c (>2–3 cm)	IA3	IIB	IIIA	IIIB
T2	T2a (Cent, Visc Pl)	IB	IIB	IIIA	IIIB
	T2a (>3–4 cm)	IB	IIB	IIIA	IIIB
	T2b (>4–5 cm)	IIA	IIB	IIIA	IIIB
T3	T3 (>5–7 cm)	IIB	IIIA	IIIB	IIIC
	T3 (Inv)	IIB	IIIA	IIIB	IIIC
	T3 (Satell)	IIB	IIIA	IIIB	IIIC
T4	T4 (>7 cm)	IIIA	IIIA	IIIB	IIIC
	T4 (Inv)	IIIA	IIIA	IIIB	IIIC
	T4 (Ipsi Nod)	IIIA	IIIA	IIIB	IIIC
M1	M1a (Pl Dissem)	IVA	IVA	IVA	IVA
	M1a (Contr Nod)	IVA	IVA	IVA	IVA
	M1b (Single)	IVA	IVA	IVA	IVA
	M1c (Multi)	IVB	IVB	IVB	IVB

Cent central, *Visc Pl* visceral pleura, *Inv* invading chest wall, pericardium, phrenic nerve, *Satell* separate tumor nodule(s) in the same lobe, *Pl Dissem* malignant pleural/pericardial effusion, or pleural/pericardial nodules, *Contr Nod* separate tumor nodule(s) in a contralateral lobe, *Single* single extrathoracic metastasis, *multi*, multiple extrathoracic metastases

ensuring precise staging, evaluating different therapeutic options, and identifying clinical trials that may benefit the patient [6, 7].

Surgery and radiation therapy are well-established local control treatment modalities, but the high incidence of distant relapse emphasizes the importance of effective systemic therapy. With recent advances in immune checkpoint inhibitors and molecularly targeted agents, research in systemic treatment has increasingly shifted to more personalized therapy based on the individual patient's immune and oncogene mutation status. Clinical trials exploring the combination of these new systemic agents with existing therapeutic approaches are ongoing and represent a paradigm change in the management of locally advanced NSCLC. In this chapter, we provide an overview of the management of stage III NSCLC, focusing on the recent incorporation of immunotherapy and molecularly targeted therapy.

Current Treatment Strategies for Stage III NSCLC

The first step to determining the treatment strategy for patients with stage III NSCLC is determining resectability through a multidisciplinary committee. Only select patients with stage III disease are resectable (e.g., T3-4 disease with limited invasion of adjacent structures without N2-3 involvement). Unresectable patients are generally those who, even following neoadjuvant treatment, cannot expect complete

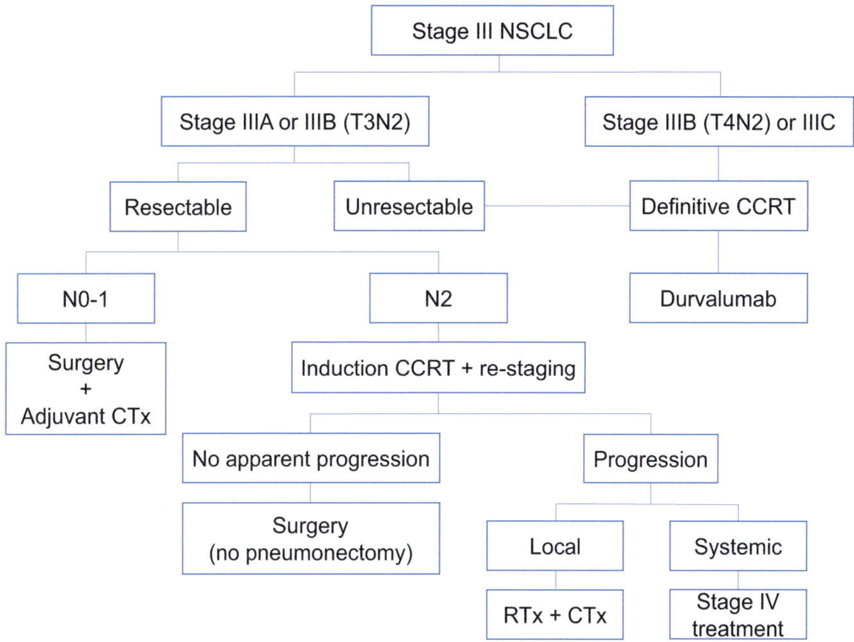

Fig. 7.1 Principles of management for stage III NSCLC. *NSCLC* non-small cell lung cancer, *CCRT* concurrent chemoradiotherapy, *CTx* chemotherapy, *RTx* radiotherapy

resection and tend to be those with bulky N2 disease, most with stages IIIB/IIIC disease, and aggressive T3-4 involvement [8, 9]. Patient-related factors also need to be considered, such as impaired pulmonary function or cardiovascular comorbidities [10]. The clinical guidelines of the National Comprehensive Cancer Network (NCCN; version 3.2022) differentiate between three situations (Fig. 7.1) [11]:

1. Resectable cT3N1/T4N0-1 IIIA: Surgical resection followed by adjuvant chemotherapy with four cycles of platinum-based doublet is recommended. In cases with positive margins, re-resection or radiotherapy is recommended.
2. Resectable cN2: Neoadjuvant chemoradiotherapy or chemotherapy alone, generally with three cycles of platinum-based doublet followed by subsequent radiological reevaluation and restaging. Complete surgical resection and subsequent assessment for adjuvant chemotherapy are recommended in cases without apparent progression.
3. Unresectable IIIA–IIIC: Definitive concurrent chemoradiation (CCRT) followed by assessment for consolidation immunotherapy.

Treatment Modalities in the Pre-immunotherapy Era

Surgery Plus Adjuvant Therapy

Stage III NSCLC represents an intermediate zone between resectable and non-resectable disease [8]. Therefore, the role of surgery as part of multimodality treatment for stage III NSCLC has been controversial. However, improvements in perioperative systemic therapy for stage III NSCLC have increased the proportion of patients eligible for curative resection. Upfront surgical resection followed by adjuvant chemotherapy can be generally considered in patients with cT3N1/T4N0-1 stage IIIA NSCLC, or cN0 patients who are unexpectedly diagnosed as pN2 postoperatively. In the adjuvant setting, the standard is four cycles of cisplatin-based doublet chemotherapy. The Lung Adjuvant Cisplatin Evaluation (LACE) Collaborative Group performed a meta-analysis where 4584 patients with completely resected NSCLC treated with adjuvant cisplatin were assessed. Cisplatin-based adjuvant chemotherapy increased OS at 5 years by 5.4% and reduced the risk of death by 11% (hazard ratio [HR]:0.89, 95% confidence interval (CI):0.82–0.96, $p = 0.0043$) [12]. A significant benefit was seen for patients with stage II (HR:0.83, 95% CI:0.73–0.95) and stage IIIA disease (HR:0.83, 95% CI:0.72–0.94). Based on phase III trials and this meta-analysis, adjuvant chemotherapy after complete resection of stage III NSCLC has been established as standard of care in patients with good performance status, smooth postoperative recovery, and adequate organ function.

T4 tumors with invasion into surrounding structures are a unique subset of patients where upfront surgical treatment can be challenging. Extensive surgical resections, including the involved structures, carry a high morbidity/mortality risk, making it imperative that only patients with good performance status be selected [13]. Achievement of complete resection is a crucial factor for survival. Complete resection is potentially possible in certain tumors, such as those invading the superior vena cava, left atrium, carina, and intrapericardial pulmonary vessels, with 5-year survival rates between 9 and 48% having been reported [14, 15]. However, 22.7% of T3-4N0-1 patients have been reported as unresectable, especially in patients with esophageal/tracheal invasion [16]. Several previous studies have demonstrated that neoadjuvant chemotherapy with or without radiation facilitates the ability to achieve complete resection (and thus better survival) in patients with T3-T4N0-1 stage III NSCLC [17, 18]. However, the benefit of neoadjuvant treatment for central T4 tumors is less clear, with some studies concluding that neoadjuvant therapy does not influence survival [19, 20]. Moreover, if pathologic N2 disease were present, the prognosis was dismal despite complete resection [21, 22]. Therefore, accurate mediastinal staging by endobronchial ultrasound-guided transbronchial needle aspiration (EBUS-TBNA) is essential to determine optimal treatment strategy.

In summary, surgery followed by adjuvant therapy is the standard of care in patients with resectable cT3N1/T4N0-1 stage III NSCLC. As complete resection and negative mediastinal lymph node involvement are crucial factors for prognosis, multidisciplinary assessment of resectability and accurate preoperative mediastinal lymph node staging are of paramount importance.

Neoadjuvant Therapy Plus Surgery

Neoadjuvant chemotherapy offers theoretical advantages such as early treatment of micrometastatic disease, downstaging to facilitate resectability, and improved tolerability (compared to postoperative delivery) [23]. However, this must be balanced with potential risks for progression in chemoresistant disease (closing the window for resection) and delay of local therapy secondary to chemotoxicity [24].

In stage III NSCLC, neoadjuvant therapy followed by surgery is generally considered either in patients with stage III superior sulcus tumors or those with potentially resectable cN2 disease [25]. Although preoperative CCRT followed by surgery is the standard treatment of superior sulcus tumors, surgical management of N2 disease remains one of the most controversial topics in managing stage III NSCLC. Involved N2 lymph nodes can be classified as either "infiltrative" or "discrete" N2 disease. Infiltrative N2 metastases refer to when individual lymph nodes can no longer be distinguished by CT imaging. In contrast, discrete N2 metastases refer to when a defined metastatic lymph node(s) is/are readily distinguishable from surrounding structures. Surgical indications largely depend on the category of N2 disease; in general, surgery is not recommended for infiltrative or multi-station N2 disease [26]. Surgical resection combined with systemic chemotherapy can have a role in carefully selected patients with discrete N2 involvement.

At present, three phase III clinical trials have reported on the role of neoadjuvant therapy followed by surgery for stage IIIA NSCLC with mediastinal lymph node metastases. In the European Organization for Research and Treatment of Cancer (EORTC) 08941 trial, patients with N2 stage IIIA NSCLC were randomly assigned to surgery or radiotherapy after response to three cycles of neoadjuvant platinum-based chemotherapy [27]. In the surgery group, only 50% of patients had complete resection, and the 5-year survival rate was low (15.7%), with no difference from radiation therapy (14%). The North American Intergroup 0139 trial randomized 429 patients with biopsy-proven N2 stage IIIA NSCLC that were potentially resectable to either neoadjuvant chemotherapy (two cycles of cisplatin and etoposide) and radiation (45 Gy) followed by surgery or definitive chemoradiation uninterrupted up to 61 Gy [28]. The 5-year survival for the surgery group was not significantly different from the completion radiotherapy group (27% versus 20%, $p = 0.10$), but progression-free survival (PFS) was significantly improved (12.8 versus 10.5 months, $p = 0.017$). In addition, pathologic downstaging after neoadjuvant chemoradiation revealed ypT0 in 20% and only microscopic residual tumor in another 20%, indicating that addition of radiotherapy to neoadjuvant chemotherapy may improve survival through better locoregional control. This could explain the subgroup analysis of lobectomy patients only, which found 5-year survival rate was significantly better with surgery than with completion radiotherapy (36% versus 18%, $p = 0.002$). Conversely, among those requiring pneumonectomy, the postoperative 30-day mortality was unacceptably high (26%). The study concluded that neoadjuvant chemotherapy followed by lobectomy might potentially improve outcomes. The third study was the ESPATUE trial, where patients with biopsy-proven N2 stage IIIA and selected patients with operable IIIB disease (anatomically and physiologically) received induction chemotherapy (cisplatin, paclitaxel, and vinorelbine) as well as CCRT to 45 Gy [29]. Patients with resectable tumors on reevaluation were randomly assigned to receive surgery or continue to definitive chemoradiation (uninterrupted dose up to 65–71 Gy). Both surgery and definitive chemoradiation following neoadjuvant therapy were associated with favorable 5-year survival rates compared to those in other clinical trials, but no significant difference was observed between the two groups (44% versus 40%, $p = 0.34$). Better outcomes in this study might be due to patient selection (whereby only responders to induction therapy were randomized) and the limited trial size (81 patients in the surgery group and 80 patients in the definitive chemoradiation group). A meta-analysis examining five randomized controlled trials and four retrospective observational studies demonstrated that neoadjuvant chemotherapy with or without radiotherapy followed by surgery was superior to definitive chemoradiation alone, particularly in patients undergoing lobectomy [30]. Although the key to optimal management of stage III N2 disease is CCRT, neoadjuvant chemoradiotherapy or chemotherapy followed by surgery has a role in carefully selected patients with response to neoadjuvant treatment and in whom lobectomy is a feasible operative approach.

Nonsurgical Treatment

For patients with unresectable stage III NSCLC, systemic cytotoxic therapy with radiation therapy is generally employed. Whether delivered alone or as part of chemoradiotherapy, neoadjuvant or adjuvant, three major combinations of platinum-based doublets treatment are generally used: cisplatin + etoposide, carboplatin + paclitaxel, and cisplatin + vinorelbine. At least two phase III trials have investigated current chemotherapy regimens with radiation for unresectable stage III NSCLC. In the study conducted by Liang et al., patients received 60–66 Gy of thoracic radiation therapy concurrent with either cisplatin and etoposide (PE therapy) or carboplatin + paclitaxel (CP therapy) [31]. There was no significant superiority of PE therapy compared with CP therapy for the primary endpoint of OS (PE 23.3 months versus CP 20.7 months, $p = 0.095$). The phase III PROCLAIM study investigated OS of concurrent pemetrexed-cisplatin and radiation therapy followed by consolidation pemetrexed (PP therapy), versus cisplatin and etoposide and radiation therapy followed by consolidation etoposide (PE therapy) in unresectable stage III non-squamous NSCLC [32]. Although the median OS was similar between the two groups (PP 25.0 months versus PE 26.8 months, $p = 0.831$), cisplatin and pemetrexed had a more favorable toxicity profile, including drug-related grade 3 or higher adverse events such as neutropenia (PP 44.5% versus PE 24.4%, $p = 0.001$).

Platinum-based chemotherapy is generally employed in conjunction with radiotherapy because randomized trials consistently demonstrated a survival benefit over radiotherapy alone [33–36]. The integration of chemotherapy can be further tailored in its timing relative to radiotherapy (e.g., chemotherapy followed by radiotherapy, CCRT, or CCRT followed by consolidation chemotherapy). A meta-analysis by the NSCLC Collaborative Group demonstrated that CCRT, as compared with sequential chemoradiotherapy, was associated with an OS benefit of 5.3% at 2 years, 5.7% at 3 years, and 4.5% at 5 years in patients with stage III NSCLC, primarily attributed to decreased locoregional progression [37]. This survival benefit of CCRT does come with an increased risk for esophageal toxicity compared with sequential treatment and radiotherapy alone [38]. According to the Radiation Therapy Oncology Group (RTOG) 7301 trial, the standard irradiation regimen for CCRT in patients with stage III NSCLC is a total dose of 60 Gy in 30 fractions over 6 weeks; this schedule has not changed over the past 30 years [39]. Dose escalation beyond 60 Gy with conventional fractionation has not been demonstrated to be of benefit based on results of the RTOG 0617 trial, which compared high-dose CCRT (weekly paclitaxel/carboplatin) at 74 Gy/37 fractions to standard-dose CCRT at 60 Gy/30 fractions, with or without cetuximab [40–42]. This phase III trial demonstrated that the 74 Gy dose was associated with a higher risk of local recurrence (34% versus 25%) and significantly shorter median OS (20.3 versus 28.7 months, $p = 0.004$) [43]. The 74 Gy dose group also experienced more treatment-related deaths and severe esophagitis. Therefore, dose escalation beyond 60 Gy with conventional fractionation is not recommended.

Additional technologies are improving the delivery of radiation therapy. This includes intensity-modulated radiation therapy (IMRT), a radiation technique that uses computer-controlled linear accelerators to deliver highly conformal doses of radiation to the treatment targets. IMRT allows higher radiation doses to be focused on the tumor while minimizing exposure to surrounding normal critical structures such as the heart, uninvolved lung, and esophagus [44]. A phase I nonrandomized clinical trial evaluated an IMRT contralateral esophagus-sparing technique of radiation delivered with concurrent chemotherapy in patients with locally advanced NSCLC within 1 cm of the esophagus [45]. The high-precision technique created a sharp dose gradient between the treatment target and contralateral esophageal wall, resulting in a reduced risk of esophagitis, including no grade 3 or higher esophagitis. In addition, secondary analysis from RTOG 0617 trial compared conventional three-dimensional conformal external beam radiation therapy (3D-CRT) and IMRT outcomes [46]. IMRT was associated with significantly less grade 3 or higher pneumonitis than 3D-CRT (3.5% versus 7.9%, $p = 0.039$). In terms of prognosis, 2-year OS and PFS were not different between IMRT and 3D-CRT. Several earlier studies similarly demonstrated that IMRT reduced the incidence of treatment interruptions and resulted in better OS among patients treated with chemoradiotherapy for stage III NSCLC compared with 3D-CRT [47, 48].

To further limit the irradiation volume and toxicity of conventional photon radiotherapy, proton beam radiotherapy (PBT) has been explored for unresectable stage III NSCLC. PBT has the advantage of a much narrower dose distribution zone than IMRT. Retrospective data and phase II studies have demonstrated that PBT at a total dose of 74 Gy equivalent (GyE) administered concurrently with platinum-based chemotherapy for stage III NSCLC was well tolerated, with a median OS of 26–49 months and low esophageal/pulmonary toxicity compared to conventional photon radiotherapy [49–51]. However, the efficacy of PBT has not yet been validated; one prospective randomized clinical trial comparing PBT with IMRT demonstrated no significant differences in treatment failure (defined as radiation pneumonitis or local recurrence) [52]. A phase III trial (RTOG 1308) comparing photon radiotherapy with PBT in chemoradiation for unresectable locally advanced NSCLC is currently underway.

In summary, radiation therapy in combination with chemotherapy is a standard treatment option for unresectable stage III NSCLC. Moreover, recent advances in radiotherapy (e.g., IMRT, PBT) allow more precise dose delivery and less treatment toxicity. These new radiotherapy approaches combined with systemic therapy may lead to better local control and survival.

Immunotherapy for Stage III NSCLC

Treatment of stage III NSCLC has substantially changed with advances in immunotherapy that may potentiate the effects of radiotherapy, and vice versa [53]. Various phase II and III trials have shown that incorporating immunotherapy into conventional treatment paradigms results in better outcomes with fewer side effects than conventional chemotherapeutics via improved locoregional control and/or induction of an abscopal effect against micrometastases [54–57].

Immunotherapy in the Neoadjuvant Setting

Immune checkpoint inhibitors in the neoadjuvant setting combined with chemotherapy provide an early opportunity to treat micrometastatic disease. Various phase II clinical trials are investigating the efficacy of neoadjuvant immunotherapy in NSCLC. The NADIM clinical trial was the first study to investigate the feasibility, safety, and efficacy of combined neoadjuvant chemotherapy and immunotherapy in resectable stage IIIA NSCLC patients [58, 59]. In this phase II, single-arm, multicenter study, patients received paclitaxel (200 mg/m^2) and carboplatin (AUC 6 mg/mL·min) plus nivolumab (360 mg) every 3 weeks for three cycles before surgical resection, followed by adjuvant nivolumab monotherapy for 1 year (240 mg every 2 weeks for 4 months, followed by 480 mg every 4 weeks for 8 months). Neoadjuvant immunotherapy combined with chemotherapy was highly effective with 3-year OS and PFS of 81.9% and 69.6%, respectively. In addition, 63% of patients who underwent surgery had a complete pathological response and 83% had at least a major pathological response (<10% viable tumor cells in resected specimens). Patients with a complete pathological response had significantly longer OS and PFS than those with an incomplete or major pathological response. Although the most common grade 3–4 toxicity was hematotoxicity, an increase in immune-mediated toxicity was not specifically described. This trial demonstrated that neoadjuvant nivolumab alone or with chemotherapy showed promise with respect to feasibility, safety, complete pathological response, and survival in patients with resectable stage IIIA NSCLC.

CheckMate-816 is the first randomized phase III trial evaluating neoadjuvant immunotherapy plus chemotherapy in patients with stage IB to IIIA NSCLC [60]. Patients were randomized 1:1 to receive nivolumab plus platinum doublet chemotherapy or platinum-based chemotherapy alone. Patients underwent surgery within 6 weeks of neoadjuvant treatment completion. There was a significantly improved event-free survival of 31.6 months with neoadjuvant nivolumab plus chemotherapy (95% CI: 30.2—not reached) compared with 20.8 months with chemotherapy alone (95% CI: 14.0–26.7). Furthermore, neoadjuvant nivolumab plus chemotherapy resulted in pathological complete response in 24% of patients (95% CI:18.0–31.0) compared with 2.2% in patients treated with chemotherapy alone (95% CI:0.6–5.6). This improvement was observed regardless of disease stage and PD-L1 expression. No significant difference in grade 3–4 toxicity was observed (34% in the combination arm versus 37% in the chemotherapy alone arm). Exploratory surgical outcome analysis showed that the length of surgery was shorter, the rate of minimally invasive surgery was higher, and pneumonectomies were less common in patients treated with neoadjuvant nivolumab plus chemotherapy than chemotherapy alone. These surgical findings were most evident in the stage IIIA cohort, who accounted for >60% of patients in both arms. A higher incidence of radiographic downstaging observed with nivolumab plus chemotherapy may have contributed to lower rates of pneumonectomy. Adverse events of grade 3 or 4 identified as surgical complications occurred in 11.4% of patients after nivolumab plus chemotherapy and in 14.8% of patients after chemotherapy alone. These results prompted the Food and Drug Administration (FDA) to approve the use of nivolumab in conjunction with platinum-based chemotherapy in the neoadjuvant setting.

Combination Immunotherapy Chemoradiotherapy

Radiotherapy is known to cause immune-mediated shrinkage of other lesions distant from the irradiated site (termed the abscopal effect), suggesting that radiotherapy may enhance host immunity [61]. Therefore, immuno-radiotherapy, which aims to leverage immune checkpoint inhibition to potentiate the abscopal effect in combination with radiotherapy's local effects, has been attracting attention.

Radiotherapy-induced cell death promotes antigen presentation and induces cytotoxic activity of cancer antigen-specific T cells. Yet, counterintuitively some inflammatory cytokines released following radiotherapy promote PD-L1 expression and suppress T-cell attack. Therefore, administration of anti-PD-L1 antibody therapy was investigated as a treatment to restore antitumor immune responses [62]. The PACIFIC trial was the main study investigating the efficacy of immunotherapy in association with radiotherapy and chemotherapy for stage III NSCLC [63, 64]. This phase III trial of CCRT with platinum doublet chemotherapy followed by maintenance durvalumab for unresectable stage III NSCLC demonstrated a remarkable benefit of durvalumab maintenance treatment. With a median follow-up time of 34.2 months, the 5-year OS for the durvalumab group was 42.9% versus 33.4% in the placebo group (HR: 0.72, 95% CI:0.59–0.89), and 5-year PFS was 33.1% versus 19.0%, respectively (HR: 0.55, 95% CI: 0.45–0.68) (Fig. 7.2). The use of immune checkpoint inhibitors after radiation therapy has been associated with an increased

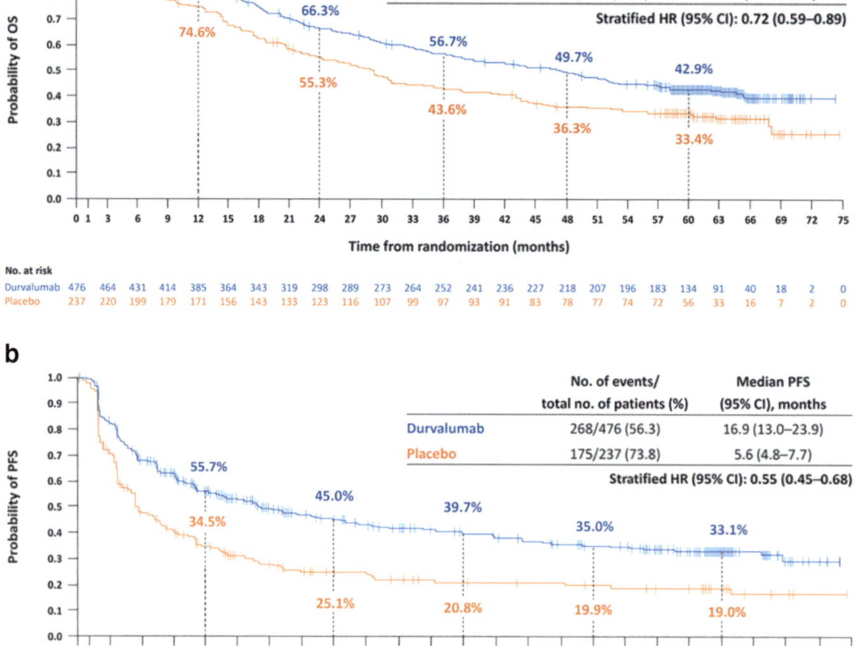

Fig. 7.2 Overall (**a**) and progression-free survival (**b**) in the PACIFIC trial [65]. The vertical dashed lines indicate yearly timepoints; the associated numerical values represent the OS and PFS rates at each timepoint. *HR* hazard ratio, *OS* overall survival, *PFS* progression-free survival

risk of toxicity, particularly radiation pneumonitis and immune-mediated pneumonia. In the study, the overall incidence of pneumonia was slightly higher in the durvalumab group (33.9%) than in the placebo group (24.8%), but there was no significant difference in severe lung inflammation of grade 3 or higher between the two groups (4.5% versus 4.3%, respectively). Following these results, the FDA approved the use of consolidation durvalumab following CCRT as standard treatment in patients with unresectable stage III NSCLC. Subsequent retrospective analyses were performed to compare efficacy relative to PD-L1 expression levels [65]. Notably, the PFS benefit with durvalumab was observed irrespective of PD-L1 expression before chemoradiotherapy (HR:0.59, 95% CI:0.43–0.82 for a PD-L1 expression level of less than 25%; HR:0.41, 95% CI:0.26–0.65 for a PD-L1 expression level of more than or equal to 25%). The only exception was OS with PD-L1 expression less than 1% (HR:1.15, 95% CI:0.75–1.75), although PFS still favored durvalumab in this subgroup (HR:0.80, 95% CI:0.53–1.20). The survival benefit of durvalumab among patients with driver mutations such as epidermal growth factor receptor (EGFR) or anaplastic lymphoma kinase (ALK) aberration-positive tumors was uncertain, considering that the number of patients with driver mutations was small (6%); EGFR and ALK status was unknown in 26.4% of randomized patients.

In summary, the PACIFIC trial demonstrated that durvalumab significantly improved PFS and OS, with manageable safety in unresectable stage III NSCLC patients without evidence of disease progression after CCRT. However, the efficacy of consolidation immune checkpoint inhibitors following CCRT in patients with PD-L1-negative or driver mutation-positive tumors remains uncertain. Further clinical studies are needed to address these subgroups and to investigate potential biomarkers that identify those with higher probability of responding to combination immunotherapy-radiotherapy.

Molecular Targeting Agents

The application of genetic testing to metastatic NSCLC led to substantial progress in the management of select patients. There was hope early on that use of tyrosine kinase inhibitor (TKI) therapy would also benefit the management of locally advanced disease. Furthermore, evidence suggested that patients with EGFR gene mutations may have lower locoregional recurrence and higher distant progression following platinum-based chemoradiotherapy compared to EGFR wild-type disease, especially brain metastases [66, 67]. The limited efficacy of chemoradiotherapy for EGFR-mutated tumors encouraged the investigation of TKIs. Various clinical studies have explored TKIs in stage III NSCLC; however, there is currently no clear evidence of benefit with the addition of TKI to current treatment paradigms. The Cancer and Leukemia Group B (CALGB) 30407 trial was a phase II study that investigated the efficacy of consolidation cetuximab after platinum-doublet chemoradiotherapy [68]. The 18-month OS were identical (58% versus 54% with and without cetuximab, respectively). The RTOG 0617 phase III trial similar found no benefit of adding cetuximab to CCRT. The efficacy of maintenance EGFR TKI in stage III NSCLC was investigated in the phase III South West Oncology Group (SWOG) S0023 trial [69]. Patients who did not progress after CCRT (cisplatin and etoposide, plus three cycles consolidation docetaxel) were randomized to maintenance treatment with the anti-EGFR therapy gefitinib or placebo for 5 years. The study was closed prematurely after a median follow-up of 27 months for perceived harm, with median OS lower with gefitinib (23 months) than placebo (35 months, $p = 0.013$). The reasons for this result remain unclear. As such, despite initial case series suggesting a benefit of targeted therapy when combined with chemoradiation for EGFR-mutated stage III NSCLC, the repeated failure of this strategy in larger phase III trials means such approaches remain outside the standard of care.

Conclusion

Stage III NSCLC is a diverse population, and there are many different treatment strategies to enhance both local and distant control. Despite the theoretical benefits of tailored therapy based on histological subtype and tumor genotype, this "personalized" therapy has thus far not outperformed concurrent chemoradiation. The emergence of immunotherapy in recent years has been a major turning point in the treatment system for locally advanced NSCLC. Maintenance durvalumab is a new standard of care for patients with unresectable stage III NSCLC based on the superior OS and PFS with minimal increased toxicity. However, patient selection remains an issue when incorporating immunotherapy into multimodality treatment. It is uncertain that patients with less than 1% PD-L1 expression and those with driver mutation-positive disease experience the same magnitude of benefit. Further research is required to better evaluate the numerous potential combinations of multimodality therapy that may ultimately offer long-term disease control, if not cure, for those with stage III NSCLC.

References

1. Detterbeck FC, Boffa DJ, Kim AW, Tanoue LT. The eighth edition lung cancer stage classification. Chest. 2017;151:193–203. https://doi.org/10.1016/j.chest.2016.10.010.
2. Amin MB, Edge S, Greene F, Byrd DR, Brookland RK, Washington MK, Gershenwald JE, Compton CC, Hess KR, et al. (Eds.). AJCC Cancer Staging Manual (8th edition). 2017.
3. Sung H, Ferlay J, Siegel R, Laversannne M, Soerjomataram I, Jemal A, et al. Global cancer statistics 2020: GLOBOCAN estimates of incidence and mortality worldwide for 36 cancers in 185 countries. CA Cancer J Clin. 2021;71:209–49. https://doi.org/10.3322/caac.21660.
4. Goldstraw P, Chansky K, Crowley J, Rami-Porta R, Asamura H, Eberhardt WE, et al. The IASLC Lung Cancer Staging Project: proposals for revision of the TNM stage groupings in

the forthcoming (eighth) edition of the TNM classification for lung cancer. J Thorac Oncol. 2016;11:39–51. https://doi.org/10.1016/j.jtho.2015.09.009.

5. Wu FZ, Kuo PL, Huang YL, Tang EK, Chen CS, Wu MT, et al. Differences in lung cancer characteristics and mortality rate between screened and non-screened cohorts. Sci Rep. 2019;9:19386. https://doi.org/10.1038/s41598-019-56025-6.

6. Postmus PE, Kerr KM, Oudkerk M, Senan S, Waller DA, Vansteenkiste J, et al. Early and locally advanced non-small-cell lung cancer (NSCLC): ESMO Clinical Practice Guidelines for diagnosis, treatment and follow-up. Ann Oncol. 2017;28(Suppl 4):1–21. https://doi.org/10.1093/annonc/mdx222.

7. Kris MG, Gaspar LE, Chaft JE, Kennedy EB, Azzoli CG, Ellis PM, et al. Adjuvant systemic therapy and adjuvant radiation therapy for stage I to IIIa completely resected non–small-cell lung cancers: American Society of Clinical Oncology/Cancer Care Ontario Clinical Practice Guideline Update. J Clin Oncol. 2017;35:2960–74. https://doi.org/10.1200/JCO.2017.72.4401.

8. Van Schil PE, Berzenji L, Yogeswaran SK, Hendriks JM, Lauwers P. Surgical management of stage IIIA non-small cell lung cancer. Front Oncol. 2017;7:249. https://doi.org/10.3389/fonc.2017.00249.

9. Patel V, Shrager JB. Which patients with stage III non-small cell lung cancer should undergo surgical resection? Oncologist. 2005;10:335–44. https://doi.org/10.1634/theoncologist.10-5-335.

10. Brunelli A, Kim AW, Berger KI, Addrizzo-Harris DJ. Physiologic evaluation of the patient with lung cancer being considered for resectional surgery: diagnosis and management of lung cancer, 3rd ed: American College of Chest Physicians evidence-based clinical practice guidelines. Chest. 2013;143(Suppl 5):e166S–90S. https://doi.org/10.1378/chest.12-2395.

11. National Comprehensive Cancer Network. NCCN Guidelines Version 2.2021 Non-Small Cell Lung Cancer. https://www.nccn.org/professionals/physician_gls/pdf/nscl.pdf.

12. Pignon JP, Tribodet H, Scagliotti GV, Douillard JY, Shepherd FA, Stephens RJ, et al. Lung adjuvant cisplatin evaluation: a pooled analysis by the LACE Collaborative Group. J Clin Oncol. 2008;26:3552–9. https://doi.org/10.1200/JCO.2007.13.9030.

13. Pitz CCM, de la Rivière AB, van Swieten HA, Westermann CJJ, Lammers J-WJ, van den Bosch JMM. Results of surgical treatment of T4 non-small cell lung cancer. Eur J Cardiothorac Surg. 2003;24:1013–8. https://doi.org/10.1016/s1010-7940(03)00493-7.

14. Chambers A, Routledge T, Bille A, Scarci M. Does surgery have a role in T4N0 and T4N1 lung cancer? Interact Cardiovasc Thorac Surg. 2010;11:473–9. https://doi.org/10.1510/icvts.2010.235119.

15. Reardon ES, Schrump DS. Extended resections of non-small cell lung cancers invading the aorta, pulmonary artery, left atrium, or esophagus: can they be justified? Thorac Surg Clin. 2014;24:457–64. https://doi.org/10.1016/j.thorsurg.2014.07.012.

16. Garrido P, Gonzalez-Larriba JL, Insa A, Provencio M, Torres A, Isla D, et al. Long-term survival associated with complete resection after induction chemotherapy in stage IIIA (N2) and IIIB (T4N0-1) non small-cell lung cancer patients: the Spanish Lung Cancer Group Trial 9901. J Clin Oncol. 2007;25:4736–42. https://doi.org/10.1200/JCO.2007.12.0014.

17. Shien K, Toyooka S, Kiura K, Matsuo K, Soh J, Yamane M, et al. Induction chemoradiotherapy followed by surgical resection for clinical T3 or T4 locally advanced non-small cell lung cancer. Ann Surg Oncol. 2012;19:2685–92. https://doi.org/10.1245/s10434-012-2302-x.

18. Daly BD, Ebright MI, Walkey AJ, Fernando HC, Zaner KS, Morelli DM, et al. Impact of neoadjuvant chemoradiotherapy followed by surgical resection on node-negative T3 and T4 non-small cell lung cancer. J Thorac Cardiovasc Surg. 2011;141:1392–7. https://doi.org/10.1016/j.jtcvs.2010.12.011.

19. Lococo F, Cesario A, Margaritora S, Dall'Armi V, Nachira D, Cusumano G, et al. Induction therapy followed by surgery for T3-T4/N0 non-small cell lung cancer: long-term results. Ann Thorac Surg. 2012;93:1633–40. https://doi.org/10.1016/j.athoracsur.2012.01.109.

20. Uramoto H, Shimokawa H, Hanagiri T, Ichiki Y, Tanaka F. Factors predicting the surgical outcome in patients with T3/4 lung cancer. Surg Today. 2014;44:2249–54. https://doi.org/10.1007/s00595-014-0861-0.
21. Rendina EA, Venuta F, De Giacomo T, et al. Induction chemotherapy for T4 centrally located non-small cell lung cancer. J Thorac Cardiovasc Surg. 1999;117:225–33.
22. De Leyn P, Dooms C, Kuzdzal J, Lardinois D, Passlick B, Rami-Porta R, et al. Revised ESTS guidelines for preoperative mediastinal lymph node staging for non-small-cell lung cancer. Eur J Cardiothorac Surg. 2014;45:787–98. https://doi.org/10.1093/ejcts/ezu028.
23. Pataer A, Kalhor N, Correa AM, Raso MG, Erasmus JJ, Kim ES, et al. Histopathologic response criteria predict survival of patients with resected lung cancer after neoadjuvant chemotherapy. J Thorac Oncol. 2012;7:825–32. https://doi.org/10.1097/JTO.0b013e318247504a.
24. Chaft JE, Shyr Y, Sepesi B, Forde PM. Preoperative and postoperative systemic therapy for operable non-small-cell lung cancer. J Clin Oncol. 2022;40:546–55. https://doi.org/10.1200/JCO.21.01589. Epub 2022 Jan 5.
25. Marulli G, Battistella L, Mammana M, Calabrese F, Rea F. Superior sulcus tumors (Pancoast tumors). Ann Transl Med. 2016;4:239. https://doi.org/10.21037/atm.2016.06.1.
26. Ramnath N, Dilling TJ, Harris LJ, Kim AW, Michaud GC, Balekian AA, et al. Treatment of stage III non-small cell lung cancer: diagnosis and management of lung cancer, 3rd ed: American College of Chest Physicians evidence-based clinical practice guidelines. Chest. 2013;143(Suppl 5):e314S–40S. https://doi.org/10.1378/chest.12-2360.
27. van Meerbeeck JP, Kramer GW, Van Schil PE, Legrand C, Smit EF, Schramel F, et al. Randomized controlled trial of resection versus radiotherapy after induction chemotherapy in stage IIIA-N2 non-small-cell lung cancer. J Natl Cancer Inst. 2007;99:442–50. https://doi.org/10.1093/jnci/djk093.
28. Albain KS, Swann RS, Rusch VW, Turrisi AT III, Shepherd FA, Smith C, et al. Radiotherapy plus chemotherapy with or without surgical resection for stage III non-small-cell lung cancer: a phase III randomised controlled trial. Lancet. 2009;374:379–86. https://doi.org/10.1016/S0140-6736(09)60737-6.
29. Eberhardt WE, Pottgen C, Gauler TC, Friedel G, Veit S, Heinrich V, et al. Phase III study of surgery versus definitive concurrent chemoradiotherapy boost in patients with resectable stage IIIA(N2) and selected IIIB non-small-cell lung cancer after induction chemotherapy and concurrent chemoradiotherapy (ESPATUE). J Clin Oncol. 2015;33:4194–201. https://doi.org/10.1200/JCO.2015.62.6812.
30. Xu XL, Dan L, Chen W, Zhu SM, Mao WM. Neoadjuvant chemoradiotherapy or chemotherapy followed by surgery is superior to that followed by definitive chemoradiation or radiotherapy in stage IIIA (N2) nonsmall-cell lung cancer : a meta-analysis and system review. Onco Targets Ther. 2016;9:845–53. https://doi.org/10.2147/OTT.S95511.
31. Liang J, Bi N, Wu S, Chen M, Lv C, Zhao L, et al. Etoposide and cisplatin versus paclitaxel and carboplatin with concurrent thoracic radiotherapy in unresectable stage III non-small cell lung cancer: a multicenter randomized phase III trial. Ann Oncol. 2017;28:777–83. https://doi.org/10.1093/annonc/mdx009.
32. Senan S, Brade A, Wang LH, Vansteenkiste J, Dakhil S, Biesma B, et al. PROCLAIM: randomized phase III trial of pemetrexed-cisplatin or etoposide-cisplatin plus thoracic radiation therapy followed by consolidation chemotherapy in locally advanced nonsquamous non-small-cell lung cancer. J Clin Oncol. 2016;34:953–62. https://doi.org/10.1200/JCO.2015.64.8824.
33. Pignon JP, Stewart LA. Randomized trials of radiotherapy alone versus combined chemotherapy and radiotherapy in stages IIIa and IIIb nonsmall cell lung cancer: a meta-analysis. Cancer. 1996;77:2413–4. https://doi.org/10.1002/(SICI)1097-0142(19960601)77:11<2413::AID-CNCR34>3.0.CO;2-Y.
34. Marino P, Preatoni A, Cantoni A. Randomized trials of radiotherapy alone versus combined chemotherapy and radiotherapy in stages IIIa and IIIb nonsmall cell lung cancer. A meta-analysis. Cancer. 1995;76:593–601. https://doi.org/10.1002/1097-0142(19950815)76:4<593::aid-cncr2820760409>3.0.co;2-n.
35. Pritchard RS, Anthony SP. Chemotherapy plus radiotherapy compared with radiotherapy alone in the treatment of locally advanced, unresectable, non-small-cell lung cancer. A

meta-analysis. Ann Intern Med. 1996;125:723–9. https://doi.org/10.7326/0003-4819-125-9 -199611010-00003.

36. Belani CP, Choy H, Bonomi P, Scott C, Travis P, Haluschak J, et al. Combined chemora-diotherapy regimens of paclitaxel and carboplatin for locally advanced non-small-cell lung cancer: a randomized phase II locally advanced multi-modality protocol. J Clin Oncol. 2005;23:5883–91. https://doi.org/10.1200/JCO.2005.55.405.

37. Aupérin A, Péchoux C, Rolland E, Curran WJ, Furuse K, Fournel P, et al. Meta-analysis of concomitant versus sequential radiochemotherapy in locally advanced non-small-cell lung cancer. J Clin Oncol. 2010;28:2181–90. https://doi.org/10.1200/JCO.2009.26.2543.

38. Zatloukal P, Petruzelka L, Zemanova M, Havel L, Janku F, Judas L, et al. Concurrent versus sequential chemoradiotherapy with cisplatin and vinorelbine in locally advanced non-small cell lung cancer: a randomized study. Lung Cancer. 2004;46:87–98. https://doi.org/10.1016/j.lungcan.2004.03.004.

39. Perez CA, Stanley K, Rubin P, Kramer S, Brady L, Perez-Tamayo R, et al. A prospective randomized study of various irradiation doses and fractionation schedules in the treatment of inoperable non-oat-cell carcinoma of the lung. Preliminary report by the Radiation Therapy Oncology Group. Cancer. 1980;45:2744–53. https://doi.org/10.1002/1097-0142(19800601)4 5:11<2744::aid-cncr2820451108>3.0.co;2-u.

40. Bradley JD, Paulus R, Komaki R, Masters G, Blumenschein G, Schild S, et al. A randomized phase III comparison of standard-dose (60 Gy) versus high-dose (74 Gy) conformal chemo-radiotherapy with or without cetuximab for stage III non-small cell lung cancer: results on radiation dose in RTOG 0617. J Clin Oncol. 2013;31(Suppl):7501. https://doi.org/10.1200/jco.2013.31.15_suppl.7501.

41. Bradley JD, Paulus R, Komaki R, Masters G, Blumenschein G, Schild S, et al. Standard-dose versus high-dose conformal radiotherapy with concurrent and consolidation carboplatin plus paclitaxel with or without cetuximab for patients with stage IIIA or IIIB non-small-cell lung cancer (RTOG 0617): a randomised, two-by-two factorial phase 3 study. Lancet Oncol. 2015;16:187–99. https://doi.org/10.1016/S1470-2045(14)71207-0.

42. Hong JC, Salama JK. Dose escalation for unresectable locally advanced non-small cell lung cancer: end of the line? Transl Lung Cancer Res. 2016;5:126–33. https://doi.org/10.3978/j.issn.2218-6751.2016.01.07.

43. Bradley JD, Hu C, Komaki R, Masters G, Blumenschein G, Schild S, et al. Long-term results of NRG Oncology RTOG 0617: standard- versus high-dose chemoradiotherapy with or without cetuximab for unresectable stage III non-small-cell lung cancer. J Clin Oncol. 2020;38:706–14. https://doi.org/10.1200/JCO.19.01162.

44. Yom SS, Liao Z, Liu HH, Tucker SL, Hu CS, Wei X, et al. Initial evaluation of treatment-related pneumonitis in advanced-stage non-small-cell lung cancer patients treated with con-current chemotherapy and intensity-modulated radiotherapy. Int J Radiat Oncol Biol Phys. 2007;68:94–102. https://doi.org/10.1016/j.ijrobp.2006.12.031.

45. Kamran SC, Yeap BY, Ulysse CA, Cronin C, Bowes C, Durgin B, et al. Assessment of a con-tralateral esophagus-sparing technique in locally advanced lung cancer treated with high-dose chemoradiation: a phase 1 nonrandomized clinical trial. JAMA Oncol. 2021;7:910–4. https://doi.org/10.1001/jamaoncol.2021.0281.

46. Chun SG, Hu C, Choy H, Komaki R, Timmerman RD, Schild SE, et al. Impact of intensity-modulated radiation therapy technique for locally advanced non-small-cell lung cancer: a sec-ondary analysis of the NRG oncology RTOG 0617 randomized clinical trial. J Clin Oncol. 2017;35:56–62. https://doi.org/10.1200/JCO.2016.69.1378.

47. Koshy M, Malik R, Spiotto M, Mahmood U, Rusthoven CG, Sher DJ. Association between intensity modulated radiotherapy and survival in patients with stage III non-small cell lung can-cer treated with chemoradiotherapy. Lung Cancer. 2017;108:222–7. https://doi.org/10.1016/j.lungcan.2017.04.006.

48. Jegadeesh N, Liu Y, Gillespie T, Fernandez F, Ramalingam S, Mikell J, et al. Evaluating intensity-modulated radiation therapy in locally advanced non-small-cell lung cancer:

results from the national cancer data base. Clin Lung Cancer. 2016;17:398–405. https://doi.org/10.1016/j.cllc.2016.01.007.

49. Chang YJ, Verma V, Li M, Zhang W, Komaki R, Lu C, et al. Proton beam radiotherapy and concurrent chemotherapy for unresectable stage III non-small cell lung cancer: final results of a phase 2 study. JAMA Oncol. 2017;3:e172032. https://doi.org/10.1001/jamaoncol.2017.2032.

50. Nguyen QN, Ly NB, Komaki R, Levy LB, Gomez DR, Chang JY, et al. Long-term outcomes after proton therapy, with concurrent chemotherapy, for stage II-III inoperable non-small cell lung cancer. Radiother Oncol. 2015;115:367–72. https://doi.org/10.1016/j.radonc.2015.05.014.

51. Oonishi K, Ishikawa H, Nakazawa K, Shiozawa T, Mori Y, Nakamura M, et al. Long-term outcomes of high-dose (74 GyE) proton beam therapy with concurrent chemotherapy for stage III non-small-cell lung cancer. Thorac Cancer. 2021;12:1320–7. https://doi.org/10.1111/1759-7714.13896.

52. Liao ZX, Lee JJ, Komaki R, Gomez DR, O'Reilly MS, Fossella FV, et al. Bayesian adaptive randomization trial of passive scattering proton therapy and intensity-modulated photon radiotherapy for locally advanced non-small-cell lung cancer. J Clin Oncol. 2018;36:1813–22. https://doi.org/10.1200/JCO.2017.74.0720.

53. Daly ME, Monjazeb AM, Kelly K. Clinical trials integrating immunotherapy and radiation for non–small-cell lung cancer. J Thorac Oncol. 2015;10:1685–93. https://doi.org/10.1097/JTO.0000000000000686.

54. Reckamp K, Radman MW, Dragnev KH, Minichiello K, Villaruz LC, Faller B, et al. Phase II randomized study of ramucirumab and pembrolizumab versus standard of care in advanced non-small-cell lung cancer previously treated with immunotherapy-Lung-MAP S1800A. J Clin Oncol. 2022;40:2295–306. https://doi.org/10.1200/JCO.22.00912.

55. Durm GA, Jabbour SK, Althouse SK, Liu Z, Sadiq AA, Zon RT, et al. A phase 2 trial of consolidation pembrolizumab following concurrent chemoradiation for patients with unresectable stage III non-small cell lung cancer: Hoosier Cancer Research Network LUN 14-179. Cancer. 2020;126:4353–61. https://doi.org/10.1002/cncr.33083.

56. Garassino M, Gadgeel S, Esteban E, Felip E, Speranza G, Domine M, et al. Patient-reported outcomes following pembrolizumab or placebo plus pemetrexed and platinum in patients with previously untreated, metastatic, non-squamous non-small-cell lung cancer (KEYNOTE-189): a multicentre, double-blind, randomised, placebo-controlled, phase 3 trial. Lancet Oncol. 2020;21:387–97. https://doi.org/10.1016/S1470-2045(19)30801-0.

57. Peters S, Spigel D, Ahn M, Tsuboi M, Chaft J, Harpole D, et al. MERMAID-1: A phase III study of adjuvant durvalumab plus chemotherapy in resected NSCLC patients with MRD+ post-surgery. J Thorac Oncol. 2021;16(Suppl 3):S258–9. https://doi.org/10.1016/j.jtho.2021.01.376.

58. Provencio M, Nadal E, Insa A, García-Campelo MR, Casal-Rubio J, Dómine M, et al. Neoadjuvant chemotherapy and nivolumab in resectable non-small-cell lung cancer (NADIM): an open-label, multicentre, single-arm, phase 2 trial. Lancet Oncol. 2020;21:1413–22. https://doi.org/10.1016/S1470-2045(20)30453-8.

59. Provencio M, Serna-Blasco R, Nadal E, Insa A, García-Campelo MR, Casal-Rubio J, et al. Overall survival and biomarker analysis of neoadjuvant nivolumab plus chemotherapy in operable stage IIIA non-small-cell lung cancer (NADIM phase II trial). J Clin Oncol. 2022;40:2924. https://doi.org/10.1200/JCO.21.02660.

60. Forde PM, Spicer J, Lu S, Provencio M, Mitsudomi T, Awad MM, et al. Neoadjuvant nivolumab plus chemotherapy in resectable lung cancer. N Engl J Med. 2022;386:1973–85. https://doi.org/10.1056/NEJMoa2202170.

61. Grimaldi AM, Simeone E, Giannarelli D, Muto P, Falivene S, Borzillo V, et al. Abscopal effects of radiotherapy on advanced melanoma patients who progressed after ipilimumab immunotherapy. Onco Targets Ther. 2014;3:e28780. https://doi.org/10.4161/onci.28780.

62. Franzi S, Mattioni G, Rijavec E, Croci GA, Tosi D. Neoadjuvant chemo-immunotherapy for locally advanced non-small-cell-lung cancer: a review of the literature. J Clin Med. 2022;11:2629. https://doi.org/10.3390/jcm11092629.

63. Antonia SJ, Villegas A, Daniel D, Vicente D, Murakami S, Hui R, et al. Durvalumab after chemoradiotherapy in stage III non-small-cell lung cancer. N Engl J Med. 2017;377:1919–29. https://doi.org/10.1056/NEJMoa1709937.
64. Antonia SJ, Villegas A, Daniel D, Vicente D, Murakami S, Hui R, et al. Overall survival with durvalumab after chemoradiotherapy in stage III NSCLC. N Engl J Med. 2018;379:2342–50. https://doi.org/10.1056/NEJMoa1809697.
65. Spigel DR, Faivre-Finn C, Gray JE, Vicente D, Planchard D, Paz-Ares L, et al. Five-year survival outcomes from the PACIFIC trial: durvalumab after chemoradiotherapy in stage III non-small-cell lung cancer. J Clin Oncol. 2022;40:1301–11. https://doi.org/10.1200/JCO.21.01308.
66. Qin Q, Peng B, Li B. The impact of epidermal growth factor receptor mutations on the efficacy of definitive chemoradiotherapy in patients with locally advanced unresectable stage III non-small cell lung cancer: a systematic review and meta-analysis. Expert Rev Anticancer Ther. 2019;19:533–9. https://doi.org/10.1080/14737140.2019.1621754.
67. Blumenschein GR Jr, Paulus R, Curran WJ, Robert F, Fossella F, Werner-Wasik M, et al. Phase II study of cetuximab in combination with chemoradiation in patients with stage IIIA/B non-small-cell lung cancer: RTOG 0324. J Clin Oncol. 2011;29:2312–8. https://doi.org/10.1200/JCO.2010.31.7875.
68. Govindan R, Bogart J, Stinchcombe T, Wang X, Hodgson L, Kratzke R, et al. Randomized phase II study of pemetrexed, carboplatin, and thoracic radiation with or without cetuximab in patients with locally advanced unresectable non-small-cell lung cancer: Cancer and Leukemia Group B trial 30407. J Clin Oncol. 2011;29:3120–5. https://doi.org/10.1200/JCO.2010.33.4979.
69. Kelly K, Chansky K, Gaspar LE, Albain KS, Jett J, Ung YC, et al. Phase III trial of maintenance gefitinib or placebo after concurrent chemoradiotherapy and docetaxel consolidation in inoperable stage III non–small-cell lung cancer: SWOG S0023. J Clin Oncol. 2008;26:2450–6. https://doi.org/10.1200/JCO.2007.14.4824.

Chapter 8
Treatment of Stage IV Non-small Cell Lung Cancer

Thomas Yang Sun and Millie Das

Introduction

Lung cancer is the leading cause of death among all cancers worldwide, with roughly two million deaths each year; the number of new lung cancer cases continues to rise [1]. In the United States, the number of deaths from lung cancer exceeds the total of those from breast, prostate, and colon cancer combined [2]. Unfortunately most lung cancers are diagnosed at stage IV, with an incidence rate of roughly 20 per 100,000 persons, representing more than twice the rate of the earlier stages [3]. The 5-year survival rate for patients with stage IV cancer has improved due to advances from new therapies, but remains below 10% [4]. The advent of immunotherapy and targeted therapies has significantly improved survival outcomes for this patient population over the last 10 years. In this chapter, we review these exciting new treatment advances for stage IV non-small cell lung cancer (NSCLC) and provide a suggested treatment algorithm.

Stage IV NSCLC remains incurable except in rare circumstances, and systemic therapy is usually the recommended approach. Current therapy options are either single agent or combinations of the following: chemotherapy, biologic agents, molecularly targeted therapy, and immunotherapy.

Historically, chemotherapy has been the only treatment option. A meta-analysis showed that chemotherapy confers roughly a 10% absolute survival benefit over

T. Y. Sun
Division of Oncology, Department of Medicine, Stanford University School of Medicine, Palo Alto, CA, USA

M. Das (✉)
Division of Oncology, Department of Medicine, Stanford University School of Medicine, Palo Alto, CA, USA

Department of Medicine, Veteran Affairs Palo Alto Healthcare System, Palo Alto, CA, USA
e-mail: mdas@stanford.edu

C. MacRosty, M. P. Rivera (eds.), *Lung Cancer*, Respiratory Medicine,
https://doi.org/10.1007/978-3-031-38412-7_8

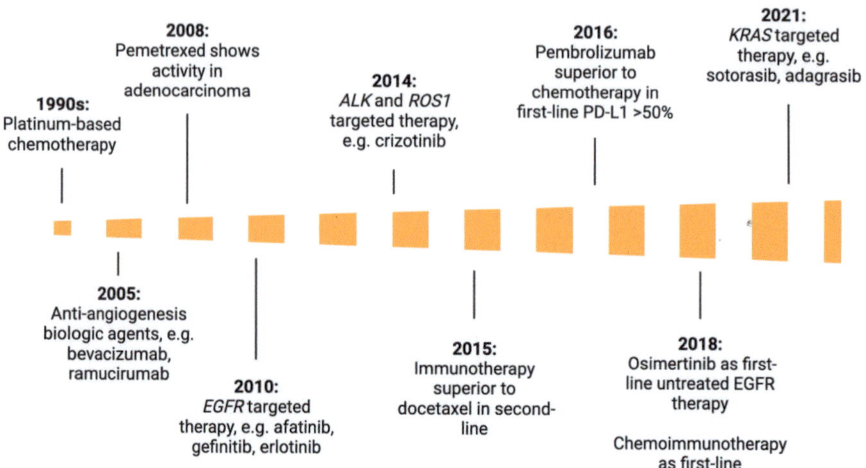

Fig. 8.1 Timeline of practice changing therapy updates for stage IV NSCLC

best supportive care [5] resulting in the adoption of platinum-based doublet chemotherapy in the 1990s. Beginning in 2005, antiangiogenic biologic agents such as bevacizumab and ramucirumab were found to provide a small but statistically significant increase in overall survival (OS) of approximately 5%, particularly in adenocarcinoma subtypes (see Fig. 8.1) [6]. The next advance in lung cancer treatment began in 2010 when the first molecularly targeted therapies became available for those NSCLC tumors with an underlying driver gene, most notably epidermal growth factor receptor (EGFR). In 2016, the first trials involving novel checkpoint inhibitors in patients with advanced NSCLC were published, and over time immunotherapy has become frontline therapy for some patients with stage IV disease, with durable responses in select patients that hint at the possibility of cure [7].

Choosing First-Line Therapy

Histology

The first step in deciding upfront treatment for stage IV NSCLC is to determine the histologic subtype of the tumor, as biological behavior and treatment options vary widely based upon this characteristic. The main subtypes of NSCLC are adenocarcinoma, squamous cell carcinoma (SCC), and large cell neuroendocrine carcinoma (LCNEC). Other rarer histologic subtypes include adenosquamous and sarcomatoid carcinoma [8]. Approximately 40% of NSCLCs are adenocarcinomas, 25–30% are SCCs, and 10–15% are LCNECs [9]. A suggested treatment algorithm is shown in Fig. 8.2.

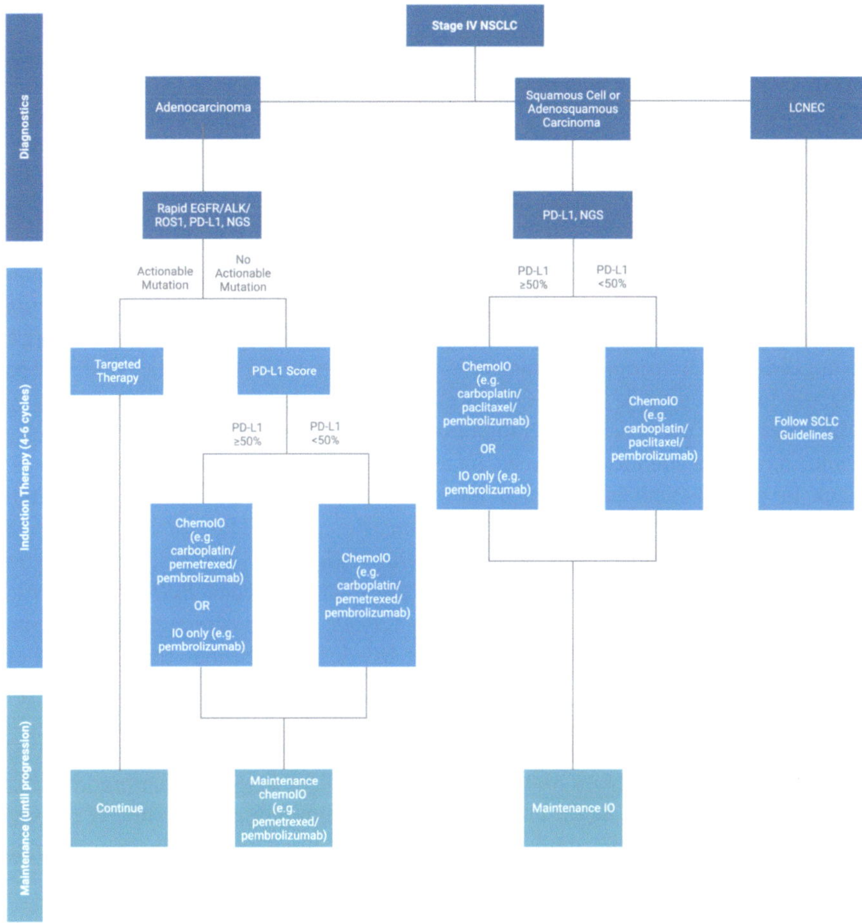

Fig. 8.2 Treatment algorithm for newly diagnosed stage IV NSCLC. *NSCLC* non-small cell lung cancer, *LCNEC* large cell neuroendocrine carcinoma, *NGS* next-generation sequencing, *IO* immunotherapy, *SCLC* small cell lung cancer

Adenocarcinoma Versus Squamous Cell Carcinoma

There are differences in the treatment approach for adenocarcinomas compared to squamous cell carcinomas. Pemetrexed is recommended and approved for the treatment of lung adenocarcinomas, but not for SCCs, due to greater efficacy and better tolerability compared to other chemotherapeutic agents [10]. A pivotal phase III trial in 2008 comparing cisplatin/gemcitabine with cisplatin/pemetrexed found that among patients with non-SCC cancers, OS was superior in the pemetrexed group (12.6 months vs. 10.9 months) but was inferior among patients with SCC cancers (9.4 months vs. 10.8 months) [11]. Patients who received pemetrexed had better tolerability with lower rates of severe neutropenia, anemia, thrombocytopenia, and alopecia. Similar trials have found greater tolerability with pemetrexed over pacli-taxel and docetaxel [12]. Pemetrexed is therefore a preferred chemotherapeutic agent in the treatment of adenocarcinomas.

Another difference lies in the use of antiangiogenic biologic agents. A random-ized phase II trial of 99 patients comparing chemotherapy with and without bevaci-zumab noted excessively high rates of life-threatening pulmonary hemorrhage in 4 of 13 patients with SCC (31%) compared to 2 of 54 patients with non-SCC (4%) [13]. Due to this increased toxicity, subsequent studies have excluded SCC histol-ogy from bevacizumab trials, and bevacizumab is avoided in patients with squa-mous histology. While bevacizumab is a monoclonal antibody targeting vascular-endothelial growth factor A (VEGF-A), ramucirumab was later developed to target the VEGF receptor. In the phase 3 REVEL trial, 1253 patients with relapsed disease, including those with SCCs, were randomized to receive either docetaxel with placebo or docetaxel with ramucirumab [14]. The rate of serious pulmonary hemorrhage was identical between patients with non-SCC and SCC (1% each). Thus, for patients who are treatment naïve, bevacizumab should only be considered for those with non-SCC histology, while ramucirumab could be considered for both SCC and non-SCC histology in the second-line setting.

Finally, actionable mutations, such as those in the genes *EGFR*, anaplastic lymphoma kinase (*ALK*), c-ros oncogene 1 (*ROS1*), and Kiersten rat sarcoma virus (*KRAS*), are more frequently present in adenocarcinomas than SCCs. For example, *EGFR* mutations occur in approximately 15% of adenocarcinomas in the United States and can be seen at an incidence rate as high as 60% in Asian populations [15, 16]. In contrast, *EGFR* mutations are present in only 0–3% of SCCs [17]. Similarly, *KRAS* mutations occur in 30% of lung adenocarcinomas but are only seen in 5% of SCCs [18]. As a result, rapid molecular testing is recom-mended for those tumors with any component of adenocarcinoma but remains optional for SCC.

Large Cell Neuroendocrine Carcinoma

Large cell neuroendocrine carcinoma (LCNEC) has historically been categorized with NSCLC, despite being a high-grade neuroendocrine neoplasm similar to small cell lung cancer (SCLC). This grouping is the result of initial gene panel sequencing studies showing LCNEC mutational patterns more closely resembling NSCLC than SCLC. In a retrospective study of 45 LCNEC samples involving testing of 241 genes, most (56%) had genomic profiles closer to a NSCLC geno-type, while fewer (40%) mirrored those of SCLC [19]. More recent comprehen-sive whole exome and transcriptome studies have demonstrated the opposite; despite sharing common gene mutations with adenocarcinomas and SCCs, LCNECs bear no transcriptional similarity to them but instead closely resemble SCLCs [20]. Clinically, survival outcomes of LCNEC are also more similar to SCLC than NSCLC [21, 22].

For these reasons, we and others recommend that the treatment of LCNEC follows that of SCLC [23]. However, treating LCNEC with a NSCLC regimen is an accepted practice as LCNEC is commonly included in NSCLC trials [11, 24]. As LCNEC is relatively rare, there is no high-quality data comparing survival outcomes between NSCLC and SCLC regimens. One retrospective analysis of 79 cases showed that cases which were *RB1* wildtype treated with a NSCLC regimen (platinum with gemcitabine or with a taxane) had longer OS (9.6 months vs. 5.8 months) than when treated with a SCLC regimen (platinum with etoposide) [25]. Notably, in this study, the LCNEC cases with *RB1* mutation had similar outcomes when treated with different regimens. This study is limited by its retrospective nature and lack of multivariable survival analysis. A test of interaction between *RB1* status and type of chemotherapy regimen was not statistically significant. Thus, in clinical practice, we currently do not routinely decide treatment based on *RB1* status and normally prescribe a SCLC regimen for patients with LCNEC histology based upon recent data indicating greater similarity in tumor biology between these two histologies.

Sarcomatoid Carcinoma

Pulmonary sarcomatoid carcinoma is a rare subtype that comprises 0.1–0.4% of all lung tumors [26]. Most patients are elderly men with a significant smoking history. Sarcomatoid carcinoma is marked by aggressive invasiveness and is associated with poor prognosis and response to treatment with 8% response rate to chemotherapy and median OS of 9.9 months [27]. There is no standard treatment regimen for this rare disease, and combinations such as platinum doublet chemotherapy with immunotherapy are reasonable. In our practice, we commonly use a taxane or gemcitabine, as opposed to pemetrexed, in combination with platinum and immunotherapy, as these two chemotherapy agents demonstrate greater activity in soft tissue sarcomas.

Actionable Mutations

Since 2010, the development of targeted therapies that could inhibit the growth of those tumors driven by the presence of a single genetic driver, also called oncogene addiction, has dramatically altered the treatment landscape and significantly prolonged survival for select groups of patients. Such tailored therapies could translate to a survival benefit of several months to years. For instance, the first-generation *EGFR* inhibitor, gefitinib, conferred an additional 6.9 months of OS on average when compared to chemotherapy in a phase III randomized controlled trial (RCT) [28]. In many instances, targeted therapy has superseded chemotherapy or chemoimmunotherapy as the preferred frontline option due to higher response rates, improved tolerance, and the convenience of oral administration.

When deciding on treatment, once the specific histology of the NSCLC is ascertained, it is next important to determine whether the subtype—usually adenocarcinoma—is associated with a high probability of harboring a driver mutation that could be amenable to targeted therapy. For any NSCLC with at least a component of adenocarcinoma, molecular testing is recommended. First-line therapies exist for gene alterations in *EGFR, ALK, ROS1, BRAF, NTRK 1/2/3, MET* exon 14 skipping mutation, and *RET* (Table 8.1).

EGFR

EGFR is a cell-surface tyrosine kinase receptor that when activated results in rapid cell division and migration thru mediation of Ras/MAPK, PI3K/AKT, and STAT pathways [29]. Mutations of this gene can be found in 15–60% of adenocarcinomas, with higher prevalence in nonsmoking Asian populations [15, 16]. Beginning in 2009, landmark trials involving *EGFR*-targeted inhibitors, such as the IPASS study, demonstrated superior efficacy of *EGFR* tyrosine kinase inhibitors (TKIs) over conventional platinum doublet chemotherapy in the first-line setting [30]. Patients who developed resistance to the first- or second-generation TKIs, and were noted to have a T790M substitution mutation in EGFR (seen in 60% cases of acquired resistance), could then be offered osimertinib, a third-generation TKI [31]. In 2018, results from the phase 3 FLAURA demonstrated that patients with previously untreated EGFR-mutation positive disease who received osimertinib had significantly improved OS compared to those treated with an earlier generation TKI (38.6 months vs. 31.8 months), despite a 31% crossover rate [32]. As a result of this pivotal trial, osimertinib is now the preferred first-line option for those patients with tumors harboring any of the following sensitizing EGFR mutations: exon 19 deletion, L858R, S768I, L861Q, and G719X. Notably, *EGFR* exon 20 insertion mutations are not susceptible to oral TKIs, and systemic platinum-based chemotherapy is usually recommended frontline.

Table 8.1 Less common actionable targets and potential targeted therapy options

Driver gene	Frequency in NSCLCs (%)	Targeted therapy
ROS1	1	Crizotinib, entrectinib
HER2	1–3	Fam-trastuzumab deruxtecan, ado-trastuzumab emtansine[a]
MET exon 14 skipping	1–3	Capmatinib, tepotinib
BRAF V600E	1–3	Dabrafenib + trametinib
RET	1–2	Selpercatinib, pralsetinib
NTRK	<1	Larotrectinib, entrectinib

[a] Not yet FDA approved for this indication

ALK

Chromosomal rearrangements involving the *ALK* gene are found in approximately 3–5% of NSCLCs, particularly in patients who have never smoked [33]. An oncogenic protein made by *ELM4-ALK* fusion is the most common [34]. Unlike *EGFR* mutations which are detected by gene sequencing methods, *ALK* alterations can also be found by fluorescence in situ hybridization (FISH) or immunohistochemistry (IHC) testing, which in some institutions can offer a more rapid turnaround time [35]. A pivotal trial in 2014 that randomized patients with *ALK* positive tumors to either the ALK inhibitor crizotinib or standard chemotherapy found that patients treated with crizotinib had a substantially higher overall response rate (ORR, 74% vs. 45%), longer progression-free survival (PFS; 10.9 months vs. 7 months), and longer OS when adjusted for crossover [36]. This trial showed impressive survival rates with most patients (56.6%) on the crizotinib arm still alive at 4 years. Superseding the first-generation crizotinib are the newer ALK TKIs alectinib, brigatinib, and lorlatinib which have all shown higher overall response rate (ORR) and substantially longer PFS when compared to crizotinib and are now FDA-approved frontline options for patients with *ALK* gene rearrangements [37–39]. In the phase III ALEX study which compared alectinib to crizotinib, ORR was 82.9% vs. 75.5%, and PFS was three times longer (34.8 months vs. 10.9 months), favoring patients treated with alectinib [40]. It is unclear which of the newer agents is the most efficacious, as there has been no trial comparing them. Alectinib is the most commonly used first-line ALK TKI given the longer-term follow-up data available and overall good tolerability of this drug. Lorlatinib is often considered as second-line therapy due to its efficacy in tumors that have developed acquired resistance to prior ALK therapy, though this drug is more frequently associated with edema and cognitive side effects that need to be considered [41].

ROS1

Approximately 1% of NSCLC is driven by chromosomal rearrangements involving the *ROS1* gene [42]. Similar to *EGFR*- and *ALK*-mutated tumors, *ROS1* tumors are often found in younger patients with no smoking history. Like *ALK*-driven NSCLC, *ROS1* translocations can be detected by FISH and IHC in addition to gene sequencing. First-line FDA-approved treatment options for patients with *ROS1*-positive NSCLC are crizotinib and entrectinib. A single-arm, international trial of 50 patients treated with crizotinib noted an impressive ORR of 72%, with a median PFS of 19.2 months and OS of 51 months [43]. In another study, patients with *ROS1*-positive NSCLC treated with entrectinib had a similar ORR of 67.1% and median PFS of 15.7 months [44]. Notably, entrectinib was associated with an impressive intracranial ORR of 79.2%. As up to a third of ROS1 patients develop intracranial metastasis, entrectinib is now the preferred frontline option in this setting given the more limited CNS penetration of crizotinib [45].

KRAS G12C

The most commonly altered driver gene in NSCLC is *KRAS*, accounting for roughly 30% of all NSCLC cases [18]. Among the various *KRAS* mutations, about half are *KRAS* G12C. For years, these mutations were considered "undruggable" due to the lack of a suitable pocket on the protein surface that could be bound by a drug molecule. Recent breakthroughs in drug design led to the development of sotorasib and adagrasib, both oral agents that specifically target *KRAS* G12C. These drugs have been tested in the second-line setting, with ORRs in the range of 30–45% and PFS of 6–8 months [46, 47]. The overall benefit of these *KRAS* G12C inhibitors appear to be less significant compared to the results seen with targeted therapies against *EGFR/ALK/ROS1*, which commonly have ORR exceeding 70% and PFS on the order of years. Sotorasib was FDA approved in May 2021 as a second-line therapy option, while adagrasib was FDA approved more recently in December 2022. There are ongoing clinical trials evaluating these agents in the first-line setting.

HER2

Human epidermal growth factor receptor 2 (ERBB2 or HER2) is altered in roughly 1–3% of NSCLC tumors [48]. *HER2* alterations could either be point mutations (most common in NSCLC), amplifications, or overexpression and primarily affect patients who have never smoked with a female predominance. Outside of a clinical trial, first-line treatment for these patients is usually systemic therapy with platinum doublet chemotherapy. The efficacy of checkpoint inhibitors in the treatment of *HER2*+ NSCLC remains controversial given poor responses seen in some studies but not all [49]. HER2-targeted antibody-drug conjugates have been studied in the second-line setting, including ado-trastuzumab and fam-trastuzumab deruxtecan which have both shown efficacy in patients with HER2+ breast cancer [50]. Ado-trastuzumab emtansine was studied in a phase II trial involving 18 patients with *HER2*-mutated NSCLC and demonstrated an ORR of 44% and a median PFS of 5 months [51]. In the DESTINY-Lung01 trial of 91 lung cancer patients with a HER2 mutation who were administered fam-trastuzumab deruxtecan, an ORR of 55% and a median PFS of 8.2 months were seen [52]. These results led to the FDA granting accelerated approval to trastuzumab deruxtecan in August 2022 in patients with *HER2*-mutated metastatic NSCLC who have received prior systemic therapy. There are also HER2-targeted oral TKIs that are being investigated in ongoing clinical trials with promising results to date. For instance, poziotinib is an oral agent shown to confer an ORR of 27% in a single-arm phase II trial [53].

MET Exon 14, RET, BRAF V600E, and NTRK

The MET (c-Met encoding) gene can be mutated in up to 3% of NSCLCs [54]. In tumors with deletions involving exon 14 (MET exon-14-skipping mutation), the oral targeted inhibitors capmatinib and tepotinib have demonstrated promising results in the first- and second-line settings with ORR ranging from 41% to 68% and median duration of response at 10–11 months [55, 56].

A number of other driver genes have been identified at lower frequencies (~1–3% of NSCLC), including *RET* (rearranged during transfection) gene rearrangements, *BRAF* (B-Raf) V600E (1–2% of NSCLC), and *NTRK* (neurotrophic tyrosine receptor kinase) fusions (<1% of NSCLC) [57]. If sequencing results are noted prior to treatment initiation, patients with these alterations could be treated with the associated targeted therapy as first-line treatment, or alternatively as part of later-line therapy. A summary of the less common molecular driver mutations with associated targeted therapies are shown in Table 8.1 [58–60].

Chemotherapy

The benefit of chemotherapy over best supportive care was conclusively demonstrated in a 2008 meta-analysis of 16 RCTs which showed an absolute improvement in OS of approximately 10% at 1 year [5]. A second meta-analysis examined trials which compared regimens comprising of one, two, or three chemotherapeutic agents and found a doublet regimen to be the most effective in terms of improving survival without undue toxicity risk [61]. A doublet regimen over single-agent chemotherapy increased response rate from 13% to 26% (13% absolute benefit) and increased survival at 1-year from 30% to 35% (5% absolute benefit). A triplet regimen, however, while increasing response rate over doublets from 23% to 31% (8% absolute benefit), showed no survival difference and was associated with greater toxicity.

Doublet regimens are therefore the standard for metastatic NSCLC, and trials examining various combinations of agents including cisplatin, carboplatin, paclitaxel, docetaxel, gemcitabine, and vinorelbine have found that platinum-based regimens have a slight survival advantage [62]. When comparing the two platinum options, a meta-analysis of 4792 patients in 17 RCTs found that cisplatin-based treatment had a higher response rate compared to carboplatin, but toxicity was greater and survival outcomes were likely similar [63]. Given that stage IV NSCLC is considered incurable and is often diagnosed in older patients, carboplatin-based regimens are often preferred due to better tolerability. However, in cases where a response is needed quickly, such as tumor obstruction causing severe end organ injury, or for younger patients, cisplatin may be a reasonable option.

Various trials have examined the ideal agent to pair with platinum [64, 65]. A cooperative group trial of 1207 patients randomized to one of four possible platinum doublet regimens (cisplatin/paclitaxel, carboplatin/paclitaxel, cisplatin/gemcitabine, or cisplatin/docetaxel) found no survival difference between the regimens [66]. Over the years, platinum/pemetrexed has emerged to be the preferred frontline regimen for patients with adenocarcinoma given that multiple trials have demonstrated noninferiority in OS of platinum/pemetrexed compared to platinum/gemcitabine, but with greater tolerability [11, 24]. In the case of SCCs, pemetrexed is not recommended due to inferior survival outcomes (hazard ratio, HR 1.2–1.5) when compared to gemcitabine or a taxane [67]. In the United States, platinum/paclitaxel or platinum/nab-paclitaxel are two commonly used regimens in patients with SCC histology. In one randomized phase 3 study of 1052 patients comparing these two regimens, nab-paclitaxel was found to result in significantly improved ORR (41% vs. 24%), longer OS (12.1 months vs. 11.2 months), and better tolerability, especially in patients over 70 years old [68]. However, this drug is more costly and requires weekly infusions.

In general, 4–6 cycles of chemotherapy is recommended, after which the platinum is discontinued due to excessive rates of toxicity, including neuropathy [69]. A meta-analysis of five trials comparing four versus six cycles of chemotherapy did not demonstrate a survival difference with more cycles, but did detect a small increase in toxicity, e.g., a 5% absolute increase in the incidence of grade 3 or higher anemia [70]. Given the concern for additional toxicity resulting from other drugs being added to platinum doublet therapy frontline, such as immunotherapy or an anti-VEGF agent, four cycles is often preferred.

Bevacizumab

Bevacizumab is an anti-VEGF-A antibody which functions by inhibiting tumor angiogenesis. Due to excessive risks of pulmonary hemorrhage noted in SCCs, particularly in more centrally located and cavitary lesions, its use has been limited to non-SCC tumors not adjacent to major blood vessels [71]. A meta-analysis of four randomized phase II and phase III trials, totaling 2194 patients who were randomized to receive chemotherapy with or without bevacizumab, found a modest absolute OS benefit of 4% at 1 year (from 51% to 55%) at the risk of increased toxicity (proteinuria, hypertension, hemorrhage, neutropenia; odds ratio 2–5) [6]. With certain exceptions, such as *EGFR* or *ALK*-driven NSCLC, which are felt to benefit less from immunotherapy, the use of bevacizumab in the first-line setting has largely been supplanted by chemoimmunotherapy due to significantly higher response rates and improved survival outcomes when comparing results across trials. Patients who have contraindications to immunotherapy, such as those with severe pre-existing autoimmune disease, may benefit from chemotherapy with bevacizumab as a frontline treatment option.

Immunotherapy

Single Agent Immunotherapy: Anti-PD1/PD-L1

The discovery of anti-PD1/PD-L1 inhibitors has drastically changed the treatment landscape for stage IV lung cancer. Successive landmark trials demonstrated the impressive efficacy of these checkpoint inhibitors, and over time these drugs have become part of the standard frontline regimen for most lung cancers [72].

The first positive trials that led to FDA approval of immunotherapy in NSCLC were published in 2015 in the relapsed setting. CheckMate017 and CheckMate057 were two phase 3 RCTs which compared the role of nivolumab, an anti-PD1 monoclonal antibody, to docetaxel in pretreated patients. In CheckMate017, which enrolled patients with SCC, median OS was superior for the nivolumab group (9.2 months vs. 6.0 months) [73]. A similar 3-month survival advantage was seen in CheckMate057 which enrolled patients with non-SCC (12.2 months vs. 9.4 months) [74]. A similar trial, KEYNOTE-010 involving pembrolizumab, another anti-PD1 antibody, was conducted in the relapsed setting for patients with a PD-L1 tumor proportion score (TPS) of at least 1%. This study also demonstrated a survival benefit in patients receiving pembrolizumab compared to those receiving docetaxel, with OS of 12.7 months vs. 8.5 months, respectively [75]. These results were replicated with atezolizumab, an anti-PD-L1 antibody, in the POPLAR and OAK trials [76, 77]. A common theme across trials was the increased OS benefit seen for patients with higher PD-L1 expression. For example, in KEYNOTE-010, the most pronounced OS benefit was seen in the subgroup of patients with PD-L1 tumor proportion score (TPS) $\geq 50\%$, with a median OS of 17.3 months compared to 8.2 months (pembrolizumab vs. docetaxel).

The initial success of immunotherapy in the PD-L1 positive population led to the design of multiple RCTs that compared checkpoint inhibitors with platinum-based chemotherapy in the first-line setting. The phase 3 RCT KEYNOTE-042 enrolled patients with no *EGFR* or *ALK* mutations and with at least a PD-L1 score of 1% and found that patients treated with pembrolizumab had an improvement in OS by 4.6–7.8 months compared to those treated with platinum doublet chemotherapy, with greater benefit seen in those with a higher PD-L1 score [78]. For patients with PD-L1 TPS of $\geq 50\%$, median OS was 20.0 months vs. 12.2 months; $\geq 20\%$ was 17.7 months vs. 13.0 months; $\geq 1\%$ was 16.7 months vs. 12.1 months, favoring pembrolizumab. Based upon this data, the FDA expanded the approval of pembrolizumab to include first-line treatment of patients with advanced stage NSCLC with PD-L1 $\geq 1\%$.

A series of other trials selectively enrolled patients with PD-L1 $\geq 50\%$ due to the higher probability of efficacy with single-agent immunotherapy. KEYNOTE-024 noted a median OS of 30.0 months with pembrolizumab compared to 14.2 months with chemotherapy [79]. IMPOWER110 investigated atezolizumab also in the frontline setting against chemotherapy and found a similar 7.1-month OS benefit in patients with PD-L1 score $\geq 50\%$ (20.2 months vs. 13.1 months) [80]. EMPOWER-Lung1 assigned patients with PD-L1 $\geq 50\%$ to receive either cemiplimab (anti-PD1 antibody) or platinum doublet chemotherapy and found improved OS in those treated with cemiplimab (median OS not reached vs. 14.2 months) [81]. Given the result of these multiple trials, single-agent immunotherapy is now one of the recommended first-line options for patients with PD-L1 $\geq 50\%$. Pembrolizumab, atezolizumab, and cemiplimab are FDA-approved for this indication.

Chemoimmunotherapy

The results of immunotherapy trials have revolutionized the treatment landscape of stage 4 NSCLCs. An initial inferior survival is seen in the immunotherapy arms of multiple trials within the first 6–12 months of treatment, before a survival benefit emerges [78, 82]. This may be explained by the slower onset of action from immunotherapy. This phenomenon, along with other preclinical data showing the ability of chemotherapy to induce PD-L1 expression on tumor cells, has suggested that the combination of chemotherapy with immunotherapy may be synergistic. Their combination became the subject of subsequent investigation in multiple landmark trials [83].

KEYNOTE-189 enrolled 616 previously untreated patients with non-squamous NSCLC and assigned them to receive platinum/pemetrexed with experimental drug (pembrolizumab or placebo) every 3 weeks for four cycles followed by maintenance treatment with pemetrexed plus pembrolizumab/placebo for up to 35 total cycles [84]. The pembrolizumab triplet arm nearly doubled the OS of the doublet arm (22.0 months vs. 10.7 months). The survival advantage was clearly seen in all patients regardless of PD-L1 score. The increase in response rate was similarly impressive: 47.6% vs. 18.9%. KEYNOTE-407 was the counterpart trial for SCC NSCLC, substituting pemetrexed with either paclitaxel or nab-paclitaxel [85]. Median OS was improved from 11.3 to 15.9 months with the addition of pembrolizumab, and ORR increased from 38.4% to 57.9%. The results of these trials led the FDA to approve pembrolizumab in combination with chemotherapy as first-line treatment for patients with metastatic NSCLC without *EGFR* or *ALK* alterations, irrespective of PD-L1 expression.

A number of trials involving atezolizumab were conducted in similar patient populations, with mixed results. IMpower130, a phase 3 RCT of treatment-naïve patients with non-SCC histology, compared carboplatin/nab-paclitaxel with or without atezolizumab [86]. Patients who received atezolizumab survived longer despite a 60% crossover rate: median OS 18.6 months vs. 13.9 months. OS benefit was preserved regardless of PD-L1 score. Notably, patients with *EGFR* or *ALK* mutation did not sustain a benefit from the addition of atezolizumab.

IMpower131 was the complementary trial which enrolled patients with SCC histology. However, the addition of atezolizumab only resulted in a small improvement in PFS (6.3 months vs. 5.6 months) and did not result in significant improvement in OS (14.2 months vs. 13.5 months), despite only 43.2% (vs. 60% crossover in IMpower130) of patients in the chemotherapy-only arm later receiving immunotherapy.

A third trial, IMpower150, added bevacizumab to the treatment arms, given preclinical evidence that anti-VEGF agents could potentiate tumor infiltration by immune cells and lead to synergy [87]. Patients with non-SCC histology who were treatment naïve were randomized to one of three arms: ABCP (atezolizumab, bevacizumab, carboplatin, paclitaxel), BCP (bevacizumab, carboplatin, paclitaxel), or ACP (atezolizumab, carboplatin, paclitaxel) [88]. In the final analysis after 3-year follow-up of patients with no *EGFR* or *ALK* mutation, ABCP outperformed BCP in

OS (19.5 months vs. 14.7 months), while ACP formally did not (19.0 months vs. 14.7 months). In contrast to the IMpower130 and KEYNOTE-189 studies, which demonstrated OS benefit with the addition of immunotherapy even in PD-L1 negative patients, IMpower150 showed no significant OS difference across the three arms in this subpopulation. This may be partly due to the comparison arm having the addition of bevacizumab to chemotherapy. As a result of the aforementioned trials, atezolizumab is approved by the FDA in the United States as first-line treatment for non-SCC NSCLC in two regimens: atezolizumab/carboplatin/nab-paclitaxel per IMpower130 or atezolizumab/bevacizumab/carboplatin/paclitaxel per IMpower150. It is not approved for use in SCC NSCLC.

In addition to chemotherapy paired with a single checkpoint inhibitor, two large trials have investigated quadruplet therapy consisting of doublet chemotherapy with dual immune blockade. CheckMate9LA is an international, phase 3 RCT which randomized patients to either ipilimumab/nivolumab/histology-based chemotherapy doublet for two cycles followed by indefinite ipilimumab/nivolumab maintenance, or four cycles of chemotherapy alone followed by indefinite pemetrexed maintenance in patients with non-SCC [89]. At 3-year follow-up, the quadruplet arm had increased OS (27% vs. 19%, median 15.8 months vs. 11.0 months, HR 0.74) [90]. OS benefit was preserved across all PD-L1 subgroups and histologies. The addition of two cycles of chemotherapy to immunotherapy successfully overrode the initial inferior survival outcomes seen in the prior studies of single agent immunotherapy, suggesting that fast tumor shrinkage from chemotherapy exerted a complementary effect. Based upon this data, this treatment regimen was subsequently approved by the FDA in May 2020.

POSEIDON was a similar quadruplet trial comparing three arms: tremelimumab/durvalumab/histology-based chemotherapy for four cycles followed by durvalumab maintenance, durvalumab/chemotherapy for four cycles followed by durvalumab maintenance, and chemotherapy [91]. OS was not significantly different between the durvalumab/chemotherapy arm and the chemotherapy arm (median OS 13.3 months vs. 11.7 months, $p = 0.07$), but OS was found to be superior in the quadruplet arm compared to the chemotherapy arm (median OS 14.0 months vs. 11.7 months, HR 0.77, $p = 0.003$). This was the second trial to demonstrate an OS benefit of quadruplet therapy over chemotherapy alone. This quadruplet regimen was FDA approved in November 2022, though it is unclear whether the results from the quadruplet regimen is superior to the data from the prior KEYNOTE-189 and KEYNOTE-407 trials.

Dual Immunotherapy: Anti-CTLA-4 with Anti-PD1/PD-L1

The addition of the anti-CTLA-4 antibody ipilimumab to first-line nivolumab was investigated in CheckMate227. The results found greater OS benefit for the ipilimumab/nivolumab combination over chemotherapy: 17.1 months vs. 14.9 months for those with PD-L1 $\geq$1% and 17.2 months vs. 12.2 months for those with PD-L1 <1% [92]. Grade 3/4 adverse events were decreased for the immunotherapy arm compared to the chemotherapy arm (32.8% vs. 36%). Based upon this data, the FDA approved the ipilimumab/nivolumab combination as a frontline treatment option in patients with metastatic NSCLC with PD-L1 ≥1% in May 2020.

Similar clinical trials involving the combination of tremelimumab (another anti-CTLA-4 antibody) and durvalumab (anti-PD-L1 antibody) have failed to demonstrate a benefit over chemotherapy [93–95]. In one study, the authors cite substantial crossover of patients in the chemotherapy arm later receiving immunotherapy as a possible explanation for the lack of appreciable OS difference [93].

One important question raised by trials with dual immune blockade is whether this confers tangible survival benefit over single agent immunotherapy, especially given that rates of immune-related adverse events can be significantly higher in patients treated with combination immunotherapy. Although the CheckMate227 trial was not powered to discern differences between the combination arm and the nivolumab only arm, the former conferred a numerical improvement in the 4-year OS rate of 29% vs. 21%, ORR of 36% vs. 28%, and median duration of response 31.8 months vs. 16.8 months. The incidence of grade 3/4 adverse events, however, was doubled in the combination immunotherapy group (18.4% vs. 8.2%), compared to the nivolumab or chemotherapy groups (18.4% vs. 19.2%).

It is also important to note that combination immunotherapy has not been compared directly against chemoimmunotherapy. Therefore, based upon available data, chemoimmunotherapy, and combination immunotherapy are both frontline treatment options for patients with metastatic NSCLC with no *EGFR* or *ALK* alterations and PD-L1 ≥1%.

Deciding on Treatment: PD-L1 ≥50% and No Actionable Mutations

For patients with NSCLC who have a PD-L1 TPS score of ≥50% (seen in approximately 30% of patients), and no driver mutation with an approved first-line therapy such as *EGFR/ALK/ROS1*, the preferred recommended treatment options are (1) single-agent checkpoint inhibitor (pembrolizumab, atezolizumab, or cemiplimab) or (2) histology-based platinum-chemotherapy doublet with a checkpoint inhibitor [8]. Additional combinations of chemotherapy with immunotherapy may be useful in certain circumstances, discussed in further detail below.

There is no clear rule for how to decide between chemoimmunotherapy and single-agent immunotherapy in this high PD-L1 patient population. Each case must be approached individually, as there have been no head-to-head comparisons between immunotherapy alone versus chemoimmunotherapy in this patient population. This question is under active investigation by ongoing clinical trials, including the phase III French PERSEE trial (NCT04547504). In general, for patients with significant symptom burden related to their disease and/or a large tumor burden with a need for more urgent treatment response, chemoimmunotherapy is often preferred given higher response rates.

On the other hand, patients with poor performance status or those who have no or minimal symptoms related to their disease may be more suitable for single agent immunotherapy. When comparing across trials with the requisite caveats, the incidence of grade 3–5 adverse events in patients receiving pembrolizumab/chemotherapy was 71.9% in KEYNOTE-189, compared to only 31.2% in patients treated with pembrolizumab only in KEYNOTE-024. The grade 3–5 adverse event rates in those patients treated with chemotherapy only were similar in both trials: 66.8% and 53.3%, respectively. Additional factors such as tumor mutation burden or smoking history have not been reliable predictors of response to either therapy option [96].

Deciding on Treatment: PD-L1 1–49% and No Actionable Mutations

For patients who have tumors with PD-L1 expression of 1–49% and no actionable mutations, first-line recommendations include chemoimmunotherapy combinations and dual immunotherapy. Regimens with high efficacy and the longest follow-up data available are derived from KEYNOTE-189 and KEYNOTE-407, for non-SCC and SCC NSCLC, respectively. For non-SCC NSCLC, four cycles of platinum/ pemetrexed/pembrolizumab is recommended, followed by maintenance treatment with pemetrexed/pembrolizumab until disease progression. For SCC NSCLC, four cycles of platinum/paclitaxel or nab-paclitaxel/pembrolizumab is recommended instead, followed by maintenance with pembrolizumab until disease progression.

Additional FDA-approved variations of chemoimmunotherapy are available, including nivolumab/ipilimumab with histology-based chemotherapy doublet or carboplatin/taxane/atezolizumab +/− bevacizumab (for details see Section "Chemoimmunotherapy"). Deciding between all of the available regimens requires consideration of formulary preference, cost, drug availability, and side effect profiles. For example, in the case of non-SCC NSCLC, a pemetrexed-containing regimen may be preferred over an equivalent taxane-based regimen due to better tolerability. Treatment with a single agent checkpoint inhibitor, instead of dual immunotherapy, may be more suitable for patients at higher risk of an immune-related adverse event. Patients with good performance status and highly aggressive disease may be treated with a quadruplet regimen. Pre-existing hypertension, thrombosis, or proteinuria could be contraindications to a bevacizumab-containing regimen.

Chemoimmunotherapy is typically recommended over immunotherapy alone, as cross-trial comparisons have shown chemoimmunotherapy to have superior OS benefit compared to chemotherapy, while immunotherapy alone has only equivalent OS outcomes to chemotherapy. The ongoing INSIGNA trial compares these two options directly (NCT03793179). However immunotherapy with a PD-1/PD-L1 inhibitor alone or in combination with an anti-CTLA-4 antibody is recommended for patients who are ineligible for or who decline chemotherapy. For those with tumors with PD-L1 expression between 1–49%, both pembrolizumab and ipilimumab/nivolumab have shown equivalent OS outcomes compared to chemotherapy in their respective trials (KEYNOTE-042 and CheckMate227) [78, 92].

Deciding on Treatment: PD-L1 <1% and No Actionable Mutations

Treatment for patients with tumor PD-L1 expression <1% is largely similar to those with PD-L1 of 1–49%. The addition of immunotherapy to chemotherapy confers survival benefit even in the PD-L1 negative patient population. In the KEYNOTE trials randomizing patients to chemotherapy in combination with either placebo or pembrolizumab, for tumors with PD-L1 <1%, there was a PFS (HR 0.64, 0.47–0.89) and OS benefit (HR 0.52, 0.36–0.74) in non-SCC histology as well as a PFS benefit (HR 0.67, 0.49–0.91) in SCC histology [97, 98]. For those who are ineligible for chemotherapy or otherwise decline chemotherapy, ipilimumab/nivolumab is an alternative option, though this combination is only approved for patients with tumors expressing PD-L1 in the United States. In CheckMate227, dual immunotherapy demonstrated favorable OS outcomes compared to chemotherapy alone (HR 0.53, 0.34–0.84) in the PD-L1 <1% subgroup [82]. At present, single-agent immunotherapy is not recommended due to the lack of proven efficacy in this patient population.

Summary

The majority of patients with newly diagnosed lung cancer have stage IV NSCLC, which has historically been associated with a prognosis of approximately 1 year with chemotherapy alone. In the past decade, major advances have significantly altered the treatment landscape and have led to improved survival outcomes for patients with this disease.

The discovery of actionable molecular biomarkers, such as *EGFR* mutations, and corresponding targeted therapies have resulted in significantly higher response rates and overall survival that can now be measured in years in some cases. For instance, patients with a sensitizing *EGFR* mutation who receive first-line osimertinib have a median overall survival of 38.6 months [32]. For those patients who lack a targetable driver mutation, immunotherapy alone or in combination with chemotherapy have now become the standard of care. Median OS in many of these trials now approaches 20 months. In the first pembrolizumab trial (KEYNOTE-001), out of the 60 patients who received more than 2 years of pembrolizumab, the 5-year OS rate was 75% [99]. Such a striking statistic suggests that cure may have been achieved in a subset of patients, a concept that was considered unfathomable years ago.

When approaching a patient with newly diagnosed stage IV NSCLC, first-line treatment depends on the tumor histology. Adenocarcinomas have a high probability of harboring an actionable mutation, and thus rapid molecular screening is recommended. When indicated, targeted therapies are recommended over other forms of systemic therapy due to higher response rates, increased convenience as many drugs are available orally, and better tolerance. In the absence of an actionable target, first-line options are based on the level of PD-L1 expression.

For those tumors with high PD-L1 expression ($\geq$50%), either chemoimmunotherapy or single-agent immunotherapy is recommended. For patients who have either bulky or fast-growing disease, or who are symptomatic from their cancer with need for rapid tumor response, we recommend chemoimmunotherapy. Patients with poor performance status or who otherwise may not tolerate chemotherapy may be offered single-agent immunotherapy.

NSCLC with low or absent PD-L1 expression (<50%) are usually treated with chemoimmunotherapy. Dual anti-CTLA-4 plus anti-PD1/PD-L1 immunotherapy or single-agent immunotherapy may offer alternative options for those patients who are considered ineligible or at high risk for chemotherapy or for those who decline chemotherapy.

Advances in treatment continue to be made on all fronts. Numerous ongoing trials are exploring novel targeted therapies and chemoimmunotherapy combinations. For instance, lymphocyte-activation gene 3 (LAG-3) is a surface molecule expressed on T cells that downregulates their proliferation and activity, acting as an immune checkpoint distinct from the PD-1/PD-L1 axis [100]. The combination of anti-LAG3 antibody relatlimab with nivolumab demonstrated significantly longer median PFS versus nivolumab alone in the treatment of advanced melanoma (10.1 months vs. 4.6 months) [101]. The combination of relatlimab/nivolumab/chemotherapy is being compared with nivolumab/chemotherapy as a first-line regimen in NSCLC in an international trial that is currently enrolling (NCT04623775).

Given the incredible strides made in the past decade, the outlook on future drug development for stage IV NSCLC is optimistic. As tumor biology is further unraveled—identifying and understanding mutations which confer resistance to targeted therapy and immunotherapies, developing markers which reliably predict response to immunotherapy, and finding new methods to unleash the immune system—treatment of metastatic lung cancer can be even more personalized, leading to improved quality of life and longer survival for patients.

References

1. Bade BC, Dela Cruz CS. Lung cancer 2020: epidemiology, etiology, and prevention. Clin Chest Med. 2020;41:1–24.
2. Siegel RL, Miller KD, Jemal A. Cancer statistics, 2019. CA Cancer J Clin. 2019;69:7–34.
3. Ganti AK, Klein AB, Cotarla I, Seal B, Chou E. Update of incidence, prevalence, survival, and initial treatment in patients with non–small cell lung cancer in the US. JAMA Oncol. 2021;7:1824–32.
4. American Cancer Society. Lung cancer survival rates. 5-Year survival rates for lung cancer. n.d.. https://www.cancer.org/cancer/lung-cancer/detection-diagnosis-staging/survival-rates.html. Accessed 27 Jun 2022.

5. NSCLC Meta-Analyses Collaborative Group. Chemotherapy in addition to supportive care improves survival in advanced non-small-cell lung cancer: a systematic review and meta-analysis of individual patient data from 16 randomized controlled trials. J Clin Oncol. 2008;26:4617–25.

6. Soria J-C, Mauguen A, Reck M, et al. Systematic review and meta-analysis of randomised, phase II/III trials adding bevacizumab to platinum-based chemotherapy as first-line treatment in patients with advanced non-small-cell lung cancer. Ann Oncol. 2013;24:20–30.

7. Herbst R, Jassem J, Abogunrin S, James D, McCool R, Belleli R, Giaccone G, De Marinis F. A network meta-analysis of cancer immunotherapies versus chemotherapy for first-line treatment of patients with non-small cell lung cancer and high programmed death-ligand 1 expression. Front Oncol. 2021;11:676732.

8. National Comprehensive Cancer Network. NCCN guidelines: non-small cell lung cancer version 3.2022. 2022.

9. Schabath MB, Cote ML. Cancer progress and priorities: lung cancer. Cancer Epidemiol Biomark Prev. 2019;28:1563–79.

10. Syrigos KN, Vansteenkiste J, Parikh P, von Pawel J, Manegold C, Martins RG, Simms L, Sugarman KP, Visseren-Grul C, Scagliotti GV. Prognostic and predictive factors in a randomized phase III trial comparing cisplatin-pemetrexed versus cisplatin-gemcitabine in advanced non-small-cell lung cancer. Ann Oncol. 2010;21:556–61.

11. Scagliotti GV, Parikh P, von Pawel J, et al. Phase III study comparing cisplatin plus gemcitabine with cisplatin plus pemetrexed in chemotherapy-naive patients with advanced-stage non-small-cell lung cancer. J Clin Oncol. 2008;26:3543–51.

12. Blais N, Hirsh V. Chemotherapy in metastatic NSCLC – new regimens (pemetrexed, nab-paclitaxel). Front Oncol. 2014;4:177.

13. Johnson DH, Fehrenbacher L, Novotny WF, et al. Randomized phase II trial comparing bevacizumab plus carboplatin and paclitaxel with carboplatin and paclitaxel alone in previously untreated locally advanced or metastatic non-small-cell lung cancer. J Clin Oncol. 2004;22:2184–91.

14. Garon EB, Ciuleanu T-E, Arrieta O, et al. Ramucirumab plus docetaxel versus placebo plus docetaxel for second-line treatment of stage IV non-small-cell lung cancer after disease progression on platinum-based therapy (REVEL): a multicentre, double-blind, randomised phase 3 trial. Lancet. 2014;384:665–73.

15. Shi Y, Au JS-K, Thongprasert S, Srinivasan S, Tsai C-M, Khoa MT, Heeroma K, Itoh Y, Cornelio G, Yang P-C. A prospective, molecular epidemiology study of EGFR mutations in Asian patients with advanced non-small-cell lung cancer of adenocarcinoma histology (PIONEER). J Thorac Oncol. 2014;9:154–62.

16. Kawaguchi T, Koh Y, Ando M, et al. Prospective analysis of oncogenic driver mutations and environmental factors: Japan Molecular Epidemiology for Lung Cancer Study. J Clin Oncol. 2016;34:2247–57.

17. Cheung AH-K, Tong JH-M, Chung L-Y, Chau S-L, Ng CS-H, Wan IYP, To K-F. EGFR mutation exists in squamous cell lung carcinoma. Pathology. 2020;52:323–8.

18. Korpanty GJ, Graham DM, Vincent MD, Leighl NB. Biomarkers that currently affect clinical practice in lung cancer: EGFR, ALK, MET, ROS-1, and KRAS. Front Oncol. 2014;4:204.

19. Rekhtman N, Pietanza MC, Hellmann MD, et al. Next-generation sequencing of pulmonary large cell neuroendocrine carcinoma reveals small cell carcinoma-like and non-small cell carcinoma-like subsets. Clin Cancer Res. 2016;22:3618–29.

20. George J, Walter V, Peifer M, et al. Integrative genomic profiling of large-cell neuroendocrine carcinomas reveals distinct subtypes of high-grade neuroendocrine lung tumors. Nat Commun. 2018;9:1048.

21. Glisson BS, Moran CA. Large-cell neuroendocrine carcinoma: controversies in diagnosis and treatment. J Natl Compr Cancer Netw. 2011;9:1122–9.

22. Asamura H, Kameya T, Matsuno Y, et al. Neuroendocrine neoplasms of the lung: a prognostic spectrum. J Clin Oncol. 2006;24:70–6.

23. Ferrara MG, Stefani A, Simbolo M, et al. Large cell neuro-endocrine carcinoma of the lung: current treatment options and potential future opportunities. Front Oncol. 2021;11:650293.
24. Grønberg BH, Bremnes RM, Fløtten O, et al. Phase III study by the Norwegian lung cancer study group: pemetrexed plus carboplatin compared with gemcitabine plus carboplatin as first-line chemotherapy in advanced non-small-cell lung cancer. J Clin Oncol. 2009;27:3217–24.
25. Derks JL, Leblay N, Thunnissen E, et al. Molecular subtypes of pulmonary large-cell neuroendocrine carcinoma predict chemotherapy treatment outcome. Clin Cancer Res. 2018;24:33–42.
26. Li X, Wu D, Liu H, Chen J. Pulmonary sarcomatoid carcinoma: progress, treatment and expectations. Ther Adv Med Oncol. 2020;12:1758835920950207.
27. Maneenil K, Xue Z, Liu M, Boland J, Wu F, Stoddard SM, Molina J, Yang P. Sarcomatoid carcinoma of the lung: the Mayo Clinic experience in 127 patients. Clin Lung Cancer. 2018;19:e323–33.
28. Maemondo M, Inoue A, Kobayashi K, et al. Gefitinib or chemotherapy for non–small-cell lung cancer with mutated EGFR. N Engl J Med. 2010;362:2380–8.
29. Lee C-S, Milone M, Seetharamu N. Osimertinib in EGFR-mutated lung cancer: a review of the existing and emerging clinical data. Onco Targets Ther. 2021;14:4579–97.
30. Mok TS, Wu Y-L, Thongprasert S, et al. Gefitinib or carboplatin-paclitaxel in pulmonary adenocarcinoma. N Engl J Med. 2009;361:947–57.
31. Mok TS, Wu Y-L, Ahn M-J, et al. Osimertinib or platinum-pemetrexed in EGFR T790M-positive lung cancer. N Engl J Med. 2017;376:629–40.
32. Ramalingam SS, Vansteenkiste J, Planchard D, et al. Overall survival with osimertinib in untreated, EGFR-mutated advanced NSCLC. N Engl J Med. 2020;382:41–50.
33. Chevallier M, Borgeaud M, Addeo A, Friedlaender A. Oncogenic driver mutations in non-small cell lung cancer: past, present and future. World J Clin Oncol. 2021;12:217–37.
34. Shaw AT, Solomon B. Targeting anaplastic lymphoma kinase in lung cancer. Clin Cancer Res. 2011;17:2081–6.
35. Weickhardt AJ, Aisner DL, Franklin WA, Varella-Garcia M, Doebele RC, Camidge DR. Diagnostic assays for identification of anaplastic lymphoma kinase-positive non-small cell lung cancer. Cancer. 2013;119:1467–77.
36. Solomon BJ, Kim D-W, Wu Y-L, et al. Final overall survival analysis from a study comparing first-line crizotinib versus chemotherapy in ALK-mutation-positive non–small-cell lung cancer. J Clin Oncol. 2018;36:2251–8.
37. Shaw AT, Bauer TM, de Marinis F, et al. First-line lorlatinib or crizotinib in advanced ALK-positive lung cancer. N Engl J Med. 2020;383:2018–29.
38. Camidge DR, Kim HR, Ahn M-J, et al. Brigatinib versus crizotinib in ALK-positive non–small-cell lung cancer. N Engl J Med. 2018;379:2027–39.
39. Peters S, Camidge DR, Shaw AT, et al. Alectinib versus crizotinib in untreated ALK-positive non–small-cell lung cancer. N Engl J Med. 2017;377:829–38.
40. Mok T, Camidge DR, Gadgeel SM, et al. Updated overall survival and final progression-free survival data for patients with treatment-naive advanced ALK-positive non–small-cell lung cancer in the ALEX study. Ann Oncol. 2020;31:1056–64.
41. Shaw AT, Solomon BJ, Besse B, et al. ALK resistance mutations and efficacy of lorlatinib in advanced anaplastic lymphoma kinase-positive non–small-cell lung cancer. J Clin Oncol. 2019;37:1370–9.
42. Sun TY, Stehr H, Suarez CJ, Wakelee HA. Tumor heterogeneity and testing discrepancy confound ROS1 detection in NSCLC. J Thorac Oncol. 2019;14:e111–3.
43. Shaw AT, Ou S-HI, Bang Y-J, et al. Crizotinib in ROS1-rearranged non–small-cell lung cancer. N Engl J Med. 2014;371:1963–71.
44. Dziadziuszko R, Krebs MG, De Braud F, et al. Updated integrated analysis of the efficacy and safety of entrectinib in locally advanced or metastatic ROS1 fusion–positive non–small-cell lung cancer. J Clin Oncol. 2021;39:1253–63.

45. Gainor JF, Tseng D, Yoda S, et al. Patterns of metastatic spread and mechanisms of resistance to crizotinib in ROS1-positive non–small-cell lung cancer. JCO Precis Oncol. 2017;2017:1–13.
46. Jänne PA, Riely GJ, Gadgeel SM, et al. Adagrasib in non–small-cell lung cancer harboring a KRASG12C mutation. N Engl J Med. 2022;387:120.
47. Skoulidis F, Li BT, Dy GK, et al. Sotorasib for lung cancers with KRAS p.G12C mutation. N Engl J Med. 2021;384:2371–81.
48. Arcila ME, Chaft JE, Nafa K, Roy-Chowdhuri S, Lau C, Zaidinski M, Paik PK, Zakowski MF, Kris MG, Ladanyi M. Prevalence, clinicopathologic associations, and molecular spectrum of ERBB2 (HER2) tyrosine kinase mutations in lung adenocarcinomas. Clin Cancer Res. 2012;18:4910–8.
49. Saalfeld FC, Wenzel C, Christopoulos P, et al. Efficacy of immune checkpoint inhibitors alone or in combination with chemotherapy in NSCLC harboring ERBB2 mutations. J Thorac Oncol. 2021;16:1952–8.
50. Zhao J, Xia Y. Targeting HER2 alterations in non–small-cell lung cancer: a comprehensive review. JCO Precis Oncol. 2020;4:411–25.
51. Li BT, Shen R, Buonocore D, et al. Ado-trastuzumab emtansine for patients with HER2-mutant lung cancers: results from a phase II basket trial. J Clin Oncol. 2018;36:2532–7.
52. Li BT, Smit EF, Goto Y, et al. Trastuzumab deruxtecan in HER2-mutant non-small-cell lung cancer. N Engl J Med. 2022;386:241–51.
53. Elamin YY, Robichaux JP, Carter BW, et al. Poziotinib for patients with HER2 exon 20 mutant non-small-cell lung cancer: results from a phase II trial. J Clin Oncol. 2022;40:702–9.
54. Champagnac A, Bringuier P-P, Barritault M, Isaac S, Watkin E, Forest F, Maury J-M, Girard N, Brevet M. Frequency of MET exon 14 skipping mutations in non-small cell lung cancer according to technical approach in routine diagnosis: results from a real-life cohort of 2,369 patients. J Thorac Dis. 2020;12:2172–8.
55. Wolf J, Seto T, Han J-Y, et al. Capmatinib in MET exon 14-mutated or MET-amplified non-small-cell lung cancer. N Engl J Med. 2020;383:944–57.
56. Paik PK, Felip E, Veillon R, et al. Tepotinib in non-small-cell lung cancer with MET exon 14 skipping mutations. N Engl J Med. 2020;383:931–43.
57. Takeuchi K, Soda M, Togashi Y, et al. RET, ROS1 and ALK fusions in lung cancer. Nat Med. 2012;18:378–81.
58. Drilon A, Laetsch TW, Kummar S, et al. Efficacy of larotrectinib in TRK fusion-positive cancers in adults and children. N Engl J Med. 2018;378:731–9.
59. Planchard D, Besse B, Groen HJM, et al. Phase 2 study of dabrafenib plus trametinib in patients with BRAF V600E-mutant metastatic NSCLC: updated 5-year survival rates and genomic analysis. J Thorac Oncol. 2022;17:103–15.
60. Drilon A, Oxnard GR, Tan DSW, et al. Efficacy of selpercatinib in RET fusion-positive non-small-cell lung cancer. N Engl J Med. 2020;383:813–24.
61. Delbaldo C, Michiels S, Syz N, Soria J-C, Le Chevalier T, Pignon J-P. Benefits of adding a drug to a single-agent or a 2-agent chemotherapy regimen in advanced non-small-cell lung cancer: a meta-analysis. JAMA. 2004;292:470–84.
62. Rajeswaran A, Trojan A, Burnand B, Giannelli M. Efficacy and side effects of cisplatin- and carboplatin-based doublet chemotherapeutic regimens versus non-platinum-based doublet chemotherapeutic regimens as first line treatment of metastatic non-small cell lung carcinoma: a systematic review of randomized controlled trials. Lung Cancer. 2008;59:1–11.
63. Hotta K, Matsuo K, Ueoka H, Kiura K, Tabata M, Tanimoto M. Meta-analysis of randomized clinical trials comparing Cisplatin to Carboplatin in patients with advanced non-small-cell lung cancer. J Clin Oncol. 2004;22:3852–9.
64. Kelly K, Crowley J, Bunn PA, et al. Randomized phase III trial of paclitaxel plus carboplatin versus vinorelbine plus cisplatin in the treatment of patients with advanced non-small-cell lung cancer: a Southwest Oncology Group trial. J Clin Oncol. 2001;19:3210–8.
65. Scagliotti GV, De Marinis F, Rinaldi M, et al. Phase III randomized trial comparing three platinum-based doublets in advanced non-small-cell lung cancer. J Clin Oncol. 2002;20:4285–91.

66. Schiller JH, Harrington D, Belani CP, Langer C, Sandler A, Krook J, Zhu J, Johnson DH. Comparison of four chemotherapy regimens for advanced non–small-cell lung cancer. N Engl J Med. 2002;346:92–8.
67. Scagliotti G, Hanna N, Fossella F, Sugarman K, Blatter J, Peterson P, Simms L, Shepherd FA. The differential efficacy of pemetrexed according to NSCLC histology: a review of two Phase III studies. Oncologist. 2009;14:253–63.
68. Socinski MA, Bondarenko I, Karaseva NA, et al. Weekly nab-paclitaxel in combination with carboplatin versus solvent-based paclitaxel plus carboplatin as first-line therapy in patients with advanced non-small-cell lung cancer: final results of a phase III trial. J Clin Oncol. 2012;30:2055–62.
69. Socinski MA, Schell MJ, Peterman A, et al. Phase III trial comparing a defined duration of therapy versus continuous therapy followed by second-line therapy in advanced-stage IIIB/IV non–small-cell lung cancer. J Clin Oncol. 2002;20:1335–43.
70. Rossi A, Chiodini P, Sun J-M, et al. Six versus fewer planned cycles of first-line platinum-based chemotherapy for non-small-cell lung cancer: a systematic review and meta-analysis of individual patient data. Lancet Oncol. 2014;15:1254–62.
71. Lauro S, Onesti CE, Righini R, Marchetti P. The use of bevacizumab in non-small cell lung cancer: an update. Anticancer Res. 2014;34:1537–45.
72. Shields MD, Marin-Acevedo JA, Pellini B. Immunotherapy for advanced non–small cell lung cancer: a decade of progress. Am Soc Clin Oncol Educ Book. 2021;41:e105–27.
73. Brahmer J, Reckamp KL, Baas P, et al. Nivolumab versus docetaxel in advanced squamous-cell non–small-cell lung cancer. N Engl J Med. 2015;373:123–35.
74. Borghaei H, Paz-Ares L, Horn L, et al. Nivolumab versus docetaxel in advanced nonsquamous non–small-cell lung cancer. N Engl J Med. 2015;373:1627–39.
75. Herbst RS, Baas P, Kim D-W, et al. Pembrolizumab versus docetaxel for previously treated, PD-L1-positive, advanced non-small-cell lung cancer (KEYNOTE-010): a randomised controlled trial. Lancet. 2016;387:1540–50.
76. Fehrenbacher L, Spira A, Ballinger M, et al. Atezolizumab versus docetaxel for patients with previously treated non-small-cell lung cancer (POPLAR): a multicentre, open-label, phase 2 randomised controlled trial. Lancet. 2016;387:1837–46.
77. Rittmeyer A, Barlesi F, Waterkamp D, et al. Atezolizumab versus docetaxel in patients with previously treated non-small-cell lung cancer (OAK): a phase 3, open-label, multicentre randomised controlled trial. Lancet. 2017;389:255–65.
78. Mok TSK, Wu Y-L, Kudaba I, et al. Pembrolizumab versus chemotherapy for previously untreated, PD-L1-expressing, locally advanced or metastatic non-small-cell lung cancer (KEYNOTE-042): a randomised, open-label, controlled, phase 3 trial. Lancet. 2019;393:1819–30.
79. Reck M, Rodríguez-Abreu D, Robinson AG, et al. Updated analysis of KEYNOTE-024: pembrolizumab versus platinum-based chemotherapy for advanced non–small-cell lung cancer with PD-L1 tumor proportion score of 50% or greater. J Clin Oncol. 2019;37:537–46.
80. Herbst RS, Giaccone G, de Marinis F, et al. Atezolizumab for first-line treatment of PD-L1-selected patients with NSCLC. N Engl J Med. 2020;383:1328–39.
81. Sezer A, Kilickap S, Gümüş M, et al. Cemiplimab monotherapy for first-line treatment of advanced non-small-cell lung cancer with PD-L1 of at least 50%: a multicentre, open-label, global, phase 3, randomised, controlled trial. Lancet. 2021;397:592–604.
82. Paz-Ares LG, Ramalingam SS, Ciuleanu T-E, et al. First-line nivolumab plus ipilimumab in advanced NSCLC: 4-year outcomes from the randomized, open-label, phase 3 CheckMate 227 part 1 trial. J Thorac Oncol. 2022;17:289–308.
83. Langer CJ, Gadgeel SM, Borghaei H, et al. Carboplatin and pemetrexed with or without pembrolizumab for advanced, non-squamous non-small-cell lung cancer: a randomised, phase 2 cohort of the open-label KEYNOTE-021 study. Lancet Oncol. 2016;17:1497–508.
84. Gandhi L, Rodríguez-Abreu D, Gadgeel S, et al. Pembrolizumab plus chemotherapy in metastatic non-small-cell lung cancer. N Engl J Med. 2018;378:2078–92.
85. Paz-Ares L, Luft A, Vicente D, et al. Pembrolizumab plus chemotherapy for squamous non-small-cell lung cancer. N Engl J Med. 2018;379:2040–51.

86. West H, McCleod M, Hussein M, et al. Atezolizumab in combination with carboplatin plus nab-paclitaxel chemotherapy compared with chemotherapy alone as first-line treatment for metastatic non-squamous non-small-cell lung cancer (IMpower130): a multicentre, randomised, open-label, phase 3 trial. Lancet Oncol. 2019;20:924–37.

87. Hegde PS, Wallin JJ, Mancao C. Predictive markers of anti-VEGF and emerging role of angiogenesis inhibitors as immunotherapeutics. Semin Cancer Biol. 2018;52:117–24.

88. Socinski MA, Jotte RM, Cappuzzo F, et al. Atezolizumab for first-line treatment of metastatic nonsquamous NSCLC. N Engl J Med. 2018;378:2288–301.

89. Paz-Ares L, Ciuleanu T-E, Cobo M, et al. First-line nivolumab plus ipilimumab combined with two cycles of chemotherapy in patients with non-small-cell lung cancer (CheckMate 9LA): an international, randomised, open-label, phase 3 trial. Lancet Oncol. 2021;22:198–211.

90. Paz-Ares LG, Ciuleanu T-E, Cobo-Dols M, et al. First-line (1L) nivolumab (NIVO) + ipilimumab (IPI) + 2 cycles of chemotherapy (chemo) versus chemo alone (4 cycles) in patients (pts) with metastatic non–small cell lung cancer (NSCLC): 3-year update from CheckMate 9LA. J Clin Oncol. 2022;40:LBA9026.

91. IASLC. Phase III POSEIDON trial shows positive results for patients taking chemotherapy plus durvalumab and tremelimumab. n.d.. https://www.iaslc.org/iaslc-news/press-release/phase-iii-poseidon-trial-shows-positive-results-patients-taking. Accessed 8 Jul 2022.

92. Hellmann MD, Paz-Ares L, Bernabe Caro R, et al. Nivolumab plus ipilimumab in advanced non-small-cell lung cancer. N Engl J Med. 2019;381:2020–31.

93. Rizvi NA, Cho BC, Reinmuth N, et al. Durvalumab with or without tremelimumab vs standard chemotherapy in first-line treatment of metastatic non-small cell lung cancer: the MYSTIC phase 3 randomized clinical trial. JAMA Oncol. 2020;6:661–74.

94. Planchard D, Reinmuth N, Orlov S, et al. ARCTIC: durvalumab with or without tremelimumab as third-line or later treatment of metastatic non-small-cell lung cancer. Ann Oncol. 2020;31:609–18.

95. Mok T, Schmid P, Arén O, Arrieta O, Gottfried M, Jazieh AR, Ramlau R, Timcheva K, Martin C, McIntosh S. 192TiP: NEPTUNE: a global, phase 3 study of durvalumab (MEDI4736) plus tremelimumab combination therapy versus standard of care (SoC) platinum-based chemotherapy in the first-line treatment of patients (pts) with advanced or metastatic NSCLC. J Thorac Oncol. 2016;11:S140–1.

96. Gainor JF, Rizvi H, Jimenez Aguilar E, et al. Clinical activity of programmed cell death 1 (PD-1) blockade in never, light, and heavy smokers with non-small-cell lung cancer and PD-L1 expression ≥50. Ann Oncol. 2020;31:404–11.

97. Gadgeel S, Rodríguez-Abreu D, Speranza G, et al. Updated analysis from KEYNOTE-189: pembrolizumab or placebo plus pemetrexed and platinum for previously untreated metastatic nonsquamous non-small-cell lung cancer. J Clin Oncol. 2020;38:1505–17.

98. Paz-Ares L, Vicente D, Tafreshi A, et al. A randomized, placebo-controlled trial of pembrolizumab plus chemotherapy in patients with metastatic squamous NSCLC: protocol-specified final analysis of KEYNOTE-407. J Thorac Oncol. 2020;15:1657–69.

99. Garon EB, Hellmann MD, Rizvi NA, et al. Five-year overall survival for patients with advanced non-small-cell lung cancer treated with pembrolizumab: results from the phase I KEYNOTE-001 study. J Clin Oncol. 2019;37:2518–27.

100. Durham NM, Nirschl CJ, Jackson CM, Elias J, Kochel CM, Anders RA, Drake CG. Lymphocyte activation gene 3 (LAG-3) modulates the ability of CD4 T-cells to be suppressed in vivo. PLoS One. 2014;9:e109080.

101. Tawbi HA, Schadendorf D, Lipson EJ, et al. Relatlimab and nivolumab versus nivolumab in untreated advanced melanoma. N Engl J Med. 2022;386:24–34.

Chapter 9
Treatment of Small Cell Lung Cancer

Russell Hales and Khinh Ranh Voong

Small cell lung cancer (SCLC) is a high-grade, neuro-endocrine-expressing tumor with kinetics that favor rapid growth and spread. It is almost exclusively associated with tobacco use [1], but its incidence in the United States (USA) has decreased with smoking cessation efforts [2]. However, in areas of the world where smoking is increasing, the incidence of SCLC is rising [3]. Currently, it accounts for ~12% of all lung cancers in the USA [2].

In this chapter, we explore the treatment of SCLC. After decades of relatively indolent growth in innovation and changes in systemic management in SCLC, the last 5 years have ushered many of the most significant changes in treatment.

Staging and Diagnosis

SCLC is usually diagnosed in locally advanced or advanced stages [4]. Although symptoms of paraneoplastic conditions can be a precursor to diagnosis [5], patients often present with symptoms of intrathoracic diseases, such as cough, shortness of breath, hemoptysis, or hoarseness related to recurrent laryngeal nerve compression from mediastinal adenopathy. Constitutional symptoms such as weight loss and fatigue are also common.

Common paraneoplastic conditions seen in SCLC include the syndrome of inappropriate diuretic hormone (SIADH), Lambert-Eaton myasthenic syndrome (LEMS), dermatomyositis, and cerebellar degeneration [5]. Although these conditions can be reversible in response to therapy, patients with central nervous system (CNS) manifestations such as cerebellar degeneration will not have restoration of

R. Hales (✉) · K. R. Voong
Johns Hopkins School of Medicine, Baltimore, MD, USA
e-mail: rhales1@jhmi.edu; kvoong1@jhmi.edu

© The Author(s), under exclusive license to Springer Nature Switzerland AG 2023
C. MacRosty, M. P. Rivera (eds.), *Lung Cancer*, Respiratory Medicine,
https://doi.org/10.1007/978-3-031-38412-7_9

function even with successful treatment. In patients with reversible paraneoplastic manifestations at diagnosis, disease surveillance once treatment is complete can be monitored in part by evaluation for relapse of the symptoms associated with the presenting syndrome [6].

Pathologic assessment is often undertaken with mediastinal lymph node biopsy, and histologic features of SCLC include positivity for TTF-1 and neuroendocrine markers such as chromogranin A, synaptophysin, CD 56+, and NCAM (neural cell adhesion molecule) [7]. In addition, a high metabolic index is a fundamental feature of SCLC [8].

Basic evaluation of SCLC includes computed tomography (CT) of the chest, abdomen, and pelvis and metabolic imaging with FDG-PET. Brain imaging is also critical and should include magnetic resonance imaging (MRI) with gadolinium contrast unless there are contraindications to MRI or gadolinium-based contrast. For these patients, a CT of the head with contrast is a reasonable alternative. Basic laboratory assessment can evaluate for some paraneoplastic conditions [9] and stratify the patient's metabolic and hematologic fitness for therapy [10]. Finally, assessment of intercurrent disease with the Charleston Comorbidity Index (CCI) or other scales and performance status evaluation is a key component of the patient's initial evaluation [11]. Given the prognosis and treatment involved, we recommend a review of goals of care in shared decision-making in initial counseling. A comprehensive discussion of code status is an important layer of informing the patient of the risks, benefits, and possible scenarios with therapy and within the disease itself.

Although SCLC can be staged with American Joint Committee on Cancer (AJCC) eighth edition staging with assessment of T (tumor), N (lymph node), and M (distant metastases) status [12], it is often simplified into being either limited stage (LS) or extensive stage (ES) [13]. Literature on SCLC will also use limited disease (LD) or extensive disease (ED). The simplification of the treatment of SCLC may relate to at least three features: (a) treatment paradigms that are less nuanced with modest nodal changes, (b) the almost exclusive use of radiation instead of surgery for local therapy, and (c) the para-central nature of intrathoracic disease. Often bulky mediastinal lymph node conglomerates can merge into a primary tumor, making a distinction between the T stage and N stage a diagnostic challenge. Limited stage disease (LD) versus extensive stage disease (ED) distinguishes the relevant therapy pathways in a clinically parsimonious way.

LD refers to a tumor limited to the thoracic cage and supraclavicular fossa. Although contralateral mediastinal or supraclavicular lymph node involvement can be included in the definition of LD, the ability to give definitive radiotherapy to a clinically reasonable field speaks to the treatment-focused nature of SCLC [14]. SCLC may be the only tumor wherein the clinician can influence the designation of LD versus ED. Disease in the contralateral lung or spread to other disease sites upstage to ED, such as the brain, adrenal glands, or bone. Pleural effusions do not necessarily denote ED, but if pathologic assessment reveals malignant cells, the disease is ED in nature [15]. Thoracentesis is critical for therapeutic and diagnostic relevance in patients with no evidence of distant spread but with a pleural effusion.

Prognosis is driven by staging and the timeliness of diagnosis and treatment. A multidisciplinary team including medical oncology, radiation oncology, pulmonary medicine, thoracic surgery, chest radiology, and pathology are key components. In patients with LD, the 2-year survival outcome using modern therapy is estimated to be 50%, with a median survival of 30 months [16]. Conversely, the median survival in ED SCLC with optimal therapy is ~12 months [17].

Treatment of Limited Stage Disease

Systemic Treatment Considerations

Early systemic treatment regimens included a cyclophosphamide foundation, although it was recognized as early as the 1940s that nitrogen mustard had antitumoral properties in SCLC [18]. Etoposide with cisplatin (EP) was shown to have activity in LS and ES disease in 1979 [19]. However, EP-based chemotherapy became an appropriate alternative to cyclophosphamide, adriamycin, and vincristine (CAP) after a study of 437 patients showed equivalence of both regimens in SCLC [20]. The investigators reported similar response and complete response rates and median overall survival.

EP-based regimen became a preferred standard for ED SCLC treatment because it can be administered safely with thoracic radiation. The two widely used regimens for LD SCLC both use cisplatin and etoposide. The historic regimen from the Turissi study [21] includes a regimen of cisplatin 60 mg/m^2 Day 1 and etoposide 120 mg/m^2 Days 1, 2, and 3 repeated on a 21–28-day cycle for four cycles [21]. The alternative regimen was used in the CONVERT study with cisplatin 75 mg/m^2 Day 1 and etoposide 100 mg/m^2 Days 1, 2, and 3 repeated on a 21-day cycle for four cycles. An alternative regimen of cisplatin 25 mg/m^2 Days 1, 2, and 3 and etoposide 100 mg/m^2 Days 1, 2, and 3 was also offered in the CONVERT study [16]. In patients with renal impairment or hearing loss, carboplatin can be an appropriate substitute, although LD systemic regimens have focused on cisplatin-based chemotherapy.

Patients who receive thoracic radiotherapy should avoid hematopoietic colony-stimulating factors during concurrent systemic therapy. In a randomized study of 230 patients with LD-SCLC who were treated with or without granulocyte-macrophage colony-stimulating factor (GM-CSF) support on Days 4–18, there were no significant differences in median survival (14 months with GM-CSF versus 17 months without GM-CSF, $p = 0.15$) or complete response rates (36% with GM-CSF support versus 44% without CM-CSF support, $p = 0.29$). However, there was more non-hematologic toxicity, more days in hospital, higher use of intravenous (IV) antibiotics, and more life-threatening thrombocytopenia in patients receiving GM-CSF [22].

Although multiple studies have explored novel treatment regimens for systemic management of SCLC, an EP-based chemotherapy regimen remains the standard of care. Although some patients will experience long-term disease control, distant relapse is a common outcome, and additional therapies are often needed. We cover second-line treatment options for patients with relapsed disease in the extensive stage section, systemic treatment considerations below.

Surgical Considerations

Whereas non-small cell lung cancer (NSCLC) management in the nonmetastatic setting incorporates surgical resection in the medically and technically operable setting, the treatment of SCLC is almost exclusively limited to radiation therapy as a primary local therapy treatment. However, surgical resection can be considered for patients with very early-stage SCLC (T1-T2N0) disease and has been shown to have good outcomes in carefully selected patients [23, 24]. In addition, the likelihood of tumor spread to intrathoracic lymph nodes and distant sites is so common in SCLC that careful pathologic assessment is important in T1-T2N0 disease to ensure that other neuro-endocrine staging tumors are not the underlying diagnosis, such as carcinoid tumors or non-small cell high-grade neuroendocrine disease. T1N0 SCLC arises in <5% of cases [25].

Some patients who undergo resection may have lymph node involvement of SCLC. In these situations, referral for adjuvant systemic therapy and radiographic staging for distant disease must be undertaken promptly. Although the role of postoperative radiotherapy in NSCLC is evolving, NCCN guidelines advocate for consideration of postoperative radiotherapy in resected N1- and N2-involved SCLC [26].

An alternative to resection in medically inoperable stage I SCLC is SBRT, which is safe and effective [27]. However, systemic therapy is critical for patients with all stages of SCLC. Systemic dissemination is the norm in stage I disease unless multi-agent chemotherapy is administered in conjunction with effective local therapy [28].

Thoracic Radiation Considerations

Systemic therapy is necessary but insufficient for long-term disease control in LD-SCLC. Two different meta-analyses further characterized the benefit of thoracic radiation given with chemotherapy. Warde et al. analyzed 11 randomized studies and reported that additional thoracic radiotherapy resulted in a 25% improvement in local control and an absolute 2-year survival benefit of 5.4% [29]. A meta-analysis of 13 trials of LD-SCLC reported a 14% reduction in mortality with an absolute survival benefit of 5.4% at 3 years (9% vs. 14%) when thoracic radiotherapy was combined with chemotherapy in comparison to chemotherapy alone [30]. The era of combined modality therapy was cemented into the legacy of LD-SCLC management with the studies that composed this meta-analysis.

Chest radiotherapy has evolved with technological advances and a better understanding of optimal therapies in SCLC. Although discrete advances have been made in different domains of thoracic radiotherapy management, they add together to create a situation that can maximize clinical outcomes. In the following sections, we explore these interconnected but distinctive facets.

Fractionation and Dose of Thoracic Radiation

The meta-analyses by Warde et al. and Pignon et al. established thoracic radiotherapy as a key component of LD-SCLC management, but fractionation and timing needed to be addressed [29, 30]. Tumors with a high proliferation index favor a more abbreviated course of radiotherapy because this allows for the complete delivery of treatment before the effects of accelerated repopulation limit treatment efficacy. Further, in vitro studies of SCLC demonstrated high radiosensitivity to treatment at relatively low therapeutic doses [31]. The in vitro findings supported the use of multiple frequent small doses of radiation. Consequently, clinical practice mirrored pre-clinical results. Current practice includes radiation given twice daily at 1.5 Gray (Gy) per fraction delivered with an interval of at least 6 h to allow for sublethal repair of normal tissues [26]. A Gray equals 100 centigray (cGy) and is a measure of the absorbed radiation dose. The lower dose per fraction is associated with a lower risk of late effects from treatment. Taken together, twice daily radiation can improve the therapeutic index by preferentially affecting tumor versus normal tissue.

The randomized study by Turrisi et al. explored the role of dose and fractionation by randomizing 417 patients with LD SCLC to 45 Gy of radiation given in standard fractionation of 1.8 Gy/day delivered over 5 weeks versus 1.5 Gy delivered twice daily over 3 weeks [21]. The radiotherapy was given with concurrent standard-of-care EP-based chemotherapy. Using a primary endpoint of overall survival, twice-daily compared to once-daily radiotherapy was associated with a statistically significant improvement in median overall survival (1.6 years vs. 1.9 years) and 5-year overall survival (26% vs. 16%). However, twice-daily radiation was associated with worsened grade 3 esophagitis, defined as an inability to swallow solids, requiring narcotic analgesics or the use of a feeding tube (11% vs. 27%, $p < 0.001$).

Although twice-daily radiotherapy became the standard of care once the mature results by Turrisi et al. were published, the study was critiqued for a comparison arm that was not at parity with the experimental arm; the study did not compare a biologically equivalent radiation dose used in the twice-daily arm in the once-daily arm. A radiation dose of >60 Gy in conventionally fractionated daily radiation is biologically more equivalent to 45 Gy in 1.5 Gy twice-daily dosing. Consequently, studies were proposed that compared the twice-daily regimen to a more biologically equivalent once-daily regimen [32].

Two randomized studies have recently evaluated the role of high-dose once-daily conventionally fractionated radiation versus twice-daily radiation given, as per Turrisi et al. Both studies showed no difference in outcomes between twice-daily versus once-daily radiotherapy [16, 33]. However, the studies were not powered to demonstrate equivalence, so twice-daily RT remains the standard of care.

The CONVERT study was a phase three study of once-daily radiation to 66 Gy in 33 fractions versus twice-daily radiation given to 45 Gy in 1.5 Gy twice-daily therapy to 30 fractions [16]. After randomization of 547 patients, the median overall survival was 30 months with twice daily radiation versus 25 months with daily radiation (p value 0.14), with a 2-year overall survival of 56% versus 51%. There was no difference in grade 3 for esophagitis rates between the two groups (19% in the twice-daily arm versus 19% in the daily arm). As the study was designed to show the superiority of once-daily high-dose radiotherapy, the authors concluded that twice-daily radiation should be considered the standard of care in LD SCLC.

Recently, the results of cancer and leukemia group B (CALGB) 30610 were published, which also compared twice-daily radiation given to 45 Gy in 30 fractions to a high-dose once-daily regimen of 70 Gy given once daily at 2 Gy/fraction for 35 fractions [33]. After randomization of 638 patients, the median survival is 26.5 months for twice-daily treatment and 30.1 months for once-daily treatment. The 5-year overall survival was not distinctly different at 29% versus 32%. The efficacy and frequency of severe adverse events were similar between both arms.

Both CALGB 30610 and CONVERT studies were designed to show the superiority of once-daily high-dose radiotherapy; the authors concluded that twice-daily radiation should be considered the standard of care in the setting of LD SCLC.

Recently, promising outcomes were reported in a phase two Scandinavian study of twice-daily radiation to 60 Gy compared with twice-daily radiation to 45 Gy [34]. Both arms gave radiation at 1.5 Gy twice daily. In this provocative phase 2 study of 167 patients, the 2-year overall survival of 74.2% versus 48.1% favored the use of twice-daily radiotherapy. Local relapse was more common in the 45 Gy arm versus the 60 Gy arm (35% versus 21%, p value 0.054). The study reported no difference in toxicity between the arms. These data are being explored in a phase 3 study of high-dose twice-daily radiotherapy versus standard-dose twice-daily radiotherapy.

Although the 60 Gy arm had much better overall survival than the CONVERT study, the 45 Gy arm of the Scandinavian study had outcomes inferior to the 45 Gy arm of the CONVERT study. Consequently, phase 3 evaluation will be necessary to explore whether high-dose twice-daily radiation will be a standard of care option in LD SCLC.

Radiation Target Volumes

Before CT-based planning, radiation treatment was delivered using large ports that included the primary tumor, ipsilateral hilum, and bilateral mediastinum. As radiation planning became more sophisticated and allowed for cross-sectional defined targets with CT, a simultaneous ability to use intensity-modulated radiotherapy ushered an era of better tissue sparing in nearby structures. Studies (undertaken initially in NSCLC) showed that treating only involved mediastinal lymph node stations resulted in a low elective nodal failure rate.

Studies were also undertaken in SCLC to evaluate the omission of elective nodal regions. An initial phase two prospective study of 27 patients with LD SCLC delivered radiation only to the primary and involved nodal stations using CT-based planning. These results showed higher-than-expected elective nodal recurrence, and caution was given to involving nodal radiation in LD SCLC using CT-based inputs [35].

The same group then evaluated the role of involved nodal radiation using PET-based imaging to guide areas of treatment. In a prospective study of 60 patients with LD disease, the isolated nodal failure rate was 3%, suggesting that involved nodal radiation can safely be administered if PET- and CT-based imaging is used to plan radiotherapy [36]. As these data were published to support the safe omission of elective nodal regions, the CONVERT and CALGB 30610 amended their protocols to allow for involved nodal irradiation. Consequently, the studies contained a chimera of patients treated with elective nodal coverage and involved mediastinal lymph node coverage. Currently, the standard of care in LD SCLC is to cover only lymph node regions that are deemed involved by (1) biopsy, (2) ^{19}F-fluorodeoxyglucose (FDG) uptake, or (3) CT enlargement.

Normal Tissue Dose Objectives

Planning radiotherapy for patients with LD SCLC will use similar principles used in NSCLC therapy. Although accelerated fractionation with twice-daily radiotherapy can result in different acute and delayed side effects profiles, dose objectives for daily versus twice-daily radiotherapy are similar. However, one notable exception is the spinal cord. Whereas most normal tissues recover from sublethal repair within 4–6 h, the spinal canal is felt to mirror other nerve structures requiring 24 h to undergo sublethal repair. Hence, twice-daily therapy of 150 cGy/fraction is biologically received to the CNS disease as a daily dose of 300 cGy/day to the spinal canal tissue. Hence, the spinal cord experiences a hypofractionated dose of approximately 3 Gy/day and a point max of 41 Gy is recommended, which mirrors the protocol guidelines for CALGB 30610 [33].

Timing of Systemic and Local Therapies

We have defined the treatment of LD-SCLC to include chest radiotherapy and chemotherapy. The timing of these treatments is also important to optimize therapeutic outcomes. Concurrent versus sequential thoracic radiotherapy was undertaken in the Japanese clinical oncology group study 9104. Of 231 patients who received twice-daily radiotherapy to a total dose of 45 Gy in 3 weeks, those treated with concurrent radiotherapy had an improvement in overall survival as well as 2-, 3-, and 5-year survival compared with those who received sequential radiotherapy. The authors note that severe esophagitis was uncommon in both arms, occurring in 9% of those treated with concurrent therapy and 4% with sequential treatment [37].

A meta-analysis that included studies of LD SCLC compared outcomes between early versus late timing of thoracic radiotherapy in relation to chemotherapy administration [38]. Early radiotherapy was defined as starting within 9 weeks of chemotherapy and before cycle 3. In the studies evaluated, the 2-year and median overall survival was significantly increased for early versus late timing of thoracic radiotherapy. Interestingly, studies that included patients with once-daily radiation showed no difference in early versus late radiotherapy. The studies suggest that the early administration of thoracic radiotherapy during definitive treatment of LD SCLC may improve outcomes.

Finally, a study explored the relationship between timing with start of therapy and end of radiation based on the hypothesis that the quick administration of radiotherapy will be positively associated with outcome. They analyzed phase 3 clinical trials of SCLC using meta-analysis methodology and introduced the concept of the interval between the start of any therapy and the end of radiotherapy, which was abbreviated as the SER interval as a marker of outcome [39]. These studies showed that shorter SER intervals were associated with a significantly higher survival rate and a higher incidence of severe esophagitis. For example, in patients with a SER less than 30 days, the 5-year overall survival was >20%.

Taken together, these studies support the early administration of thoracic radiotherapy given in conjunction with chemotherapy. Unless the volume of the treated area is not safe for therapeutic radiation treatment, our practice is to attempt concurrent chemoradiotherapy on cycle 1 of treatment.

Particle-Based Therapy

The two dominant modalities for radiation delivery use either photons or protons. Most patients treated worldwide are administered radiation with photon (or X-ray)-based therapy. Proton therapy is unique because the radiation dose does not have an exit dose beyond the targeted area. In contrast, photon-based treatment continues to scatter low-dose therapy beyond the target. Using techniques to modulate the depth of the treatment, proton therapy can result in less radiation dose to normal tissues and, in dosimetric studies, better tissue sparing.

Whether proton-based therapy improves outcomes in treating tumors in the chest is unclear. A randomized study of protons versus photons in NSCLC failed to show a reduction in clinical toxicity or an improvement in tumor control, but this study used earlier forms of proton-based therapy that may have compromised results [40]. Consequently, an NRG study is currently exploring proton-based therapy in inoperable stage 3 NSCLC.

Proton-based therapy does have limitations. Whereas photon-based therapy is resilient to anatomic changes such as target motion, shrinkage, or changes in tissue density, proton-based therapy can have dramatic differences in target coverage with even modest changes. Hence, adaptive planning is critical to ensure evolving coverage in tumors such as SCLC that are brisk responders to therapy.

Tumors of the chest, including SCLC, are more mobile than targets in other non-thoracic anatomic sites. Consequently, proton-based therapy needs to be optimized to account for motion, and motion itself needs to be minimized to achieve predictable therapeutic dose for target coverage. Lastly, SCLC specifically may pose a particular challenge. Response to therapy can be brisk and use twice daily radiotherapy; the treatment course is temporarily short. In addition, notable tumor size reductions during therapy are often seen, and real-time accounting for and adaption to these changes is vital.

Further, as noted above, thoracic radiotherapy and chemotherapy timing can influence outcomes. For example, holding chest radiotherapy until chemotherapy results in target volume reduction and stability may allow for a safer and more predictable course of proton-based therapy, but this delay may also adversely affect clinical outcomes [38, 39]. These limitations are seen in photon-based treatment but not nearly to the degree seen with protons. Consequently, the practical limitations noted above can attenuate the physical advantages of protons.

Early clinical experience with proton-based therapy in SCLC in dosimetric and limited patient studies have suggested a theoretic improvement with protons [41]. Further, this technique is safe, but further studies are needed to establish the technique as standard clinical therapy in SCLC.

Treatment of Extensive Stage Disease

Systemic Therapy Considerations

Initial Systemic Treatment

Extensive stage SCLC has therapeutic parallels to LD SCLC in systemic management. SCLC is considered a disseminated disease regardless of stage, but in ES disease, the primary focus is on effective systemic management. Both stages use a backbone of EP-based chemotherapy. However, the ED SCLC treatment paradigms focus on carboplatin chemotherapy instead of cisplatin [26]. Carboplatin AUC 5–6 Day 1 and etoposide 100 mg/m^2 Days 1, 2, and 3 are safe and effective in elderly patients (seven NCCN guidelines), repeated every 21–28 days, and given for 4–6 cycles [42]. Other variations of this regimen are also used in some centers.

In patients for which etoposide-based chemotherapy is not feasible or tolerated, an alternative regimen of irinotecan 50 mg/m^2 on Days 1, 8, and 15 with concurrent carboplatin (AUC 5) has been shown to be equivalent and may have less toxicity in some patients [43].

Despite multiple clinical trials in ED SCLC, studies from the 1980s through the early 2010s failed to improve the backbone of EP for management established in the 1980s until recently. However, immunotherapy is transforming the field of ED SCLC treatment. The first immunotherapy shown to improve outcomes in ED SCLC is atezolizumab, a PD-L1 inhibitor. The IMpower 133 study group conducted a randomized phase 3 study of 403 patients with ED SCLC randomized 1:1 to either carboplatin-based chemotherapy with etoposide or similar EP-based chemotherapy with concurrent atezolizumab given with each cycle and then as maintenance therapy at the completion of upfront treatment [17]. Carboplatin was administered at an AUC of 5 on Day 1, etoposide 100 mg/m^2 on Days 1–3, and atezolizumab 1200 mg/m^2 on Day 1. The study had a primary endpoint of progression-free and overall survival using intent to treat. With a median follow-up of 13.9 months, the atezolizumab arm had improved median overall survival (OS) (12.3 months vs. 10.3 months, $p = 0.007$) and improved median PFS (5.2 months vs. 4.3 months, $p = 0.02$).

More recently, the CASPIAN study explored the use of durvalumab, a programmed death ligand-1 (PD-L1) inhibitor, and tremelimumab, a cytotoxic T-lymphocyte-associated protein-4 (CTLA-4) inhibitor [44]. In this three-arm study, 805 patients were randomly assigned to (a) durvalumab + tremelimumab + platinum-etoposide, (b) durvalumab + platinum-etoposide, or (c) platinum-etoposide alone. The etoposide was administered at 80–100 mg/m^2 on Days 1–3, and the platinum was either carboplatin (AUC 5–6) or cisplatin 75–80 mg/m^2 on Day 1 of each cycle. The durvalumab was given at 1500 mg and tremelimumab at 75 mg. In those patients randomized to immunotherapy, maintenance durvalumab was administered every 4 weeks (1500 mg). The co-primary endpoints were (a) overall survival for durvalumab + EP versus EP alone and (b) overall survival for durvalumab-tremelimumab + EP vs. EP alone. With a median follow-up of 25.1 months, durvalumab + tremelimumab + platinum-etoposide did not improve overall survival versus platinum-etoposide alone (10.4 months vs. 10.5 months, $p = 0.045$). However, durvalumab + platinum-etoposide did show an improved overall survival versus platinum-etoposide alone (12.9 months vs. 10.5 months, $p = 0.0032$).

Consequently, the upfront systemic management of ES SCLC includes EP-based chemotherapy with concurrent PD-L1 inhibition (either atezolizumab or durvalumab) followed by maintenance PDL-L1 inhibition until progression or intolerance.

Systemic Treatment for Relapsed Disease

Whereas patients have a high objective response rate in both LS and ES SCLC using first-line treatment regimens, the response of SCLC in the relapsed setting can be modest. Patients are considered EP responsive if they have a disease-free interval of >6 months. In these patients, re-introducing EP-based chemotherapy can be a reasonable treatment option. This option is also a reasonable second-line option in patients with a disease-free interval of 3–6 months (NCCN guidelines). Other treatment options in relapsed disease include topotecan, lurbinectedin, metronomic chemotherapy, cyclophosphamide/doxorubicin/vincristine (CAV), temozolomide, or alternative immunotherapy agents, including pembrolizumab. However, second-line systemic therapy options have limited efficacy, and outcomes are generally poor.

Topotecan

Topotecan is an inhibitor of topoisomerase 1, a nuclear enzyme. Oral and IV administrations of topotecan are available and have efficacy in disease relapse. For example, in a randomized study of relapse ED SCLC in patients not candidates for IV chemotherapy, 141 patients were enrolled in a comparison of best supportive care (BSC) versus BSC + oral topotecan (BSC) [45]. The oral topotecan was given at 2.3 mg/m^2 on Days 1–5 every 21 days. A median survival of 13.9 weeks was seen with BSC versus 25.9 weeks with topotecan. Stable disease was seen in 44% of patients and a partial response in 7% of patients given topotecan. The therapy was well tolerated by most patients.

Lurbinectedin

Lurbinectedin decreases tumor cell proliferation by inhibiting mitosis through RNA polymerase II inhibition. In a phase II study of relapsed SCLC, 3.2 mg/m^2 of lurbinectedin was administered in 3-week cycles until disease progression or unacceptable toxicity [46]. With a median follow-up of 17.1 months, 105 patients were treated, with an overall response in 35% of patients. Although hematologic toxicity is common, given treatment efficacy, lurbinectedin was granted accelerated FDA approval in 2020 [47].

Metronomic Chemotherapy

The frequent administration of chemotherapy at low doses to avoid the dose-limiting toxicities often with a combination of therapies has been explored in relapsed SCLC. In a study of 180 patients randomized to topotecan versus metronomic chemotherapy consisting of cisplatin, etoposide, and irinotecan, overall survival was improved with the metronomic chemotherapy (18.2 months vs. 12.5 months, $p = 0.0079$) [48]. However, this regimen poses significant hematologic toxicity (grades 3–4: neutropenia, 83%; anemia, 84%; leucopenia, 80%; thrombocytopenia, 41%), and febrile neutropenia, grades 3–4, was seen in 31% of patients.

Cyclophosphamide, Doxorubicin, and Vincristine (CAV)

CAV-based chemotherapy was historically a first-line treatment option until EP-based chemotherapy was shown to be equally effective. The ability to co-administer EP with thoracic RT made it a preferred therapy, as co-administration is not feasible with CAV. However, CAV-based chemotherapy can be an attractive option in relapsed disease. In a randomized study of IV topotecan versus CAV (cyclophosphamide 1000 mg/m^2, doxorubicin 45 mg/m^2, and vincristine 2 mg) given in a once-daily cycle every 21 days, 107 patients given CAV had a response rate of 24.3% in comparison to topotecan (18.3%) [49]. There were no differences in time to progression or overall survival

Temozolomide

Temozolomide is an alkylating agent and has the added benefit of being an oral therapy. Its use in high-grade gliomas illustrates the CNS penetration of this therapy. Consequently, it can be an attractive option for relapse SCLC with brain metastases. In a study of 64 patients with relapsed SCLC, patients were assigned to O^6-methylguanine-DNA methyltransferase (*MGMT*) promoter methylation status, which is associated with sensitivity to temozolomide-based therapy [50]. Of the 48 patients deemed sensitive to MGMT expression by immunohistochemistry, one had a complete response, and ten had a partial response. In the 16 patients that were predicted to be refractory by MGMT expression, two partial responses were seen. In patients with brain metastases, complete or partial response incidence was 38%. The MGMT-methylated group had a response in comparison to the unmethylated MGMT patients (38% vs. 7%, $p = 0.08$).

Pembrolizumab

In a pooled analysis of two studies that explored the use of the PD-L1 inhibitor pembrolizumab after receiving two or more lines of prior therapy (KEYNOTE-028 and KEYNOTE-158), 83 patients had an objective response rate of 19.3% with two complete responses and 14 partial responses [51]. Of those who were responders, 61% had responses >18 months, with the median duration of response not reached.

Other Systemic Regimens

Patients with relapsed SCLC who are candidates for additional therapy should be encouraged to enroll in a clinical trial. Further advances will require ongoing commitment to clinical investigation. Other regimens have also been shown to be active in the relapsed SCLC setting, including docetaxel, oral etoposide, nivolumab, paclitaxel, gemcitabine, vinorelbine, and irinotecan [26].

Thoracic Radiation Considerations

Whereas all stages of SCLC are systemic, ED SCLC is a clinical scenario where the role of local therapy is limited. However, the importance of primary tumor control, even in metastatic disease, has been shown to confer benefit. Jeremic and colleagues explored the role of chest radiotherapy in a 5-arm randomized study involving 210 patients [52]. Patients who underwent three cycles of EP-based chemotherapy and had a complete response in metastatic sites of disease and at least a partial response in the chest-based disease were randomized to (a) two additional cycles of chemotherapy with definitive chest radiotherapy using accelerated hyperfractionation to a total dose of 54 Gy given in 1.5 Gy daily twice-daily fractionation in 36 treatments or (b) four additional cycles of chemotherapy alone. For patients randomized to radiotherapy with chemotherapy instead of chemotherapy alone, the median survival was 17 months versus 11 months, with a 5-year overall survival of 13% versus 4% (vs. 4% for which treatment?), which improved with those treated with thoracic radiotherapy ($p = 0.041$). Of note, all patients were treated with prophylactic cranial irradiation.

Local Therapy for Oligometastatic SCLC

Despite the favorable outcomes of the study by Jeremic et al., studies still need to replicate the favorable findings of definitive radiotherapy in ED SCLC. For example, RTOG 0937 randomized patients with oligometastatic SCLC (defined as three or fewer sites of distant disease) to either prophylactic cranial irradiation (PCI) alone or PCI and consolidative chest radiotherapy with the option of consolidative radiation to distant areas of disease as well [53]. Patients were randomized after undergoing four cycles of carboplatin and etoposide, achieving either a partial or complete response to therapy. Consolidative radiotherapy was given to the chest and 45 Gy at 3 Gy/fraction. Distant sites of disease were consolidated and 30–40 Gy in 3–4 Gy/fraction. All patients received PCI with 25 Gy in 10 fractions. At interim analysis, the study was closed early for futility. With a median overall survival of 9.1 months, the 1-year overall survival was 60.1% (PCI) versus 50.8% (PCI + RT) ($p = 0.208$). However, the time to progression favored those who received consolidative radiotherapy to the chest ($p = 0.0102$). Taken together, the results of RTOG

0937 and the study by Jeremic et al. do not support routine use of definitive radio-therapy in patients with ED SCLC.

Palliative, Attenuated Dose Radiotherapy in ED SCLC

In a randomized study of prophylactic cranial irradiation in patients with ED SCLC, the rate of chest relapse was over 90% [54]. Consequently, Slotman et al. hypothesized that non-definitive doses of radiotherapy might delay the time to intrathoracic progression resulting in an improvement in progression-free and overall survival.

A total of 498 patients with ED SCLC were randomized in a phase 3 study of thoracic radiotherapy versus standard-of-care treatment [55]. Standard-of-care treatment was defined as platinum-based chemotherapy with etoposide followed by PCI. Chest radiotherapy was delivered to a total dose of 30 Gy in 10 fractions. Target volumes included residual gross disease in the primary and mediastinum and initially involved nodal stations. A 3D conformal technique was used for treatment planning and optimization. With a median follow-up of 24 months, the primary outcome of overall survival at 1 year was not different between the groups. In those who underwent thoracic radiotherapy, the 1-year survival was 33% versus 28% in those in the control group (p value 0.066). However, the authors note that in exploratory 2-year overall survival showed an improvement in outcome with chest radiotherapy, 13% versus 3% ($p = 0.004$). Additionally, at 6 months, the progression-free survival favored chest radiotherapy, 24% versus 7%, p value 0.001.

Given a favorable toxicity profile to 30 Gy of chest radiotherapy in 10 fractions, the use of consolidative chest therapy in ED SCLC is an appropriate option in patients who have a response to initial therapy.

Prophylactic Cranial Irradiation (PCI)

Patients with SCLC have a high risk for intracranial metastasis. Studies have estimated that the lifetime risk exceeds 50% in LD and ED SCLC [56, 57]. In addition, autopsy series report the risk of CNS involvement may be seen in up to 60–70% of patients [58]. Given that CNS spread will render LD patients incurable and can often lead to a cause of morbidity and death in patients with SCLC, studies have explored the role of prophylactic endeavors to decrease the risk of brain metastasis. The most studied of these interventions includes prophylactic cranial irradiation (PCI).

PCI involves the administration of whole-brain radiotherapy to attenuated doses. The assumption is that treating the brain before evidence of macroscopic disease is seen either influences the seed (tumor cells) or the soil (the brain parenchyma). Hence, PCI decreases CNS spread by treating micrometastatic disease already in the brain or creating an environment where the primary tumor is less likely to spread.

PCI in Limited Stage Disease

Although no single randomized study has shown a survival benefit to using PCI in LD SCLC, the meta-analysis by Auperin et al. included patients in seven clinical trials with LD SCLC who had a complete remission [59]. In this meta-analysis, a relative risk of death in those who underwent PCI was statistically lower than those who did not, corresponding to a 5.4% improvement in the survival rate at 3 years (20.7% in the PCI group versus 15.3% in the control group). Notably, the incidence of brain metastasis was still approximately 33% at 3 years in those treated with PCI.

The meta-analysis by Auperin and colleagues included a spectrum of doses for PCI from 8 Gy in 1 fraction to 40 Gy in 20 fractions. A study of 720 patients who had a complete response to upfront therapy with LD disease was undertaken to define the optimal dose of PCI dose [60]. Patients were randomly assigned to (a) 25 Gy in 10 fractions versus (b) two different comparison arms of 36 Gy using either 2 Gy/fraction or twice-daily radiation at 1.5 Gy/fraction. Using a primary endpoint of brain metastasis at 2 years, the study showed no improvement in 2-year incidence of brain metastasis between the standard dose (29%) and high-dose (23%) PCI groups. However, the 2-year overall survival trended toward improvement in those receiving standard dose radiotherapy (42%) versus those receiving higher-dose radiotherapy (37%) ($p = 0.05$).

Although studies are again exploring the role of PCI in LD SCLC, standard of care in patients with a good response to upfront therapy includes PCI delivered to the whole brain in 25 Gy in 10 fractions. However, notable exceptions may be made for patients with a contraindication for whole brain radiation, including age and neurocognitive deficits.

PCI in Extensive Stage Disease

Researchers hypothesized that if PCI is beneficial and LD SCLC, there may be a role for PCI in ED SCLC because the risk of CNS spread is even higher in the latter. In a study of 286 patients with ED SCLC randomized to PCI versus no further therapy, patients who underwent PCI had a lower rate of symptomatic brain metastasis [54]. At 1 year, 14.6% of patients in the PCI group developed brain metastasis versus 40.4% in the control group. The 1-year survival of 27.1% in the PCI group was improved from those without further therapy, 13.3%.

The study was critiqued for several limitations. First, patients were not pre-screened with brain imaging before enrolling in the study. Up to 15% of patients may have asymptomatic brain metastases at diagnosis [61, 62]. Hence, the favorable outcomes may have been driven by those patients randomized to observation who had macrometastatic disease at enrollment. Second, the routine use of CNS radiographic screening was not undertaken unless symptoms warranted evaluation. While the co-primary endpoint of symptomatic brain metastases is practical, the implication is that patients with asymptomatic brain metastasis were not receiving therapy until symptoms arose, delaying brain-directed treatment in the observation group that can be associated with improved outcomes.

Given the limitations of the study, a companion study was undertaken in Japan to explore the use of PCI and ED SCLC. This study randomized patients after pre-screening enrollment imaging showed no CNS metastases [63]. Those patients who were randomized to observation as well as those who underwent PCI had brain imaging every 3 months. The study was terminated after 224 patients were randomized because of futility on interim analysis. The median overall survival was 11.6 months for those who underwent PCI versus 13.7 months for those who underwent observation. The cumulative risk of brain metastasis at 6, 12, and 24 months supported the use of PCI (6 months, 15% vs. 46%; 12 months, 33% vs. 59%; 18 months, 40% vs. 64%). Of note, radiation was given to 83% of patients who eventually developed brain metastasis in the observation group. Taken together, these data suggest that PCI can be safely omitted in patients with ED SCLC who undergo brain imaging every 3 months. Further, these data suggest that the role of brain radiation may have more to do with the timing of therapy. Said another way, patients with ED SCLC may safely receive whole-brain radiation instead of adjuvant PCI if close surveillance imaging and clinical evaluation are included in survivorship.

Hippocampal Avoidance PCI

Chest radiotherapy in ED SCLC has gained greater uptake in clinical practice than PCI in part because of the differences in toxicity profiles between brain and chest radiation. In addition, early studies in patients with metastatic cancer of all types to the brain show a possible benefit to the avoidance of the hippocampal areas of the brain when whole-brain radiation is given [64]. Consequently, researchers investigated whether PCI given with hippocampal avoidance is safe while also reducing the long-term morbidity of whole-brain radiotherapy.

Redmond et al. explored hippocampal avoidance PCI in 20 patients with LD SCLC [65]. The 2-year overall survival was 88%, and using Hopkins verbal learning test revised delayed recall at 6 months as a primary endpoint, there was no significant decline in performance. These results were replicated at 12 months. MRI surveillance showed asymptomatic brain metastasis in 20% of patients. In patients who developed brain metastasis, these occurred in underdosed areas proximal to the hippocampal regions.

Three randomized studies have further explored the role of hippocampal avoidance in both LD and ED SCLC. The PREMER study enrolled 150 patients and used a primary outcome of delayed free recall (DFR) on the free and cued selective reminding test at 3 months [66]. With a median follow-up of 40.4 months, the DFR decline at 3 months was lower in those treated with hippocampal avoidance (5.8%) versus those treated with the standard PCI (23.5%). The authors report no difference in the incidence of brain metastasis, quality of life, or overall survival.

An NK/Dutch study of hippocampal avoidance PCI in SCLC used an alternative outcome of changes on the Hopkins verbal learning test at 4 months [67]. One hundred sixty-eight patients were enrolled, of whom 70% had LD SCLC. Patients were randomized to hippocampal avoidance versus standard PCI, and the rate of HVLT decline at 4 months was not different between the groups. Additionally, there was no difference in the incidence of brain metastasis (20% PCI vs. 16% HA-PCI) or overall survival.

A third study by the NRG (CC 003) completed enrollment of 304 patients in July 2022 [68]. Using a primary outcome of Hopkins verbal learning test recall at 6 months using the Reliable Change Index (RCI), we await the report of these results. These data, in conjunction with the NK/Dutch and PREMIER data, may help to further define whether hippocampal avoidance PCI can improve the therapeutic outcome and carefully selected patients with SCLC. At present, hippocampal avoidance PCI can be administered but should be offered on a clinical trial.

Summary of Recommendations

In patients with LD SCLC, treatment with concurrent EP given in four 21-day cycles is the standard of care (see Table 9.1). Definitive, twice-daily radiotherapy using 150 cGy/fraction to a total planned dose of 45–60 Gy is administered concurrently with systemic therapy. The use of thoracic radiation earlier in the course of therapy is associated with improved outcomes. PCI in patients with a good response to therapy can be offered to complete therapy. Careful assessment of imaging of both brain and extracranial sites with clinical assessment of constitutional, pulmonary, or recrudescence of paraneoplastic symptoms complete the comprehensive survivorship assessment.

In patients with ED SCLC, treatment with 4–6 cycles of carboplatin, etoposide, and atezolizumab in 21-day cycles followed by maintenance atezolizumab in 28-day cycles is standard of care. Thoracic radiotherapy to initially involved nodal sites and residual gross disease to 30 Gy in 10 fractions can reduce intrathoracic recurrence. An alternative to PCI in ED SCLC is surveillance brain imaging every 3 months. Disease assessment between every two cycles of initial therapy and every 8–12 weeks with maintenance therapy can ensure that ongoing treatment is adjusted to the current disease state. Eventual tumor relapse is anticipated in most patients within 6 months of initial therapy, and second- and third-line options are available, although their efficacy and durability are limited.

Finally, the role of consolidative chest RT in ED SCLC with immunotherapy has not been defined. Still, ongoing studies will merge these two treatment strategies to optimize outcomes for this patient population.

Table 9.1 Current treatment guidelines in small cell lung cancer

Limited stage disease
• Concurrent cisplatin- and etoposide-based chemotherapy × 4 cycles[a]
• Chest radiotherapy[a] to initially involved sites
– 45 Gy in 1.5 Gy/fraction delivered twice daily
– Incorporation of concurrent RT as quickly as is reasonably feasible with chemotherapy
• Restaging with brain and body imaging
• Prophylactic cranial irradiation to 25 Gy at 2.5 Gy/fraction[b]
Extensive stage disease
• Concurrent carboplatin- and etoposide-based chemotherapy[c] × 4 cycles
• Restaging with brain and body imaging
• Chest radiotherapy[c] to residual gross disease and initially involved lymph node areas[b]
– 30 Gy at 3 Gy/fraction given once daily
• Maintenance immunotherapy with Atezolizumab
• Serial brain imaging every 3 months[d]

[a] Chemotherapy and radiation are delivered concurrently
[b] Offered if restaging shows no new areas of concern for progressive disease
[c] Chemotherapy and radiation are delivered sequentially
[d] If serial brain imaging is not feasible, consider prophylactic cranial irradiation

References

1. Ettinger DS, Aisner J. Changing face of small-cell lung cancer: real and artifact. J Clin Oncol. 2006;24(28):4526–7. https://doi.org/10.1200/JCO.2006.07.3841. PMID: 17008688.
2. Govindan R, Page N, Morgensztern D, Read W, Tierney R, Vlahiotis A, Spitznagel EL, Piccirillo J. Changing epidemiology of small-cell lung cancer in the United States over the last 30 years: analysis of the surveillance, epidemiologic, and end results database. J Clin Oncol. 2006;24(28):4539–44. https://doi.org/10.1200/JCO.2005.04.4859. PMID: 17008692.
3. van Meerbeeck JP, Fennell DA, De Ruysscher DK. Small-cell lung cancer. Lancet. 2011;378(9804):1741–55. https://doi.org/10.1016/S0140-6736(11)60165-7. Epub 2011 May 10. PMID: 21565397.

4. Gazdar AF, Bunn PA, Minna JD. Small-cell lung cancer: what we know, what we need to know and the path forward. Nat Rev Cancer. 2017;17(12):725–37. https://doi.org/10.1038/nrc.2017.87. Epub 2017 Oct 27. Erratum in: Nat Rev Cancer. 2017; PMID: 29077690.

5. Marchioli CC, Graziano SL. Paraneoplastic syndromes associated with small cell lung cancer. Chest Surg Clin N Am. 1997;7(1):65–80. PMID: 9001756.

6. Gandhi L, Johnson BE. Paraneoplastic syndromes associated with small cell lung cancer. J Natl Compr Cancer Netw. 2006;4(6):631–8. https://doi.org/10.6004/jnccn.2006.0052. PMID: 16813730.

7. Rudin CM, Brambilla E, Faivre-Finn C, Sage J. Small-cell lung cancer. Nat Rev Dis Prim. 2021;7(1):3. https://doi.org/10.1038/s41572-020-00235-0. PMID: 33446664; PMCID: PMC8177722.

8. Travis WD, Brambilla E, Burke AP, Marx A, Nicholson AG. Introduction to the 2015 World Health Organization Classification of tumors of the lung, pleura, thymus, and heart. J Thorac Oncol. 2015;10(9):1240–2. https://doi.org/10.1097/JTO.0000000000000663. PMID: 26291007.

9. Pelosof LC, Gerber DE. Paraneoplastic syndromes: an approach to diagnosis and treatment. Mayo Clin Proc. 2010;85(9):838–54. https://doi.org/10.4065/mcp.2010.0099. Erratum in: Mayo Clin Proc. 2011;86(4):364. Dosage error in article text. PMID: 20810794; PMCID: PMC2931619.

10. Hazell SZ, Mai N, Fu W, Hu C, Friedes C, Negron A, Voong KR, Feliciano JL, Han P, Myers S, McNutt TR, Hales RK. Hospitalization and definitive radiotherapy in lung cancer: incidence, risk factors and survival impact. BMC Cancer. 2020;20(1):334. https://doi.org/10.1186/s12885-020-06843-z. PMID: 32306924; PMCID: PMC7169027.

11. Okamoto H, Watanabe K, Kunikane H, Yokoyama A, Kudoh S, Asakawa T, Shibata T, Kunitoh H, Tamura T, Saijo N. Randomised phase III trial of carboplatin plus etoposide vs split doses of cisplatin plus etoposide in elderly or poor-risk patients with extensive disease small-cell lung cancer: JCOG 9702. Br J Cancer. 2007;97(2):162–9. https://doi.org/10.1038/sj.bjc.6603810. Epub 2007 Jun 19. PMID: 17579629; PMCID: PMC2360311.

12. Shepherd FA, Crowley J, Van Houtte P, Postmus PE, Carney D, Chansky K, Shaikh Z, Goldstraw P. International Association for the Study of Lung Cancer International Staging Committee and Participating Institutions. The International Association for the Study of Lung Cancer lung cancer staging project: proposals regarding the clinical staging of small cell lung cancer in the forthcoming (seventh) edition of the tumor, node, metastasis classification for lung cancer. J Thorac Oncol. 2007;2(12):1067–77. https://doi.org/10.1097/JTO.0b013e31815bdc0d. PMID: 18090577.

13. Micke P, Faldum A, Metz T, Beeh KM, Bittinger F, Hengstler JG, Buhl R. Staging small cell lung cancer: Veterans Administration Lung Study Group versus International Association for the Study of Lung Cancer--what limits limited disease? Lung Cancer. 2002;37(3):271–6. https://doi.org/10.1016/s0169-5002(02)00072-7. PMID: 12234695.

14. Zelen M. Keynote address on biostatistics and data retrieval. Cancer Chemother Rep 3. 1973;4(2):31–42. PMID: 4580860.

15. Goldstraw P, Chansky K, Crowley J, Rami-Porta R, Asamura H, Eberhardt WE, Nicholson AG, Groome P, Mitchell A, Bolejack V. International Association for the Study of Lung Cancer Staging and Prognostic Factors Committee, Advisory Boards, and Participating Institutions; International Association for the Study of Lung Cancer Staging and Prognostic Factors Committee Advisory Boards and Participating Institutions. The IASLC lung cancer staging project: proposals for revision of the TNM stage groupings in the forthcoming (eighth) edition of the TNM classification for lung cancer. J Thorac Oncol. 2016;11(1):39–51. https://doi.org/10.1016/j.jtho.2015.09.009. PMID: 26762738.

16. Faivre-Finn C, Snee M, Ashcroft L, Appel W, Barlesi F, Bhatnagar A, Bezjak A, Cardenal F, Fournel P, Harden S, Le Pechoux C, McMenemin R, Mohammed N, O'Brien M, Pantarotto J, Surmont V, Van Meerbeeck JP, Woll PJ, Lorigan P, Blackhall F, CONVERT Study Team. Concurrent once-daily versus twice-daily chemoradiotherapy in patients with limited-stage

small-cell lung cancer (CONVERT): an open-label, phase 3, randomised, superiority trial. Lancet Oncol. 2017;18(8):1116–25. https://doi.org/10.1016/S1470-2045(17)30318-2. Epub 2017 Jun 20. PMID: 28642008; PMCID: PMC5555437.

17. Horn L, Mansfield AS, Szczęsna A, Havel L, Krzakowski M, Hochmair MJ, Huemer F, Losonczy G, Johnson ML, Nishio M, Reck M, Mok T, Lam S, Shames DS, Liu J, Ding B, Lopez-Chavez A, Kabbinavar F, Lin W, Sandler A, Liu SV, IMpower133 Study Group. First-line atezolizumab plus chemotherapy in extensive-stage small-cell lung cancer. N Engl J Med. 2018;379(23):2220–9. https://doi.org/10.1056/NEJMoa1809064. Epub 2018 Sep 25. PMID: 30280641.

18. Haddadin S, Perry MC. History of small-cell lung cancer. Clin Lung Cancer. 2011;12(2):87–93. https://doi.org/10.1016/j.cllc.2011.03.002. Epub 2011 Apr 8. PMID: 21550554.

19. Sierocki JS, Hilaris BS, Hopfan S, Martini N, Barton D, Golbey RB, Wittes RE. cis-Dichlorodiammineplatinum(II) and VP-16-213: an active induction regimen for small cell carcinoma of the lung. Cancer Treat Rep. 1979;63(9–10):1593–7. PMID: 227598.

20. Roth BJ, Johnson DH, Einhorn LH, Schacter LP, Cherng NC, Cohen HJ, Crawford J, Randolph JA, Goodlow JL, Broun GO, et al. Randomized study of cyclophosphamide, doxorubicin, and vincristine versus etoposide and cisplatin versus alternation of these two regimens in extensive small-cell lung cancer: a phase III trial of the Southeastern Cancer Study Group. J Clin Oncol. 1992;10(2):282–91. https://doi.org/10.1200/JCO.1992.10.2.282. PMID: 1310103.

21. Turrisi AT III, Kim K, Blum R, Sause WT, Livingston RB, Komaki R, Wagner H, Aisner S, Johnson DH. Twice-daily compared with once-daily thoracic radiotherapy in limited small-cell lung cancer treated concurrently with cisplatin and etoposide. N Engl J Med. 1999;340(4):265–71. https://doi.org/10.1056/NEJM199901283400403. PMID: 9920950.

22. Bunn PA Jr, Crowley J, Kelly K, Hazuka MB, Beasley K, Upchurch C, Livingston R, Weiss GR, Hicks WJ, Gandara DR, et al. Chemoradiotherapy with or without granulocyte-macrophage colony-stimulating factor in the treatment of limited-stage small-cell lung cancer: a prospective phase III randomized study of the Southwest Oncology Group. J Clin Oncol. 1995;13(7):1632–41. https://doi.org/10.1200/JCO.1995.13.7.1632. Erratum in: J Clin Oncol 1995;13(11):2860. PMID: 7602352.

23. Lad T, Piantadosi S, Thomas P, Payne D, Ruckdeschel J, Giaccone G. A prospective randomized trial to determine the benefit of surgical resection of residual disease following response of small cell lung cancer to combination chemotherapy. Chest. 1994;106(6 Suppl):320S–3S. https://doi.org/10.1378/chest.106.6_supplement.320s. PMID: 7988254.

24. Lim E, Belcher E, Yap YK, Nicholson AG, Goldstraw P. The role of surgery in the treatment of limited disease small cell lung cancer: time to reevaluate. J Thorac Oncol. 2008;3(11):1267–71. https://doi.org/10.1097/JTO.0b013e318189a860. PMID: 18978561.

25. Ignatius Ou SH, Zell JA. The applicability of the proposed IASLC staging revisions to small cell lung cancer (SCLC) with comparison to the current UICC 6th TNM Edition. J Thorac Oncol. 2009;4(3):300–10. https://doi.org/10.1097/JTO.0b013e318194a355. PMID: 19156001.

26. NCCN. Guidelines for small cell lung cancer. n.d.. https://www.nccn.org/professionals/physician_gls/pdf/sclc.pdf.

27. Mercier SL, Moore SM, Akurang D, Tiberi D, Wheatley-Price P. Stereotactic body radiotherapy (SBRT) in very limited-stage small cell lung cancer (VLS-SCLC). Curr Oncol. 2022;30(1):100–9. https://doi.org/10.3390/curroncol30010008. PMID: 36661657; PMCID: PMC9858162.

28. Verma V, Simone CB II, Allen PK, Gajjar SR, Shah C, Zhen W, Harkenrider MM, Hallemeier CL, Jabbour SK, Matthiesen CL, Braunstein SE, Lee P, Dilling TJ, Allen BG, Nichols EM, Attia A, Zeng J, Biswas T, Paximadis P, Wang F, Walker JM, Stahl JM, Daly ME, Decker RH, Hales RK, Willers H, Videtic GM, Mehta MP, Lin SH. Multi-institutional experience of stereotactic ablative radiation therapy for stage I small cell lung cancer. Int J Radiat Oncol Biol Phys. 2017;97(2):362–71. https://doi.org/10.1016/j.ijrobp.2016.10.041. Epub 2016 Nov 2. PMID: 28011047.

29. Warde P, Payne D. Does thoracic irradiation improve survival and local control in limited-stage small-cell carcinoma of the lung? A meta-analysis. J Clin Oncol. 1992;10(6):890–5. https://doi.org/10.1200/JCO.1992.10.6.890. PMID: 1316951.
30. Pignon JP, Arriagada R, Ihde DC, Johnson DH, Perry MC, Souhami RL, Brodin O, Joss RA, Kies MS, Lebeau B, et al. A meta-analysis of thoracic radiotherapy for small-cell lung cancer. N Engl J Med. 1992;327(23):1618–24. https://doi.org/10.1056/NEJM199212033272302. PMID: 1331787.
31. Carney DN, Mitchell JB, Kinsella TJ. In vitro radiation and chemotherapy sensitivity of established cell lines of human small cell lung cancer and its large cell morphological variants. Cancer Res. 1983;43(6):2806–11. PMID: 6303568.
32. Abadir R, Orton C. Radiotherapy for small-cell lung cancer. N Engl J Med. 1999;340(25): 2002–3; author reply 2003-4. PMID: 10383278.
33. Bogart J, Wang X, Masters G, Gao J, Komaki R, Gaspar LE, Heymach J, Bonner J, Kuzma C, Waqar S, Petty W, Stinchcombe TE, Bradley JD, Vokes E. High-dose once-daily thoracic radiotherapy in limited-stage small-cell lung cancer: CALGB 30610 (Alliance)/RTOG 0538. J Clin Oncol. 2023;41:2394. https://doi.org/10.1200/JCO.22.01359. PMID: 36623230.
34. Grønberg BH, Killingberg KT, Fløtten Ø, Brustugun OT, Hornslien K, Madebo T, Langer SW, Schytte T, Nyman J, Risum S, Tsakonas G, Engleson J, Halvorsen TO. High-dose versus standard-dose twice-daily thoracic radiotherapy for patients with limited stage small-cell lung cancer: an open-label, randomised, phase 2 trial. Lancet Oncol. 2021;22(3):321–31. https://doi.org/10.1016/S1470-2045(20)30742-7. PMID: 33662285.
35. De Ruysscher D, Bremer RH, Koppe F, Wanders S, van Haren E, Hochstenbag M, Geeraedts W, Pitz C, Simons J, ten Velde G, Dohmen J, Snoep G, Boersma L, Verschueren T, van Baardwijk A, Dehing C, Pijls M, Minken A, Lambin P. Omission of elective node irradiation on basis of CT-scans in patients with limited disease small cell lung cancer: a phase II trial. Radiother Oncol. 2006;80(3):307–12. https://doi.org/10.1016/j.radonc.2006.07.029. Epub 2006 Sep 1. PMID: 16949169.
36. van Loon J, De Ruysscher D, Wanders R, Boersma L, Simons J, Oellers M, Dingemans AM, Hochstenbag M, Bootsma G, Geraedts W, Pitz C, Teule J, Rhami A, Thimister W, Snoep G, Dehing-Oberije C, Lambin P. Selective nodal irradiation on basis of (18)FDG-PET scans in limited-disease small-cell lung cancer: a prospective study. Int J Radiat Oncol Biol Phys. 2010;77(2):329–36. https://doi.org/10.1016/j.ijrobp.2009.04.075. Epub 2009 Sep 24. PMID: 19782478.
37. Takada M, Fukuoka M, Kawahara M, Sugiura T, Yokoyama A, Yokota S, Nishiwaki Y, Watanabe K, Noda K, Tamura T, Fukuda H, Saijo N. Phase III study of concurrent versus sequential thoracic radiotherapy in combination with cisplatin and etoposide for limited-stage small-cell lung cancer: results of the Japan Clinical Oncology Group Study 9104. J Clin Oncol. 2002;20(14):3054–60. https://doi.org/10.1200/JCO.2002.12.071. PMID: 12118018.
38. Fried DB, Morris DE, Poole C, Rosenman JG, Halle JS, Detterbeck FC, Hensing TA, Socinski MA. Systematic review evaluating the timing of thoracic radiation therapy in combined modality therapy for limited-stage small-cell lung cancer. J Clin Oncol. 2004;22(23):4837–45. https://doi.org/10.1200/JCO.2004.01.178. Erratum in: J Clin Oncol. 2005;23(1):248. PMID: 15570087.
39. De Ruysscher D, Pijls-Johannesma M, Bentzen SM, Minken A, Wanders R, Lutgens L, Hochstenbag M, Boersma L, Wouters B, Lammering G, Vansteenkiste J, Lambin P. Time between the first day of chemotherapy and the last day of chest radiation is the most important predictor of survival in limited-disease small-cell lung cancer. J Clin Oncol. 2006;24(7):1057–63. https://doi.org/10.1200/JCO.2005.02.9793. PMID: 16505424.
40. Liao Z, Lee JJ, Komaki R, Gomez DR, O'Reilly MS, Fossella FV, Blumenschein GR Jr, Heymach JV, Vaporciyan AA, Swisher SG, Allen PK, Choi NC, DeLaney TF, Hahn SM, Cox JD, Lu CS, Mohan R. Bayesian adaptive randomization trial of passive scattering proton therapy and intensity-modulated photon radiotherapy for locally advanced non-small-cell lung

cancer. J Clin Oncol. 2018;36(18):1813–22. https://doi.org/10.1200/JCO.2017.74.0720. Epub 2018. Erratum in: J Clin Oncol. 2018;36(24):2570. PMID: 29293386; PMCID: PMC6008104.

41. Rwigema JM, Verma V, Lin L, Berman AT, Levin WP, Evans TL, Aggarwal C, Rengan R, Langer C, Cohen RB, Simone CB II. Prospective study of proton-beam radiation therapy for limited-stage small cell lung cancer. Cancer. 2017;123(21):4244–51. https://doi.org/10.1002/cncr.30870. Epub 2017 Jul 5. PMID: 28678434.

42. Okamoto H, Watanabe K, Nishiwaki Y, Mori K, Kurita Y, Hayashi I, Masutani M, Nakata K, Tsuchiya S, Isobe H, Saijo N. Phase II study of area under the plasma-concentration-versus-time curve-based carboplatin plus standard-dose intravenous etoposide in elderly patients with small-cell lung cancer. J Clin Oncol. 1999;17(11):3540–5. https://doi.org/10.1200/JCO.1999.17.11.3540. PMID: 10550152.

43. Schmittel A, von Weikersthal LF, Sebastian M, Martus P, Schulze K, Hortig P, Reeb M, Thiel E, Keilholz U. A randomized phase II trial of irinotecan plus carboplatin versus etoposide plus carboplatin treatment in patients with extended disease small-cell lung cancer. Ann Oncol. 2006;17(4):663–7. https://doi.org/10.1093/annonc/mdj137. Epub 2006 Jan 19. PMID: 16423848.

44. Goldman JW, Dvorkin M, Chen Y, Reinmuth N, Hotta K, Trukhin D, Statsenko G, Hochmair MJ, Özgüroğlu M, Ji JH, Garassino MC, Voitko O, Poltoratskiy A, Ponce S, Verderame F, Havel L, Bondarenko I, Każarnowicz A, Losonczy G, Conev NV, Armstrong J, Byrne N, Thiyagarajah P, Jiang H, Paz-Ares L, CASPIAN Investigators. Durvalumab, with or without tremelimumab, plus platinum-etoposide versus platinum-etoposide alone in first-line treatment of extensive-stage small-cell lung cancer (CASPIAN): updated results from a randomised, controlled, open-label, phase 3 trial. Lancet Oncol. 2021;22(1):51–65. https://doi.org/10.1016/S1470-2045(20)30539-8. Epub 2020 Dec 4. PMID: 33285097.

45. O'Brien ME, Ciuleanu TE, Tsekov H, Shparyk Y, Cuceviá B, Juhasz G, Thatcher N, Ross GA, Dane GC, Crofts T. Phase III trial comparing supportive care alone with supportive care with oral topotecan in patients with relapsed small-cell lung cancer. J Clin Oncol. 2006;24(34):5441–7. https://doi.org/10.1200/JCO.2006.06.5821. PMID: 17135646.

46. Trigo J, Subbiah V, Besse B, Moreno V, López R, Sala MA, Peters S, Ponce S, Fernández C, Alfaro V, Gómez J, Kahatt C, Zeaiter A, Zaman K, Boni V, Arrondeau J, Martínez M, Delord JP, Awada A, Kristeleit R, Olmedo ME, Wannesson L, Valdivia J, Rubio MJ, Anton A, Sarantopoulos J, Chawla SP, Mosquera-Martinez J, D'Arcangelo M, Santoro A, Villalobos VM, Sands J, Paz-Ares L. Lurbinectedin as second-line treatment for patients with small-cell lung cancer: a single-arm, open-label, phase 2 basket trial. Lancet Oncol. 2020;21(5):645–54. https://doi.org/10.1016/S1470-2045(20)30068-1. Epub 2020 Mar 27. Erratum in: Lancet Oncol. 2020;21(12): e553. PMID: 32224306.

47. FDA. n.d.. https://www.fda.gov/drugs/drug-approvals-and-databases/fda-grants-accelerated-approval-lurbinectedin-metastatic-small-cell-lung-cancer.

48. Goto K, Ohe Y, Shibata T, Seto T, Takahashi T, Nakagawa K, Tanaka H, Takeda K, Nishio M, Mori K, Satouchi M, Hida T, Yoshimura N, Kozuki T, Imamura F, Kiura K, Okamoto H, Sawa T, Tamura T, JCOG0605 Investigators. Combined chemotherapy with cisplatin, etoposide, and irinotecan versus topotecan alone as second-line treatment for patients with sensitive relapsed small-cell lung cancer (JCOG0605): a multicentre, open-label, randomised phase 3 trial. Lancet Oncol. 2016;17(8):1147–57. https://doi.org/10.1016/S1470-2045(16)30104-8. Epub 2016 Jun 14. PMID: 27312053.

49. von Pawel J, Schiller JH, Shepherd FA, Fields SZ, Kleisbauer JP, Chrysson NG, Stewart DJ, Clark PI, Palmer MC, Depierre A, Carmichael J, Krebs JB, Ross G, Lane SR, Gralla R. Topotecan versus cyclophosphamide, doxorubicin, and vincristine for the treatment of recurrent small-cell lung cancer. J Clin Oncol. 1999;17(2):658–67. https://doi.org/10.1200/JCO.1999.17.2.658. PMID: 10080612.

50. Pietanza MC, Kadota K, Huberman K, Sima CS, Fiore JJ, Sumner DK, Travis WD, Heguy A, Ginsberg MS, Holodny AI, Chan TA, Rizvi NA, Azzoli CG, Riely GJ, Kris MG, Krug LM. Phase II trial of temozolomide in patients with relapsed sensitive or refractory small

cell lung cancer, with assessment of methylguanine-DNA methyltransferase as a potential biomarker. Clin Cancer Res. 2012;18(4):1138–45. https://doi.org/10.1158/1078-0432. CCR-11-2059. Epub 2012 Jan 6. PMID: 22228633.

51. Chung HC, Piha-Paul SA, Lopez-Martin J, Schellens JHM, Kao S, Miller WH Jr, Delord JP, Gao B, Planchard D, Gottfried M, Zer A, Jalal SI, Penel N, Mehnert JM, Matos I, Bennouna J, Kim DW, Xu L, Krishnan S, Norwood K, Ott PA. Pembrolizumab after two or more lines of previous therapy in patients with recurrent or metastatic SCLC: results from the KEYNOTE-028 and KEYNOTE-158 studies. J Thorac Oncol. 2020;15(4):618–27. https://doi.org/10.1016/j.jtho.2019.12.109. Epub 2019 Dec 20. PMID: 31870883.

52. Jeremic B, Shibamoto Y, Nikolic N, Milicic B, Milisavljevic S, Dagovic A, Aleksandrovic J, Radosavljevic-Asic G. Role of radiation therapy in the combined-modality treatment of patients with extensive disease small-cell lung cancer: a randomized study. J Clin Oncol. 1999;17(7):2092–9. https://doi.org/10.1200/JCO.1999.17.7.2092. PMID: 10561263.

53. Gore EM, Hu C, Sun AY, Grimm DF, Ramalingam SS, Dunlap NE, Higgins KA, Werner-Wasik M, Allen AM, Iyengar P, Videtic GMM, Hales RK, McGarry RC, Urbanic JJ, Pu AT, Johnstone CA, Stieber VW, Paulus R, Bradley JD. Randomized phase II study comparing prophylactic cranial irradiation alone to prophylactic cranial irradiation and consolidative extracranial irradiation for extensive-disease small cell lung cancer (ED SCLC): NRG oncology RTOG 0937. J Thorac Oncol. 2017;12(10):1561–70. https://doi.org/10.1016/j.jtho.2017.06.015. Epub 2017 Jun 23. PMID: 28648948; PMCID: PMC5610652.

54. Slotman B, Faivre-Finn C, Kramer G, Rankin E, Snee M, Hatton M, Postmus P, Collette L, Musat E, Senan S, EORTC Radiation Oncology Group and Lung Cancer Group. Prophylactic cranial irradiation in extensive small-cell lung cancer. N Engl J Med. 2007;357(7):664–72. https://doi.org/10.1056/NEJMoa071780. PMID: 17699816.

55. Slotman BJ, van Tinteren H, Praag JO, Knegjens JL, El Sharouni SY, Hatton M, Keijser A, Faivre-Finn C, Senan S. Use of thoracic radiotherapy for extensive stage small-cell lung cancer: a phase 3 randomised controlled trial. Lancet. 2015;385(9962):36–42. https://doi.org/10.1016/S0140-6736(14)61085-0. Epub 2014 Sep 14. Erratum in: Lancet. 2015;385(9962):28. PMID: 25230595.

56. Komaki R. Prophylactic cranial irradiation for small cell carcinoma of the lung. Cancer Treat Symp. 1985;2:1.

57. Arriagada R, Le Chevalier T, Borie F, Rivière A, Chomy P, Monnet I, Tardivon A, Viader F, Tarayre M, Benhamou S. Prophylactic cranial irradiation for patients with small-cell lung cancer in complete remission. J Natl Cancer Inst. 1995;87(3):183–90. https://doi.org/10.1093/jnci/87.3.183. PMID: 7707405.

58. Hirsch FR, Paulson OB, Hansen HH, Vraa-Jensen J. Intracranial metastases in small cell carcinoma of the lung: correlation of clinical and autopsy findings. Cancer. 1982;50(11):2433–7. https://doi.org/10.1002/1097-0142(19821201)50:11<2433::aid-cncr2820501131>3.0.co;2-e. PMID: 6182974.

59. Aupérin A, Arriagada R, Pignon JP, Le Péchoux C, Gregor A, Stephens RJ, Kristjansen PE, Johnson BE, Ueoka H, Wagner H, Aisner J. Prophylactic cranial irradiation for patients with small-cell lung cancer in complete remission. Prophylactic Cranial Irradiation Overview Collaborative Group. N Engl J Med. 1999;341(7):476–84. https://doi.org/10.1056/NEJM199908123410703. PMID: 10441603.

60. Le Péchoux C, Dunant A, Senan S, Wolfson A, Quoix E, Faivre-Finn C, Ciuleanu T, Arriagada R, Jones R, Wanders R, Lerouge D, Laplanche A, Prophylactic Cranial Irradiation (PCI) Collaborative Group. Standard-dose versus higher-dose prophylactic cranial irradiation (PCI) in patients with limited-stage small-cell lung cancer in complete remission after chemotherapy and thoracic radiotherapy (PCI 99-01, EORTC 22003-08004, RTOG 0212, and IFCT 99-01): a randomised clinical trial. Lancet Oncol. 2009;10(5):467–74. https://doi.org/10.1016/S1470-2045(09)70101-9. Epub 2009 Apr 20. PMID: 19386548.

61. Hochstenbag MM, Twijnstra A, Wilmink JT, Wouters EF, ten Velde GP. Asymptomatic brain metastases (BM) in small cell lung cancer (SCLC): MR-imaging is useful at initial diagnosis.

J Neuro-Oncol. 2000;48(3):243–8. https://doi.org/10.1023/a:1006427407281. PMID: 11100822.

62. Seute T, Leffers P, Wilmink JT, ten Velde GP, Twijnstra A. Response of asymptomatic brain metastases from small-cell lung cancer to systemic first-line chemotherapy. J Clin Oncol. 2006;24(13):2079–83. https://doi.org/10.1200/JCO.2005.03.2946. PMID: 16648509.

63. Takahashi T, Yamanaka T, Seto T, Harada H, Nokihara H, Saka H, Nishio M, Kaneda H, Takayama K, Ishimoto O, Takeda K, Yoshioka H, Tachihara M, Sakai H, Goto K, Yamamoto N. Prophylactic cranial irradiation versus observation in patients with extensive-disease small-cell lung cancer: a multicentre, randomized, open-label, phase 3 trial. Lancet Oncol. 2017;18(5):663–71. https://doi.org/10.1016/S1470-2045(17)30230-9. Epub 2017 Mar 23. PMID: 28343976.

64. Gondi V, Pugh SL, Tome WA, Caine C, Corn B, Kanner A, Rowley H, Kundapur V, DeNittis A, Greenspoon JN, Konski AA, Bauman GS, Shah S, Shi W, Wendland M, Kachnic L, Mehta MP. Preservation of memory with conformal avoidance of the hippocampal neural stem-cell compartment during whole-brain radiotherapy for brain metastases (RTOG 0933): a phase II multi-institutional trial. J Clin Oncol. 2014;32(34):3810–6. https://doi.org/10.1200/JCO.2014.57.2909. Epub 2014 Oct 27. PMID: 25349290; PMCID: PMC4239303.

65. Redmond KJ, Hales RK, Anderson-Keightly H, Zhou XC, Kummerlowe M, Sair HI, Duhon M, Kleinberg L, Rosner GL, Vannorsdall T. Prospective study of hippocampal-sparing prophylactic cranial irradiation in limited-stage small cell lung cancer. Int J Radiat Oncol Biol Phys. 2017;98(3):603–11. https://doi.org/10.1016/j.ijrobp.2017.03.009. Epub 2017 Mar 14. PMID: 28581401.

66. Rodríguez de Dios N, Couñago F, Murcia-Mejía M, Rico-Oses M, Calvo-Crespo P, Samper P, Vallejo C, Luna J, Trueba I, Sotoca A, Cigarral C, Farré N, Manero RM, Durán X, Gispert JD, Sánchez-Benavides G, Rognoni T, Torrente M, Capellades J, Jiménez M, Cabada T, Blanco M, Alonso A, Martínez-San Millán J, Escribano J, González B, López-Guerra JL. Randomized phase III trial of prophylactic cranial irradiation with or without hippocampal avoidance for small-cell lung cancer (PREMER): a GICOR-GOECP-SEOR study. J Clin Oncol. 2021;39(28):3118–27. https://doi.org/10.1200/JCO.21.00639. Epub 2021 Aug 11. PMID: 34379442.

67. Belderbos JSA, De Ruysscher DKM, De Jaeger K, Koppe F, Lambrecht MLF, Lievens YN, Dieleman EMT, Jaspers JPM, Van Meerbeeck JP, Ubbels F, Kwint MH, Kuenen MA, Deprez S, De Ruiter MB, Boogerd W, Sikorska K, Van Tinteren H, Schagen SB. Phase 3 randomized trial of prophylactic cranial irradiation with or without hippocampus avoidance in SCLC (NCT01780675). J Thorac Oncol. 2021;16(5):840–9. https://doi.org/10.1016/j.jtho.2020.12.024. Epub 2021 Feb 2. PMID: 33545387.

68. NRG Oncology. n.d.. https://www.nrgoncology.org/Home/News/Post/nrg-oncology-ncorp-trial-of-hippocampal-avoidance-for-small-cell-lung-cancer-patients-receiving-prophylactic-cranial-irradiation-reaches-accrual-goal.

Chapter 10
Management of Malignant Pleural Effusion

Benjamin DeMarco and Christina R. MacRosty

Introduction

Malignancy involving the pleura is the second most common cause of exudative pleural effusion, following parapneumonic effusion [1]. Malignant pleural effusion (MPE) is a marker of advanced disease. It is associated with worse outcomes and a high burden of care, accounting for more than 125,000 hospital admissions with annual hospital charges of more than $5 billion in the United States (USA) [2]. Epidemiological studies in MPE are limited, but there are an estimated 150,000 cases in the USA and 50,000 in the United Kingdom per year [3, 4]. MPE's incidence and associated costs are expected to rise as the global cancer rate increases and advances in cancer-directed therapies contribute to improved survival rates [5].

Epidemiology

Most MPEs are caused by lung cancer, and [6, 7] approximately 15% of patients with lung cancer have MPE at the time of diagnosis [1, 6, 7]. The frequency of MPE by cancer type is seen in Table 10.1. Metastatic breast cancer and lymphoma are the second and third leading causes of MPE, respectively [3].

B. DeMarco
Division of Pulmonary and Critical Care Medicine, Johns Hopkins University,
Baltimore, United States
e-mail: bdemarc4@jh.edu

C. R. MacRosty (✉)
Division of Pulmonary Diseases and Critical Care Medicine, University of North Carolina,
Chapel Hill, NC, USA
e-mail: christina_macrosty@med.unc.edu

© The Author(s), under exclusive license to Springer Nature
Switzerland AG 2023
C. MacRosty, M. P. Rivera (eds.), *Lung Cancer*, Respiratory Medicine,
https://doi.org/10.1007/978-3-031-38412-7_10

MPE is associated with significant cancer-associated mortality, with current guidelines reporting a median survival ranging from 3 to 12 months [9, 11–13]. Several factors, including tumor type and stage and Eastern Cooperative Oncology Group Performance Status (ECOG-PS), are independent prognostic factors in MPE [13–15]. Survival in MPE varies according to tumor type due to the underlying malignancy's sensitivity to treatment. Lung cancer carries the worst prognosis, while gynecologic and breast cancers have more favorable survival times [9, 13, 15–17].

Effusion size, specifically a massive effusion (fluid occupying the entire hemithorax), is associated with significantly worse survival in smaller non-randomized studies [13]. Pleural fluid markers, including pH, glucose, and lactate dehydrogenase (LDH), have been investigated as prognostic tools, but none have consistently reported utility or validity [13, 18]. The LENT score (LDH, ECOG, blood neutrophil-lymphocyte ratio, and tumor type) was the first externally validated prognostic scoring system for MPE, separating patients into low-, moderate-, and high-risk groups with median survival of 319 days, 130 days, and 44 days, respectively [19, 20]. A more recent prospectively validated score (PROMISE) combines biological markers and clinical parameters to stratify patients based on a 3-month mortality risk, but its complexity limits routine application [21]. The Brims' decision tree is the most well-validated prognostic model for mesothelioma [22]. While validated in study populations, the clinical utility of these scores is not yet established, and further research is needed to determine their generalizability and association with patient-centered outcomes. Available prognostic information should be factored into treatment decisions to expedite definitive pleural intervention for patients with more prolonged survival while aiming to maximize time outside the hospital for those with shorter life expectancy [9, 13].

Table 10.1 MPE by tumor type

Primary tumor type	Total (%)
Lung cancer	15–38
Breast cancer	7–17
Lymphoma	6–11
Ovarian cancer	3–7
Other	6–15
Unknown primary	4–12

Adapted from Antony [3] Light [8] Roberts [9] and Merlo et al. [10]

The Cause of Malignant Pleural Effusion by Cancer Type

Clinical Presentation

Dyspnea is the most common symptom occurring in over 50% of patients with MPE [7]. It is caused by a combination of factors, including caudal displacement of the diaphragm resulting in suboptimal length-tension relationship in the work of respiration, contralateral mediastinal shift, and decrease in ipsilateral lung volume [23, 24]. Symptoms related to the primary tumor are common such as weight loss, malaise, and anorexia. Chest pain, commonly associated with mesothelioma, is usually ipsilateral to the effusion and dull rather than pleuritic [25]. On plain chest radiography, MPE is most often unilateral but can present bilaterally in about 11% of cases [12]. MPEs are the most common cause of large (occupying more than two-thirds of the hemithorax) and massive (complete opacification of hemithorax) pleural effusions [26, 27].

Pathophysiology

Several poorly understood direct and indirect mechanisms underlie the development of MPE. Lung carcinomas may translocate to the ipsilateral visceral pleura via the pulmonary circulation or undergo hematogenous spread [4, 28]. In non-bronchogenic carcinomas not involving the lung, tumor cells metastasize to the parietal pleura via hematogenous spread [28]. Tumors may reach the parietal pleura by various mechanisms, including seeding along adhesions, lymphangitic spread, or direct extension along adjacent structures (chest wall, mediastinum, diaphragm) [4]. The complex interaction between tumor and host within the pleural space remains unclear. In vivo observations suggest defective recruitment, activation, and cytotoxicity of CD8+ lymphocytes and macrophages against autologous tumor cells [4].

Increased fluid production due to fluid extravasation from a hyper-permeable parietal and/or visceral pleura is thought to be the predominant mechanism underlying the development of MPE with impaired lymphatic outflow and decreased clearance contributing in a secondary role [4, 29, 30]. The molecular mechanism of increased pleural permeability is driven by host-tumor interplay in which paracrine and autocrine signaling stimulates pleural inflammation, tumor angiogenesis, and vascular permeability [4, 30]. Tumor-derived vascular endothelial growth factor (VEGF) and tumor necrosis factor (TNF) directly stimulate inflammatory cell influx and vascular changes, which are amplified by host inflammatory signals resulting in a positive feedback loop leading to fluid accumulation and tumor growth [4, 30].

Several secondary mechanisms can contribute. Tumor cells may obstruct the thoracic duct resulting in a chylothorax, most common in lymphomas. Malignant airway obstruction with distal atelectasis can contribute to pleural fluid accumulation [8], and pericardial involvement from metastatic malignancies can result in elevated hydrostatic pressures in both systemic and pulmonary circulation, resulting in a transudative effusion [8].

Diagnosis

Imaging

A variety of imaging modalities have a well-established role in the diagnostic workup of patients with suspected MPE. Thoracic ultrasound (TUS) is now routinely used in clinical care and is strongly supported by guideline recommendations for guidance of pleural interventions [31]. Pleural or diaphragmatic thickening and nodularity appreciated on TUS are highly specific for malignancy and can guide suspicion for MPE [32, 33]. The use of contrast-enhanced TUS to differentiate benign effusions from MPE remains under investigation. Contrast-enhanced computed tomography (CT) of the chest may demonstrate nodular pleural thickening, parietal pleural thickening greater than 1 cm, or circumferential pleural thickening, which are highly specific for malignant involvement of the pleura [33]. However, there are no data reliably correlating CT characteristics to histopathology [34, 35]. ^{18}F-fluorodeoxyglucose positron emission tomography (^{18}F-FDG-PET, PET) is widely used in oncology for characterization of malignancy and evaluation of suspected metastatic disease. However, the specificity of PET is limited in evaluating MPE due to false positivity from nonmalignant forms of pleural disease such as tuberculous pleuritis [36]. Recent meta-analyses have suggested that PET integrated with CT imaging may play a limited role in the guidance of workup for suspected MPE [37]. Magnetic resonance imaging (MRI) performs similarly to chest CT in differentiating nonmalignant from malignant pleural disease. However, availability and cost remain barriers to use, and MRI lacks a defined role in initial diagnostic workup of a suspected MPE [33]. Altogether, advanced imaging modalities may heighten suspicion for MPE and can serve a role in triage and diagnostic workup, but they lack the sensitivity and specificity to provide conclusive evidence of MPE. Direct sampling from the pleural space is required to confirm the diagnosis.

Pleural Fluid Analysis

Ultrasound-guided thoracentesis with pleural fluid analysis is the initial procedure for diagnosing suspected MPE. Standard pleural fluid analytic studies of MPE will classically reveal exudative fluid with mononuclear cell predominance. Grossly bloody pleural fluid (RBC count >100,000/mm^3), low pleural fluid glucose (<60 mg/

dL), and low pleural fluid pH (less than 7.30) have all been associated with malignant pleural disease [8, 33, 34], although none are diagnostic. In addition, low pleural fluid pH has been associated with greater cytology yield, reduced pleurodesis success, and shorter survival [35, 38, 39]. Caution must be employed when interpreting the significance of low pleural fluid pH given the possibility of confounding from commonly clinically utilized medications such as lidocaine and heparin and from other causes of inflammatory pleural effusion such as infection and autoimmune pleuritis [40].

The diagnosis of MPE is confirmed by demonstrating malignant cells in the pleural space on cytologic examination. Diagnostic yield of pleural fluid cytology varies widely in the published literature, with reported accuracy ranging from 40% to 90%, with maximal yield from two separate samples [8, 13, 33, 41, 42]. In one of the largest modern case series ($n = 831$), Porcel and colleagues demonstrated an initial cytology yield of 51% which increased to 59% with second and third cytological specimens [41]. In subgroup analysis, of the 214 patients with negative first cytology results, 55 additional patients (26%) were diagnosed with MPE on second pleural fluid aspiration. Additionally, 52 patients with two negative cytology results underwent a third thoracentesis, and 12 (23%) of these were diagnostic for MPE, suggesting serial pleural fluid cytology offers benefit if clinical suspicion for malignancy is high [33, 41]. Yield does plateau around the third sample [33, 43]. Primary tumor type has a significant effect on the pleural fluid cytology yield. Exfoliative cell types such as ovarian cancer or metastatic adenocarcinoma demonstrate significantly higher yields compared to lower yields of squamous cell carcinoma, mesothelioma, and sarcomas [8, 33, 41, 42, 44]. The volume of pleural fluid aliquots submitted and the preparation method (direct smear/cytospin versus addition of cell block) can affect diagnostic yield. A fluid sample volume of >75 mL is required to eliminate the influence of specimen size on diagnostic adequacy, while upward of 150 mL is required to maximize the yield of preparations involving cell block and direct smear [45, 46]. Higher volumes may provide additional incremental value if extensive immunohistochemical testing or genetic analysis of fluid is anticipated, although this is not well studied outside of lung cancer-related MPE [33, 47]. Flow cytometry can establish the diagnosis in cases of pleural lymphoma and should be considered in the evaluation of lymphocytic pleural effusion, where lymphoma is a diagnostic consideration. A variety of tumor markers have been studied, both individually and in combination, in efforts to guide diagnosis of MPE in cytology-negative effusions; however, they lack the specificity to establish the diagnosis of MPE in isolation [33, 48]. The role of serum biomarkers such as circulating tumor DNA (ctDNA) in diagnosing MPE remains investigational due to similar sensitivity limitations [33, 49].

Pleural Biopsy

Nonimage-guided closed needle biopsy (commonly referred to as Abrams' needle biopsy) of the pleura is no longer recommended in the diagnostic workup of MPE, given low yield compared to pleural fluid cytology, save for situations where suspicion for mesothelioma is high and thoracoscopy is unavailable [8, 33]. Ultrasound-guided biopsy targeting areas of pleural thickening greater than 1 cm or pleural nodularity has shown increased yield in patients with previously undiagnosed exudates [50, 51]. CT-guided pleural biopsy provides improved diagnostic sensitivity compared to both Abrams' needle and ultrasound-assisted biopsy [52, 53].

Medical thoracoscopy (also referred to as local anesthetic thoracoscopy and pleuroscopy) is a minimally invasive ambulatory procedure performed under local anesthesia and moderate sedation that allows for direct visualization of the pleural space and subsequent forceps biopsies of any abnormal sites on the parietal pleura. Multiple studies have demonstrated diagnostic sensitivity of greater than 90% for medical thoracoscopy for both pleural malignancy and mesothelioma [54–56]. One randomized controlled trial ($n = 124$) comparing medical thoracoscopy to CT-guided closed pleural needle biopsy demonstrated a small but not statistically significant advantage in diagnostic sensitivity of the former (95% versus 87%, respectively) [57]. With appropriate patient selection, medical thoracoscopy is a well-tolerated procedure with a favorable risk profile, demonstrating overall low rates of complication (1.6% for major events such as empyema or hemorrhage and 7.3% for minor events such as skin infection) [54, 58].

In the modern era, surgical thoracoscopy, increasingly performed via video-assisted thoracoscopic surgery (VATS), is the gold standard but the most invasive method of diagnosing pleural malignancy. In contrast to medical thoracoscopy, it requires general anesthesia and single lung positive pressure ventilation. Diagnostic yield of VATS in MPE ranges from 89% to 95% with a reported major complication rate of 15–26% in available series [33]. A 2018 retrospective study comparing VATS and medical thoracoscopy found similar diagnostic yield and safety profiles of the two procedures but a significantly higher procedural cost and hospital length of stay (LOS) with VATS [59].

Management

The optimal therapy for MPE would relieve dyspnea, improve quality of life, be minimally invasive, affordable, have a low complication rate, and minimize or eliminate the need for time in the hospital. In recent years, clinical practice guidelines have been published by several major respiratory societies [11, 13], but given the heterogeneity in the presentation of MPE, management should be individualized to patient preferences, symptoms, and quality of life. Our approach to the management of MPE is seen in Fig. 10.1. The foundation of MPE management is palliative; thus,

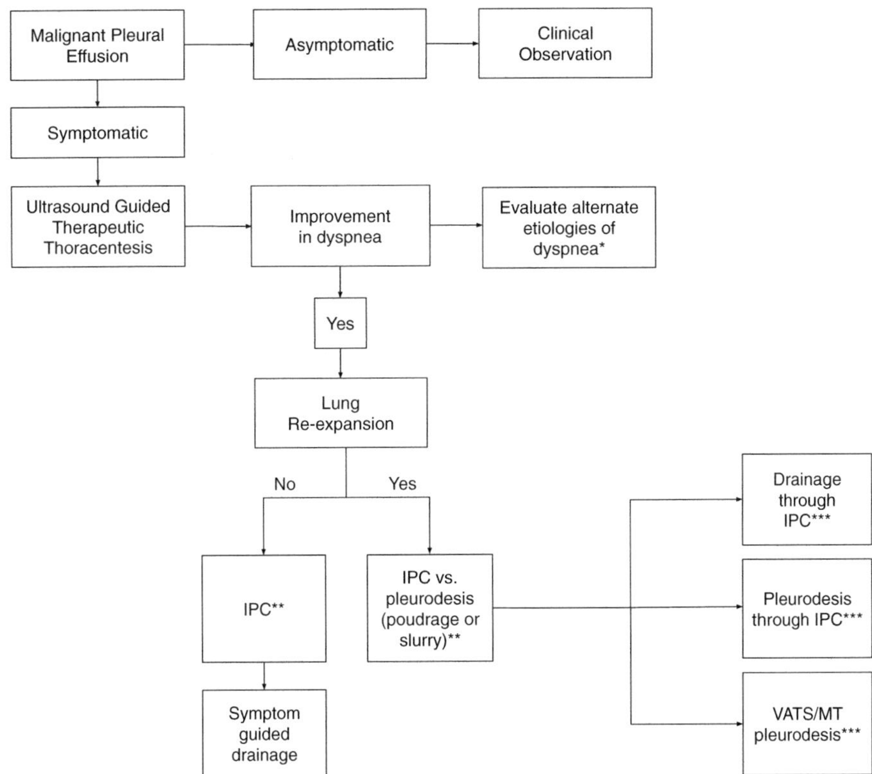

Fig. 10.1 Management of MPE (adapted from Feller-Kopman et al. [11] and Jacobs et al. [18]). IPC = indwelling pleural catheter, VATS = video-assisted thoracoscopic surgery, MT = medical thoracoscopy *Lymphangitic spread of cancer, pulmonary embolus, deconditioning, CHF (congestive heart failure), etc. **If prognosis is weeks or less, consider palliative treatment with opioids, oxygen, and serial thoracentesis. ***Decision should be individualized based on patient preferences and risk/benefit discussion of individual procedures

the first step in management is determining the effusion's impact on the patient's quality of life. In a prospective study of patients with lung cancer-related MPE by Porcel and colleagues [12], 40% of patients developed a pleural effusion during their disease course, half of which were too small for sampling or intervention. Of those patients with small, asymptomatic effusions, none became symptomatic or required drainage. In a more recent multicenter retrospective study of non-small cell lung cancer (NSCLC), 41% of patients with initially asymptomatic MPE became symptomatic within 1 year, with median time to symptom development of 4 months [60]. Given the paucity of data to support benefit, current guidelines recommend that therapeutic pleural interventions not be performed in asymptomatic patients with known or suspected MPE unless a prevailing diagnostic clinical indication exists [9, 11].

Therapeutic Thoracentesis

In patients with symptomatic MPE, large-volume thoracentesis is the first step in management [11, 31]. Therapeutic drainage before definitive pleural intervention can serve dual purposes: confirming symptomatic improvement after effusion drainage and identifying the presence of nonexpendable lung (discussed below) to elucidate further management options. Routine ultrasound guidance is recommended for all thoracentesis as multiple studies have demonstrated the role of ultrasound in enhancing safety and lowering costs [11, 31, 61]. If the patient does not demonstrate symptomatic benefit after thoracentesis, this should prompt investigation of other causes of dyspnea (pulmonary embolism, lymphangitic parenchymal spread, congestive heart failure, etc.) and defer further attempts at palliative pleural intervention. Lastly, a large volume thoracentesis (defined as draining the pleural effusion until it is fully drained or until the patient has symptoms of chest pressure or discomfort indicating nonexpandable lung) allows assessment of the rate of fluid reaccumulation after drainage. A retrospective multicenter study of 1000 patients with MPE found that 30% experienced recurrence after 15 days and 48% by 90 days, while other data suggest that as many as 60% of patients required additional fluid drainage within 10 days [62, 63]. While larger effusion size and higher pleural fluid LDH correlate with an increased recurrence rate, risk factors associated with recurrence of a MPE have not been defined well enough to be clinically useful at present [63].

Definitive Pleural Intervention

Most patients with MPE will experience fluid reaccumulation after initial therapeutic thoracentesis. Therefore, a management strategy to achieve long-term symptom relief, also termed "definitive pleural intervention," is recommended [9]. Patients undergoing definitive pleural intervention procedures need fewer additional pleural procedures, fewer procedures performed in the emergency department, and experience fewer complications than those patients undergoing serial thoracentesis [62]. The most common definitive pleural interventions will be reviewed here.

Chemical Pleurodesis

Pleurodesis is the artificial obliteration of the pleural space by inducing inflammation to cause adhesions, scarring, and fusion of the visceral and parietal pleura, thus preventing fluid reaccumulation. This can be accomplished mechanically (via surgical abrasion) or chemically (via injecting a drug or material into the pleural space). The most utilized chemical agents are graded talc, tetracycline, doxycycline, and bleomycin. However, multiple meta-analyses and head-to-head trials have demonstrated graded talc to be the most effective pleurodesis agent [64–67]. Furthermore, the use of graded (large particle size) talc is recommended over ungraded (mixed particle size) to reduce the risk of pleurodesis-induced acute respiratory distress syndrome (ARDS) [64, 66, 68]. Talc can be administered into the pleural space in two ways: a poudrage which involves insufflation of a dry powder preparation via thoracoscopy, or as a slurry in suspension with sterile fluid, which is instilled through a chest tube [9, 11].

The comparative effectiveness of talc poudrage versus talc slurry has been examined in multiple studies of varying quality with a statistically insignificant trend toward improved pleurodesis rates but more adverse events with talc poudrage [66, 69]. Given inconclusive evidence in available comparators, the 2018 American Thoracic Society (ATS), Society of Thoracic Surgeons (STS), and Society of Thoracic Radiology clinical practice guidelines suggest the use of either talc poudrage or talc slurry in patients with symptomatic MPE and expandable lung guided by local factors such as availability of thoracoscopy expertise or need for additional diagnostic tissue [11]. After these guidelines, the TAPPS (evaluating the efficacy of thoracoscopy and talc poudrage versus pleurodesis using talc slurry) multicenter randomized clinical trial was published. This trial ($n = 330$) found no statistically significant difference in pleurodesis failure at 90 days (22% in thoracoscopic talc poudrage and 24% in talc slurry) or in any of the 24 prespecified secondary outcomes, including the length of hospital stay (LOS), dyspnea, quality of life, pleurodesis failure rate at 30 and 180 days, and mortality [70]. Notably, the talc slurry arm of this trial employed small bore (12–14 Fr) chest tubes, which had previously been thought to have been less effective than large bore ($\geq$24 Fr) chest tubes in achieving pleurodesis [13, 70]. The choice of chest tube size in practice depends on the comfort of the treating physician. The use of thoracic ultrasonography was studied specifically in pleurodesis care pathways by a recent randomized controlled trial in Britain, which found that thoracic ultrasound-guided care resulted in shorter hospital stays with no reduction in the 90-day procedure success rate (median difference in LOS of 1 day) [71].

Indwelling Pleural Catheter

An indwelling pleural catheter (IPC) is a 15.5 Fr silicone tube tunneled under the skin before being inserted into the pleural space, designed for the long-term management of MPE in the outpatient setting via regular home drainage of the fluid. Initially approved by the FDA in 1997, IPCs have significantly increased in use since the late 2000s [72]. Multiple studies have demonstrated efficacy of IPCs in improving dyspnea and quality of life and low complication-related removal rate [73–76].

Infection is the most common IPC-associated complication, with an overall rate of 6% and infection-related mortality of 0.3% [77, 78]. IPC-related infections represent a spectrum of diseases ranging from local infection at the exit site to tunnel infections to deeper pleural space infections. Most cases of cellulitis can be managed with outpatient oral antibiotic therapy, while pleural space infections require the addition of intravenous antibiotics, continuous drainage, and consideration of instillation of fibrinolytics in the setting of loculated infected pleural space [77–79]. Catheter removal is considered only in the setting of antibiotic failure [11, 78, 79]. Given the lack of data supporting optimal treatment methods and the variety of available approaches (oral vs. intravenous antibiotics, treating through catheter vs. removal, etc.), treatment decisions should be made individually. Current guidelines suggest considerations should include the clinical status of the patient; the type of infection; the resources available to the patient, such as their proximity to care and local support network; and the risks of symptomatic fluid reaccumulation if the catheter is removed [11].

Less common complications include obstruction of the portion of the catheter within the pleural space (internal catheter obstruction) by fibrin, clot, or debris, obstruction of the portion outside the pleural space (extrinsic catheter obstruction) from tract metastasis or blood clot and catheter fracture. Internal catheter blockage incidence is approximately 5% and is managed by instillation of saline and then fibrinolytics if saline is unsuccessful [78, 79]. Extrinsic obstruction from catheter tract metastasis is a rare complication in non-mesothelioma-related IPC insertion. Management is palliative with analgesia and considering radiotherapy without needing to remove the IPC [77, 80]. Catheter fracture occurs primarily at the time of IPC removal. It is an underreported complication, but limited available data suggest an incidence of around 10% [81, 82]. Retained IPC fragments can be left in place without aggressive retrieval attempts [77, 81, 82].

Drainage frequency is a common question with IPC management, and two randomized controlled trials have provided data. The 2017 Randomized Trial of Pleural Fluid Drainage Frequency in Patients with Malignant Pleural Effusions Trial (ASAP Trial) compared daily drainage to alternating day drainage with auto-pleurodesis (complete or partial based on symptoms and radiographic changes) as the primary outcome. At 12 weeks, auto-pleurodesis was greater in the aggressive drainage arm than the standard arm (47% vs. 24%), with similar adverse events between groups [83]. Importantly, this trial excluded patients with nonexpandable lung, a patient population who may experience more pain with more frequent drainage. The 2018 Australasian Malignant Pleural Effusion (AMPLE-2) Trial compared aggressive (daily) drainage to symptom-guided drainage with mean daily breathlessness scores as the primary outcome. There was no difference in breathlessness scores between the two groups, but a higher rate of spontaneous pleurodesis (defined as <50 mL of fluid drained at three consecutive drainages or at least two attempts 2 weeks apart in the absence of residual fluid on imaging) at 60 days and 6 months in the daily drainage group compared to the symptom-guided group (37% and 44% vs. 11% and 16%) [84]. Although a daily drainage strategy may lead to faster pleurodesis and catheter liberation in patients with expandable lung, this strategy is more labor intensive and may be associated with increased healthcare costs [85, 86]. Thus, decisions about IPC drainage frequency should be individualized based on patient preferences, available resources, and cost burden.

Comparator Trials and Combination Approaches

Putnam et al. published the first randomized controlled trial comparing IPC to pleurodesis (with doxycycline) in 1999, demonstrating a significant decrease in LOS in the IPC group with similar degrees of symptomatic improvement and quality-of-life measures between groups [87]. The multicenter Therapeutic Intervention in Malignant Effusion (TIME-2) trial compared IPC to chest tube and talc slurry pleurodesis with a primary outcome of dyspnea (measured via visual analog scale) and found no difference in dyspnea at 6 weeks. The IPC group did demonstrate lower dyspnea score at 6 months and shorter hospital LOS. There was no significant difference in chest pain, quality of life, serious adverse events, or mortality between the two groups [88]. The recent AMPLE trial compared IPC to talc slurry pleurodesis and examined hospitalization days as the primary outcome. The IPC group had a shorter LOS (10 days vs. 12 days) and required fewer subsequent pleural interventions, but complications were higher in the IPC group, most common of which were worsening breathlessness and procedure-related pain [89]. Given the significance of the reduced LOS associated with IPC placement in available randomized controlled trials, the recent European Respiratory Society (ERS) statement and ATS clinical practice guideline support the use of IPC or pleurodesis as first-line definitive pleural intervention in patients with symptomatic MPE with expandable lung [11, 13]. The benefit of reduced LOS associated with IPCs must be balanced with the increased risk of infection (cellulitis). Clinicians should individualize management choices to patients' specific values and priorities [11].

With growing evidence supporting IPC use in MPE, there is a burgeoning interest in combined procedures, i.e., talc pleurodesis through IPC, to preserve ambulatory management of MPE while still considering pleurodesis as an option. The IPC-plus trial was a randomized controlled trial that demonstrated the combination of IPC and talc slurry pleurodesis resulted in higher pleurodesis rates and improved quality of life compared to IPC and saline with no increase in adverse events [90]. A currently recruiting study (ASAP-II) is randomizing patients with MPE to IPC with talc and daily drainage versus daily drainage alone [91]. The Early Pleurodesis via IPC with Talc for Malignant Effusion (EPIToME) observational trial evaluated the efficacy of using IPC as first-line definitive therapy for all patients, followed by talc slurry pleurodesis and daily home drainage if feasible. Using this protocol, pleurodesis was achieved in 74% of patients at a median of 20 days; however, a significant percentage of the patients were not candidates for pleurodesis through the IPC [92].

Surgical Management

Surgical approaches to MPE (pleurectomy and abrasion pleurodesis) are limited to mesothelioma. There is a paucity of high-quality data, and the existing randomized trials suggest VATS pleurectomy is associated with more complications and longer hospital stays with no additional benefit in terms of pleurodesis success compared to talc pleurodesis [13, 93].

Special Situations

Nonexpandable Lung

Nonexpandable lung refers to the situation in which the lung cannot completely expand to fill the thorax, leaving the visceral and parietal pleura unopposed. Elsewhere in the literature, this may be referred to as "trapped lung," "entrapped lung," or "unexpandable lung" [9, 11, 13]. Nonexpandable lung occurs in as many as 30% of patients with MPE, but there is a dearth of quality evidence regarding the management of MPE in this scenario [68]. The ability to predict nonexpandable lung via pleural manometry, motion over time (M-mode) thoracic ultrasonography, and patient symptoms during therapeutic thoracentesis is an area of ongoing study, but there is insufficient evidence to support change in current clinical practice [94–98]. Considering chemical pleurodesis is rarely effective in the setting of nonexpandable lung, the high morbidity of surgical approaches such as pleurectomy or pleuroperitoneal shunt, and the low observed incidence of complications associated with IPCs, each of the major respiratory medicine societies recommend IPC as the treatment of choice in MPE with nonexpandable lung [9, 11, 13].

Loculated or Septated MPE

MPEs divided into multiple separate pockets of fluid (i.e., *loculated* or *septated*) can prevent complete drainage of the pleural space and may limit lung expansion, complicating pleurodesis, or limiting the symptomatic relief provided by IPCs. There are few studies examining the role of intrapleural fibrinolytics for loculated MPE, and several prioritize nonpatient-centered outcomes such as reduced radiologic effusion size [13]. The most recent related trial (TIME-3) randomized patients with non-draining MPE due to fibrinous adhesions to either urokinase or placebo, followed by talc slurry pleurodesis. There was no difference between groups in mean dyspnea or pleurodesis failure rates over 12 months. The study, however, was marked by extremely poor overall survival (median survival of 69 days in the urokinase group and 48 days in the placebo group) [99]. Further research is needed to define the role of fibrinolytics in symptomatic locations, and current data are insufficient to support or refute their use in routine clinical practice. Current guidelines recommend use of IPC over chemical pleurodesis in this challenging situation [11].

Conclusion

MPE is a common complication of advanced malignancy associated with significant morbidity, mortality, and cost. The management of MPE has advanced significantly in recent years, considering high-quality randomized controlled trials and clinical practice guidelines focused on patient-centered outcomes. The evidence supports that both IPCs and chemical pleurodesis with talc slurry or poudrage are highly effective at improving symptoms; thus, each approach's specific risks and benefits should be discussed in detail with the patient and their caregiver(s) to individualize the decision. MPE remains a heterogenous disease both within and between primary tumor types, and investigations of novel therapies based on deeper understanding of pathogenesis or combination pleurodesis approaches based on patient-centered outcomes are promising future research directions [100–102]. For now, multidisciplinary discussions centering on patient preferences and palliation remain paramount in the optimal management of MPE [103].

References

1. Ingelfinger JR, Feller-Kopman D, Light R. Pleural disease. N Engl J Med. 2018;378: 740–51.
2. Taghizadeh N, Fortin M, Tremblay A. US Hospitalizations for Malignant Pleural Effusions Data From the 2012 National Inpatient Sample. Chest. 2017;151:845–54.
3. Antony V, Loddenkemper R, Astoui P, Boutin C, Goldstraw P. American thoracic society management of malignant pleural effusions. Am J Respir Crit Care Med. 2000;162:1987–2001.
4. Psallidas I, Kalomenidis I, Porcel JM, Robinson BW, Stathopoulos GT. Malignant pleural effusion: from bench to bedside Number 1 in the Series "Pleural Diseases" Edited by Najib Rahman and Ioannis Psallidas. Eur Respir Rev. 2016;25:189–98.
5. Asciak R, Hallifax RJ, Mercer RM, Hassan M, Wigston C, Wrightson JM, Psallidas I, Rahman NM. The hospital and patient burden of indwelling pleural catheters: a retrospective case series of 210 indwelling pleural catheter insertions. Respiration. 2019;97:70–7.
6. Johnston WW. The malignant pleural effusion. A review of cytopathologic diagnoses of 584 specimens from 472 consecutive patients. Cancer. 1985;56:905–9.
7. Chernow B, Sahn SA. Carcinomatous involvement of the pleura. An analysis of 96 patients. Am J Med. 1977;63:695–702.
8. Light R. Pleural diseases. 6th ed. Philadelphia, PA: Lippincott Williams & Wilkins; 2013.
9. Roberts ME, Neville E, Berrisford RG, Antunes G, Ali NJ. Management of a malignant pleural effusion: British Thoracic Society pleural disease guideline 2010. Thorax. 2010;65:ii32.

10. Merlo A, Strassle P, Gaber C, Mody GN. Time to malignant pleural effusion by cancer type and stage at presentation - an analysis of the surveillance, epidemiology and end results (SEER) Medicare database. J Am Coll Surg. 2020;231:S295.
11. Feller-Kopman DJ, Reddy CB, Decamp MM, et al. Management of malignant pleural effusions. An official ATS/STS/STR clinical practice guideline. Am J Respir Crit Care Med. 2018;198:839–49.
12. Porcel JM, Gasol A, Bielsa S, Civit C, Light RW, Salud A. Clinical features and survival of lung cancer patients with pleural effusions. Respirology. 2015;20:654–9.
13. Bibby AC, Dorn P, Psallidas I, et al. ERS/EACTS statement on the management of malignant pleural effusions. Eur Respir J. 2018;52:1800349.
14. Anevlavis S, Kouliatsis G, Sotiriou I, Koukourakis MI, Archontogeorgis K, Karpathiou G, Giatromanolaki A, Froudarakis ME. Prognostic factors in patients presenting with pleural effusion revealing malignancy. Respiration. 2014;87:311–6.
15. Zamboni MM, da Silva CT, Baretta R, Cunha ET, Cardoso GP. Important prognostic factors for survival in patients with malignant pleural effusion. BMC Pulm Med. 2015;15:29. https://doi.org/10.1186/s12890-015-0025-z.
16. Rusch VW, Chansky K, Kindler HL, et al. The IASLC mesothelioma staging project: proposals for the M descriptors and for revision of the TNM stage groupings in the forthcoming (eighth) edition of the TNM classification for mesothelioma. J Thorac Oncol. 2016;11:2112–9.
17. Amin MB, Edge SB, Greene FL, et al. AJCC cancer staging manual. Cham: Springer; 2017.
18. Jacobs B, Sheikh G, Youness HA, Keddissi JI, Abdo T. Diagnosis and management of malignant pleural effusion: a decade in review. Diagnostics (Basel). 2022;12:1016. https://doi.org/10.3390/diagnostics12041016.
19. Clive AO, Kahan BC, Hooper CE, et al. Predicting survival in malignant pleural effusion: development and validation of the LENT prognostic score. Thorax. 2014;69:1098–104.
20. Psallidas I, Kannelakis N, Yousuf A, Corcoran J, Hallifax R, Wrightson J, Mercer R, Talwar A, Rahman N. Lent score validation on patients with malignant pleural effusion. Eur Respir J. 2016;48:PA3385.
21. Psallidas I, Kanellakis NI, Gerry S, et al. Development and validation of response markers to predict survival and pleurodesis success in patients with malignant pleural effusion (PROMISE): a multicohort analysis. Lancet Oncol. 2018;19:930–9.
22. Brims FJH, Meniawy TM, Duffus I, de Fonseka D, Segal A, Creaney J, Maskell N, Lake RA, de Klerk N, Nowak AK. A novel clinical prediction model for prognosis in malignant pleural mesothelioma using decision tree analysis. J Thorac Oncol. 2016;11:573–82.
23. Estenne M, Yernault JC, de Troyer A. Mechanism of relief of dyspnea after thoracocentesis in patients with large pleural effusions. Am J Med. 1983;74:813–9.
24. Thomas R, Jenkins S, Eastwood PR, Gary Lee YC, Singh B. Physiology of breathlessness associated with pleural effusions. Curr Opin Pulm Med. 2015;21:338.
25. Marel M, Stastny B, Melinova L, Svandova E, Light RW. Diagnosis of pleural effusions: experience with clinical studies, 1986 to 1990. Chest. 1995;107:1598–603.
26. Porcel JM, Vives M. Etiology and pleural fluid characteristics of large and massive effusions. Chest. 2003;124:978–83.
27. Maher GG, Berger HW. Massive pleural effusion: malignant and nonmalignant causes in 46 patients. Am Rev Respir Dis. 1972;105:458–60.
28. Meyer PC. Metastatic carcinoma of the pleura. Thorax. 1966;21:437–43.
29. Light RW, Hamm H. Malignant pleural effusion: would the real cause please stand up? Eur Respir J. 1997;10:1701–2.
30. Stathopoulos GT, Kalomenidis I. Malignant pleural effusion: tumor-host interactions unleashed. Am J Respir Crit Care Med. 2012;186:487–92.
31. Havelock T, Teoh R, Laws D, Gleeson F. Pleural procedures and thoracic ultrasound: British Thoracic Society Pleural Disease Guideline 2010. Thorax. 2010;65:i61–76.
32. Bugalho A, Ferreira D, Dias SS, Schuhmann M, Branco JC, Marques Gomes MJ, Eberhardt R. The diagnostic value of transthoracic ultrasonographic features in predicting malig-

nancy in undiagnosed pleural effusions: a prospective observational study. Respiration. 2014;87:270–8.

33. Kaul V, Mccracken DJ, Rahman NM, Epelbaum O. FOCUSED REVIEW contemporary approach to the diagnosis of malignant pleural effusion. atsjournals.org. Ann Am Thorac Soc. 2019;16:1099–106.

34. Rodriguez-Panadero F, Lopez Mejias J. Low glucose and pH levels in malignant pleural effusions. Diagnostic significance and prognostic value in respect to pleurodesis. Am Rev Respir Dis. 1989;139:663–7.

35. Heffner JE, Nietert PJ, Barbieri C. Pleural fluid pH as a predictor of pleurodesis failure: analysis of primary data. Chest. 2000;117:87–95.

36. Porcel JM, Hernández P, Martínez-Alonso M, Bielsa S, Salud A. Accuracy of fluorodeoxyglucose-PET imaging for differentiating benign from malignant pleural effusions: a meta-analysis. Chest. 2015;147:502–12.

37. Fjaellegaard K, Koefod Petersen J, Reuter S, Malene Fischer B, Gerke O, Porcel JM, Frost Clementsen P, Laursen CB, Bhatnagar R, Bodtger U. Positron emission tomography-computed tomography (PET-CT) in suspected malignant pleural effusion. An updated systematic review and meta-analysis. Lung Cancer. 2021;162:106–18.

38. Heffner JE, Nietert PJ, Barbieri C. Pleural fluid pH as a predictor of survival for patients with malignant pleural effusions. Chest. 2000;117:79–86.

39. Sahn SA, Good JT. Pleural fluid pH in malignant effusions. Diagnostic, prognostic, and therapeutic implications. Ann Intern Med. 1988;108:345–9.

40. Rahman NM, Mishra EK, Davies HE, Davies RJO, Lee YCG. Clinically important factors influencing the diagnostic measurement of pleural fluid pH and glucose. Am J Respir Crit Care Med. 2008;178:483–90.

41. Porcel JM, Esquerda A, Vives M, Bielsa S. Etiology of pleural effusions: analysis of more than 3,000 consecutive thoracenteses. Arch Bronconeumol. 2014;50:161–5.

42. Arnold DT, De Fonseka D, Perry S, Morley A, Harvey JE, Medford A, Brett M, Maskell NA. Investigating unilateral pleural effusions: the role of cytology. Eur Respir J. 2018;52:1801254.

43. Garcia LW, Ducatman BS, Wang HH. The value of multiple fluid specimens in the cytological diagnosis of malignancy. Mod Pathol. 1994;7:665–8.

44. Naylor B, Schmidt RW. The case for exfoliative cytology of serous effusions. Lancet. 1964;1:711–2.

45. Swiderek J, Morcos S, Donthireddy V, Surapaneni R, Jackson-Thompson V, Schultz L, Kini S, Kvale P. Prospective study to determine the volume of pleural fluid required to diagnose malignancy. Chest. 2010;137:68–73.

46. Rooper LM, Ali SZ, Olson MT. A minimum fluid volume of 75 mL is needed to ensure adequacy in a pleural effusion: a retrospective analysis of 2540 cases. Cancer Cytopathol. 2014;122:657–65.

47. Liu X, Lu Y, Zhu G, Lei Y, Zheng L, Qin H, Tang C, Ellison G, McCormack R, Ji Q. The diagnostic accuracy of pleural effusion and plasma samples versus tumour tissue for detection of EGFR mutation in patients with advanced non-small cell lung cancer: comparison of methodologies. J Clin Pathol. 2013;66:1065–9.

48. Light RW. Tumor markers in undiagnosed pleural effusions. Chest. 2004;126:1721–2.

49. Tang Y, Wang Z, Li Z, Kim J, Deng Y, Li Y, Heath JR, Wei W, Lu S, Shi Q. High-throughput screening of rare metabolically active tumor cells in pleural effusion and peripheral blood of lung cancer patients. Proc Natl Acad Sci U S A. 2017;114:2544–9.

50. Koegelenberg CFN, Irusen EM, von Groote-Bidlingmaier F, Bruwer JW, Batubara EMA, Diacon AH. The utility of ultrasound-guided thoracentesis and pleural biopsy in undiagnosed pleural exudates. Thorax. 2015;70:995–7.

51. Qureshi NR, Rahman NM, Gleeson F. Thoracic ultrasound in the diagnosis of malignant pleural effusion. Thorax. 2009;64:139–43.

52. Maskell NA, Gleeson F, Davies RJO. Standard pleural biopsy versus CT-guided cutting-needle biopsy for diagnosis of malignant disease in pleural effusions: a randomised controlled trial. Lancet. 2003;361:1326–30.

53. Metintas M, Yildirim H, Kaya T, Ak G, Dundar E, Ozkan R, Metintas S. CT scan-guided Abrams' needle pleural biopsy versus ultrasound-assisted cutting needle pleural biopsy for diagnosis in patients with pleural effusion: a randomized, controlled trial. Respiration. 2016;91:156–63.

54. Rahman NM, Ali NJ, Brown G, et al. Local anaesthetic thoracoscopy: British Thoracic Society Pleural Disease Guideline 2010. Thorax. 2010;65:54–60.

55. Rozman A, Camlek L, Marc Malovrh M, Kern I, Schönfeld N. Feasibility and safety of parietal pleural cryobiopsy during semi-rigid thoracoscopy. Clin Respir J. 2016;10:574–8.

56. Boutin C, Rey F. Thoracoscopy in pleural malignant mesothelioma: a prospective study of 188 consecutive patients part 1: diagnosis. Cancer. 1993;72:389–93.

57. Metintas M, Ak G, Dundar E, Yildirim H, Ozkan R, Kurt E, Erginel S, Alatas F, Metintas S. Medical thoracoscopy vs CT scan-guided Abrams pleural needle biopsy for diagnosis of patients with pleural effusions: a randomized, controlled trial. Chest. 2010;137:1362–8.

58. Murthy V, Bessich JL. Medical thoracoscopy and its evolving role in the diagnosis and treatment of pleural disease. J Thorac Dis. 2017;9:S1011–21.

59. McDonald CM, Pierre C, de Perrot M, Darling G, Cypel M, Pierre A, Waddell T, Keshavjee S, Yasufuku K, Czarnecka-Kujawa K. Efficacy and cost of awake thoracoscopy and video-assisted thoracoscopic surgery in the undiagnosed pleural effusion. Ann Thorac Surg. 2018;106:361–7.

60. Roh J, Ahn HY, Kim I, Son JH, Seol HY, Kim MH, Lee MK, Eom JS, Lei G. Clinical course of asymptomatic malignant pleural effusion in non-small cell lung cancer patients: a multicenter retrospective study. Medicine. 2021;100:E25748.

61. Mercaldi CJ, Lanes SF. Ultrasound guidance decreases complications and improves the cost of care among patients undergoing thoracentesis and paracentesis. Chest. 2013;143:532–8.

62. Ost DE, Niu J, Zhao H, Grosu HB, Giordano SH. Quality gaps and comparative effectiveness of management strategies for recurrent malignant pleural effusions. Chest. 2018;153:438.

63. Grosu HB, Molina S, Casal R, et al. Risk factors for pleural effusion recurrence in patients with malignancy. Respirology. 2019;24:76.

64. Clive AO, Jones HE, Bhatnagar R, Preston NJ, Maskell N. Interventions for the management of malignant pleural effusions: a network meta-analysis. Cochrane Database Syst Rev. 2016;2016:CD010529. https://doi.org/10.1002/14651858.CD010529.pub2.

65. Diacon AH, Wyser C, Bolliger CT, Tamm M, Pless M, Perruchoud AP, Solèr M. Prospective randomized comparison of thoracoscopic talc poudrage under local anesthesia versus bleomycin instillation for pleurodesis in malignant pleural effusions. Am J Respir Crit Care Med. 2000;162:1445–9.

66. Dipper A, Jones HE, Bhatnagar R, Preston NJ, Maskell N, Clive AO. Interventions for the management of malignant pleural effusions: a network meta-analysis. Cochrane Database Syst Rev. 2020;2016:CD010529. https://doi.org/10.1002/14651858.CD010529.pub3.

67. Tan C, Sedrakyan A, Browne J, Swift S, Treasure T. The evidence on the effectiveness of management for malignant pleural effusion: a systematic review. Eur J Cardiothorac Surg. 2006;29:829–38.

68. Dresler CM, Olak J, Herndon JE, et al. Phase III intergroup study of talc poudrage vs talc slurry sclerosis for malignant pleural effusion. Chest. 2005;127:909.

69. Mummadi S, Kumbam A, Hahn PY. Malignant pleural effusions and the role of talc poudrage and talc slurry: a systematic review and meta-analysis. F1000Research. 2014;3:254. https://doi.org/10.12688/f1000research.5538.2.

70. Bhatnagar R, Piotrowska HEG, Laskawiec-Szkonter M, et al. Effect of thoracoscopic talc poudrage vs talc slurry via chest tube on pleurodesis failure rate among patients with malignant pleural effusions: a randomized clinical trial. JAMA. 2020;323:60–9.

71. Psallidas I, Hassan M, Yousuf A, et al. Role of thoracic ultrasonography in pleurodesis pathways for malignant pleural effusions (SIMPLE): an open-label, randomised controlled trial. Lancet Respir Med. 2022;10:139–48.

72. Wilshire CL, Chang SC, Gilbert CR, et al. Temporal trends in tunneled pleural catheter utilization in patients with malignancy: a multicenter review. Chest. 2021;159:2483–7.
73. Ost DE, Jimenez CA, Lei X, et al. Quality-adjusted survival following treatment of malignant pleural effusions with indwelling pleural catheters. Chest. 2014;145:1347–56.
74. Sabur NF, Chee A, Stather DR, MacEachern P, Amjadi K, Hergott CA, Dumoulin E, Gonzalez A, Tremblay A. The impact of tunneled pleural catheters on the quality of life of patients with malignant pleural effusions. Respiration. 2013;85:36–42.
75. Gilbert CR, Lee HJ, Skalski JH, et al. The use of indwelling tunneled pleural catheters for recurrent pleural effusions in patients with hematologic malignancies: a multicenter study. Chest. 2015;148:752–8.
76. van Meter MEM, McKee KY, Kohlwes RJ. Efficacy and safety of tunneled pleural catheters in adults with malignant pleural effusions: a systematic review. J Gen Intern Med. 2011;26:70–6.
77. Sundaralingam A, Bedawi EO, Harriss EK, Munavvar M, Rahman NM. The frequency, risk factors, and management of complications from pleural procedures. Chest. 2022;161:1407–25.
78. Miller RJ, Chrissian AA, Lee YCG, et al. AABIP evidence-informed guidelines and expert panel report for the management of indwelling pleural catheters. J Bronchol Interv Pulmonol. 2020;27:229–45.
79. Gilbert CR, Wahidi MM, Light RW, et al. Management of indwelling tunneled pleural catheters: a modified Delphi consensus statement. Chest. 2020;158:2221–8.
80. Frost N, Brünger M, Ruwwe-Glösenkamp C, Raspe M, Tessmer A, Temmesfeld-Wollbrück B, Schürmann D, Suttorp N, Witzenrath M. Indwelling pleural catheters for malignancy-associated pleural effusion: report on a single centre's ten years of experience. BMC Pulm Med. 2019;19:1–10.
81. Fysh ETH, Wrightson JM, Lee YCG, Rahman NM. Fractured indwelling pleural catheters. Chest. 2012;141:1090–4.
82. Matus I, Colt H. Pleural catheter fracture during IPC removal: an under-reported Complication. J Bronchol Interv Pulmonol. 2021;28:E1–3.
83. Wahidi MM, Reddy C, Yarmus L, et al. Randomized trial of pleural fluid drainage frequency in patients with malignant pleural effusions. The ASAP trial. Am J Respir Crit Care Med. 2017;195:1050–7.
84. Muruganandan S, Azzopardi M, Fitzgerald DB, et al. Aggressive versus symptom-guided drainage of malignant pleural effusion via indwelling pleural catheters (AMPLE-2): an open-label randomised trial. Lancet Respir Med. 2018;6:671–80.
85. Shafiq M, Frick KD, Lee H, Yarmus L, Feller-Kopman DJ. Management of malignant pleural effusion: a cost-utility analysis. J Bronchol Interv Pulmonol. 2015;22:215–25.
86. Gilbert CR, Akulian JA, Gorden JA. The impact of the ASAP trial: maybe we shouldn't act so quickly. Am J Respir Crit Care Med. 2018;197:142–3.
87. Putnam JB, Light RW, Michael Rodriguez R, Ponn R, Olak J, Pollak JS, Lee RB, Keith D, Graeber G, Kovitz KL. A randomized comparison of indwelling pleural catheter and doxycycline pleurodesis in the management of malignant pleural effusions. Cancer. 1999;86:1992–9.
88. Davies HE, Mishra EK, Kahan BC, et al. Effect of an indwelling pleural catheter vs chest tube and talc pleurodesis for relieving dyspnea in patients with malignant pleural effusion: the TIME2 randomized controlled trial. JAMA. 2012;307:2383–9.
89. Thomas R, Fysh ETH, Smith NA, et al. Effect of an indwelling pleural catheter vs talc pleurodesis on hospitalization days in patients with malignant pleural effusion: the AMPLE randomized clinical trial. JAMA. 2017;318:1903–12.
90. Bhatnagar R, Keenan EK, Morley AJ, et al. Outpatient talc administration by indwelling pleural catheter for malignant effusion. N Engl J Med. 2018;378:1313–22.
91. ClinicalTrials.gov. Duke University randomized controlled trial of talc instillation in addition to daily drainage through a tunneled pleural catheter to improve rates of outpatient pleurodesis in patients with malignant pleural effusion. n.d.. https://clinicaltrials.gov/ct2/show/NCT04792970. Accessed 13 Aug 2022.

92. Fitzgerald DB, Muruganandan S, Stanley C, Badiei A, Murray K, Read CA, Lee YCG. EPIToME (early pleurodesis via IPC with talc for malignant effusion): evaluation of a new management algorithm. Eur Respir J. 2019;54:OA493.

93. Rintoul RC, Ritchie AJ, Edwards JG, Waller DA, Coonar AS, Bennett M, Lovato E, Hughes V, Fox-Rushby JA, Sharples LD. Efficacy and cost of video-assisted thoracoscopic partial pleurectomy versus talc pleurodesis in patients with malignant pleural mesothelioma (MesoVATS): an open-label, randomised, controlled trial. Lancet. 2014;384:1118–27.

94. Martin GA, Tsim S, Kidd AC, Foster JE, McLoone P, Chalmers A, Blyth KG. Pre-EDIT: a randomized feasibility trial of elastance-directed intrapleural catheter or talc pleurodesis in malignant pleural effusion. Chest. 2019;156:1204–13.

95. Chopra A, Judson MA, Doelken P, Maldonado F, Rahman NM, Huggins JT. The relationship of pleural manometry with postthoracentesis chest radiographic findings in malignant pleural effusion. Chest. 2020;157:421–6.

96. Salamonsen MR, Lo AKC, Ng ACT, Bashirzadeh F, Wang WYS, Fielding DIK. Novel use of pleural ultrasound can identify malignant entrapped lung prior to effusion drainage. Chest. 2014;146:1286–93.

97. Feller-Kopman D, Walkey A, Berkowitz D, Ernst A. The relationship of pleural pressure to symptom development during therapeutic thoracentesis. Chest. 2006;129:1556–60.

98. Psallidas I, Yousuf A, Talwar A, Hallifax RJ, Mishra EK, Corcoran JP, Ali N, Rahman NM. Assessment of patient-reported outcome measures in pleural interventions. BMJ Open Respir Res. 2017;4:e000171. https://doi.org/10.1136/BMJRESP-2016-000171.

99. Mishra EK, Clive AO, Wills GH, et al. Randomized controlled trial of urokinase versus placebo for nondraining malignant pleural effusion. Am J Respir Crit Care Med. 2018;197:502–8.

100. Murthy P, Ekeke CN, Russell KL, Butler SC, Wang Y, Luketich JD, Soloff AC, Dhupar R, Lotze MT. Making cold malignant pleural effusions hot: driving novel immunotherapies. Oncoimmunology. 2019;8:e1554969. https://doi.org/10.1080/2162402X.2018.1554969.

101. Aggarwal C, Haas AR, Metzger S, et al. Phase I study of intrapleural gene-mediated cytotoxic immunotherapy in patients with malignant pleural effusion. Mol Ther. 2018;26:1198.

102. Fitzgerald DB, Sidhu C, Budgeon C, et al. Australasian Malignant PLeural Effusion (AMPLE)-3 trial: study protocol for a multi-centre randomised study comparing indwelling pleural catheter (±talc pleurodesis) versus video-assisted thoracoscopic surgery for management of malignant pleural effusion. Trials. 2022;23:530.

103. Rivera MP. Management of malignant pleural effusions: round and round we go. Ann Am Thorac Soc. 2019;16:59–61.

Chapter 11
Pulmonary Complications of Lung Cancer Treatment

Kathleen A. McAvoy and Jennifer D. Possick

Introduction

As innovations in lung cancer therapies improve patient survival, treatment histories become more complex. Treatment has shifted to include systemic therapies at earlier stages of disease and in novel combinations. Tolerability profiles of newer therapies allow for use in older, more comorbid patients, and for many, cancer is becoming a chronic disease. Consequently, patients encounter more therapy types over time, increasing the possibility of sequential complications, synergistic toxicities, and delayed-onset events. Growing survivorship highlights the importance of pulmonologists in recognizing complications, addressing treatment, and providing longitudinal care.

Patients with lung cancer are at risk for many types of pulmonary complications arising from their underlying malignancy, treatments they receive, or their comorbidities. Treatment-related complications must be rapidly distinguished from other causes to avoid undue morbidity and mortality [1]. Conversely, inappropriately invoking oncologic treatments as the cause of a patient's symptoms may lead to discontinuation of effective therapies. Nonspecific clinical features and lack of gold standard diagnostic criteria pose significant challenges to treating physicians. Fundamentally, diagnosis of treatment-related complications is one of exclusion. Here we present a general approach to evaluating a patient with lung cancer presenting with new pulmonary symptoms, before considering the nuances of toxicities related to individual therapies.

K. A. McAvoy · J. D. Possick (✉)
Section of Pulmonary, Critical Care, and Sleep Medicine, Yale School of Medicine, New Haven, CT, USA
e-mail: kathleen.mcavoy@yale.edu; jennifer.possick@yale.edu

C. MacRosty, M. P. Rivera (eds.), *Lung Cancer*, Respiratory Medicine,
https://doi.org/10.1007/978-3-031-38412-7_11

Approach to the Patient with Lung Cancer and New Pulmonary Symptoms

Dyspnea and cough are the most common presenting symptoms of treatment-related lung disease but are common symptoms in lung cancer and chronic lung diseases. Advent or exacerbation of such symptoms must be thoroughly investigated before definitive attribution is made. Patients with baseline lung function impairments or cardiopulmonary comorbidities have diminished reserve to tolerate superimposed processes, so precipitating cause(s) may be subtle. The presence of concurrent non-pulmonary symptoms might invoke alternative causes or implicate a therapy with extrapulmonary toxidromes. Though radiographic abnormalities are relevant to diagnosis, examining longitudinal changes and referencing baseline imaging is essential.

General Approach to Evaluation

Systematic evaluation should emphasize exclusion of alternative causes [2]. Conventional computed tomography (CT) imaging is helpful in assessing for malignancy progression and evaluating for most treatment-related complications unless pulmonary embolism is suspected, in which case CT angiography is required. Pulmonary function tests (PFTs) can establish the presence of obstructive or restrictive ventilatory defects and diffusion impairments but require comparison to prior data to be instructive. Bronchoscopy with bronchoalveolar lavage (BAL) helps exclude infection, especially in immunocompromised patients, and transbronchial biopsy can assess for disease progression. Failure to consider all possible explanations for new symptoms may lead to misdiagnoses, delays in appropriate care, and inappropriate discontinuation of therapies.

Multidisciplinary lung cancer care, including pulmonologists, medical oncologists, radiation oncologists, thoracic surgeons, radiologists, and palliative medicine specialists, is known to improve patient outcomes [3]. Evaluation of complications during lung cancer treatment is no different, and collaborative discussion of cases may improve diagnostic confidence.

Pulmonary Complications of Radiation Therapy

Though modern radiation techniques have evolved to minimize effects on surrounding tissues, radiation-induced complications including radiation pneumonitis, fibrosis, and recall phenomena impact a significant number of patients [4].

Epidemiology, Risk Factors, and Risk Reduction

In classic radiation pneumonitis associated with whole-lung radiation, incidence was reported as high as 20% and increased predictably with escalating total dose [5]. Modern techniques such as stereotactic body radiation therapy (SBRT) decreased incidence, though reported rates vary [6]. SBRT carries a 9.4% risk of clinically significant radiation pneumonitis, with less than 5% of patients developing high-grade toxicity [4, 7]. The exception is in patients with history of prior thoracic radiation receiving subsequent palliative SBRT; in these instances, the risk of high-grade pneumonitis is as high as 20% [8].

Additional treatment-related factors influence the incidence and severity of radiation pneumonitis. In traditional radiation therapy, morbidity and mortality from radiation pneumonitis increase sharply over a narrow dose range once a threshold dose is exceeded [6]. The distribution of a given radiation dose to surrounding normal lung tissue is important. The volume of normal lung receiving 20 Gy or more during treatment, or V20, is a strong predictor of clinically significant radiation pneumonitis—V20 less than 22% yields 0% risk, versus 36% risk for V20 over 40% [9]. In SBRT, the dose-toxicity relationship is not as well-established, but V10, V20, and mean lung dose can all help predict toxicity; fractionating radiation into smaller doses allows normal tissues a period of recovery.

Several factors, including older age, female sex, poor performance status, comorbid lung disease, and abnormal baseline lung function, are associated with increased risk for radiation pneumonitis [5, 6, 10]. Patients who actively smoke may have lower risk of radiation pneumonitis [9]. The presence of preexisting radiographic interstitial lung disease (ILD), including subclinical disease, increases the incidence, severity, and mortality from radiation pneumonitis [4]. Patients with preexisting ILD are more likely to have uncommon presentations of pneumonitis, often with extensive radiographic changes outside the treatment field [11].

As guidelines for lung cancer treatment evolve to include neoadjuvant and adjuvant systemic therapies in earlier stages of disease, and as the complement of potential systemic therapies expands, the potential for synergistic toxicity augmenting radiation pneumonitis risk increases. Radiation recall pneumonitis, a delayed inflammatory reaction in previously irradiated tissue triggered by antineoplastic agents, is a well-recognized phenomenon [12]. Several drugs shown to increase or carry risk of radiation or radiation recall pneumonitis include bevacizumab, *BRAF* inhibitors, epidermal growth factor receptor-tyrosine kinase inhibitors (EGFR-TKIs), gemcitabine, immune checkpoint inhibitors (ICIs), pemetrexed, taxanes, topoisomerase I inhibitors, and vinorelbine [9, 12–16]. These drugs can cause drug-induced pneumonitis in the absence of radiation therapy, making discrimination between radiation-recall and drug-induced pneumonitis difficult, and estimation of incidence less precise [13].

Phases of Radiation-Induced Lung Injury

As radiation passes through tissues, free radical injury causes microscopic changes in the lung parenchyma apparent within hours of treatment [9]. While microscopic injury is ubiquitous in radiation treatment, not every patient develops clinically significant radiation pneumonitis [9, 17]. Within 3–12 weeks following treatment, it is common to observe faint ground glass opacities within the radiation field which may not conform to anatomic boundaries ("in-field"). In the 3–6 months following treatment completion, this may progress to a more dense, consolidative appearance with air bronchograms, traction bronchiectasis, and volume loss. While subsequent fibrosis and scarring should correspond to the shape of the "radiation portal," anatomic distortion, and mediastinal shift may make identification of treatment field boundaries more difficult [17]. Fibrosis is insidious, taking up to 2 years to stabilize (Fig. 11.1).

Evaluation of Suspected Radiation-Induced Lung Injury

Identifying clinically significant radiation pneumonitis is important, as those with severe toxicity have worse survival [6]. Diagnosis is circumstantial based on symptoms, therapy characteristics, compatible imaging, and exclusion of alternative causes [9].

Patients may first demonstrate cough and thickened secretions from ciliary dysfunction [17]. Symptoms of acute radiation pneumonitis typically present 3–12 weeks after completion of treatment and include fever, nonproductive cough, dyspnea, and malaise [9]. Though physical exam is frequently normal, rales, rhonchi, dullness to percussion, or pleural rub may be observed [17, 18]. Laboratory

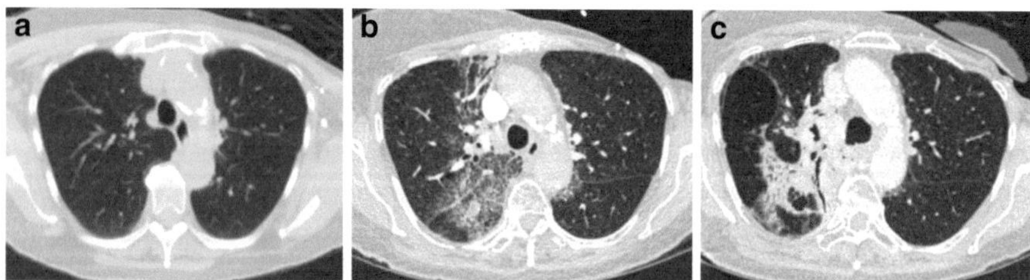

Fig. 11.1 Evolution of radiographic changes following thoracic radiation. A 74-year-old with stage IIIA adenocarcinoma of the right upper lobe received concurrent chemoradiation with platinum-doublet chemotherapy and 60 Gy in 30 fractions to the right upper lung and mediastinum. (**a**) Pre-treatment imaging without preexisting interstitial lung disease; primary tumor is excluded from this image. (**b**) Eight weeks after radiation, ground glass opacities consistent with radiation pneumonitis appear within the treatment field. (**c**) Eight months later, consolidative changes, traction bronchiectasis, and volume loss consistent with radiation fibrosis appear in the same region

studies may demonstrate a modest elevation in white blood cells (WBC) and elevation in erythrocyte sedimentation rate or C-reactive protein [9].

Establishing a diagnosis of radiation pneumonitis can be challenging in patients receiving concurrent systemic treatments that could also result in lung injury. Identification of "in-field" changes on CT imaging can help differentiate direct cytotoxic effect from systemic insult; reviewing treatment field maps with the radiation oncologist is instructive [9, 18]. Ground glass opacities outside of the radiation field in a pattern more consistent with organizing pneumonia may be observed, possibly due to a systemic immunologic response to the initial local injury [9].

No test can confirm or exclude a diagnosis of radiation pneumonitis [18]. Bronchoscopy with BAL +/− transbronchial biopsy can help rule out alternative causes such as infection or progression of tumor and may demonstrate increased leukocytes, CD4+ lymphocytes, or nonspecific inflammatory patterns [9, 18]. PFTs typically remain unchanged during and 4–8 weeks following radiation treatment; in the setting of radiation pneumonitis or fibrosis, declines in diffusion capacity, forced vital capacity, and total lung capacity may be observed [6].

Management of Radiation-Related Pulmonary Toxicity

Treatment for radiation pneumonitis is stratified by clinical severity [18]. The Common Terminology Criteria for Adverse Events (CTCAE) scale (Table 11.1) defines the grading schema used to classify severity for both radiation pneumonitis and drug-induced lung disease [19].

Patients with mild symptoms (grade ≤ 2) may be observed or may consider a trial of inhaled corticosteroids [9]. For patients with severe pneumonitis (grade ≥ 3), oral corticosteroids (prednisone 1 mg/kg/day for 2–4 weeks followed by a 6–12-week taper) are the mainstay of treatment despite a lack of randomized controlled trials demonstrating efficacy [6]. Relapse can occur when treatment is stopped or tapered, though inhaled corticosteroids may mitigate recrudescence [20]. Azathioprine can be considered as a steroid-sparing agent if required [6]. Prognosis is good, and symptoms typically resolve in 6–8 weeks without long-term sequelae [9, 17].

Systemic steroids are ineffective once lung fibrosis is established, and supportive care should be provided to mitigate chronic symptoms [18]. Those who develop radiation fibrosis have minimal chronic symptoms if injury is confined to less than 50% of one lung. Chronic respiratory failure due to radiation fibrosis is rare [17].

Table 11.1 The National Cancer Institute Common Terminology Criteria for Adverse Events (CTCAE) grading scale for pneumonitis and suggested approach to management of ICI pneumonitis

CTCAE grade: definition Radiographic findings	Suggested management for ICI pneumonitis
CTCAE grade 1: asymptomatic; clinical or diagnostic observations only; intervention not indicated	• Hold ICI or continue with close clinical monitoring (including pulse oximetry)
Radiographic changes: one lobe or <25% of lung parenchyma	• Short interval radiographic follow up recommended (~4 weeks)
	• Consider repeat PFTs for those with baseline testing available
	• If no improvement, or if symptoms develop, treat as grade 2
CTCAE grade 2: symptomatic; medical intervention needed; limiting instrumental ADL[a]	• Hold ICI until improvement to grade ≤1
Radiographic changes: >1 lobe or 25–50% of lung parenchyma	• Consider bronchoscopy with BAL +/− transbronchial biopsy after less invasive workup[b]
	• Prednisone 1–2 mg/kg/day; taper over 4–6 weeks based on clinical and radiographic improvement
	• Consider empiric broad-spectrum antibiotics
	• If no improvement after 48–72 h, treat as grade 3
CTCAE grade 3: severe symptoms; limiting self-care ADL[c]; oxygen indicated	• Permanently discontinue ICI
Radiographic changes: all lobes or >50% of lung parenchyma	• Hospitalization indicated
or	• Consider bronchoscopy with BAL +/− transbronchial biopsy after less invasive workup[b], as patient able to tolerate
CTCAE grade 4: life-threatening respiratory compromise; urgent intervention indicated (e.g., tracheotomy or intubation)	• Methylprednisolone IV 1–2 mg/kg/day; taper over ≥4–6 weeks based on clinical and radiographic improvement
	• Consider empiric broad-spectrum antibiotics
	• If no improvement after 48 h, consider secondary immunosuppressive agent[d]

Adapted from: Common Terminology Criteria for Adverse Events (CTCAE), Version 5.0, November 2017; Management of Immunotherapy-Related Toxicities, V 1.2022, NCCN Clinical Practice Guidelines; Schneider et al. 2021

ICI immune checkpoint inhibitor, *PFTs* pulmonary function tests, *ADL* activity of daily living, *BAL* bronchoalveolar lavage, *IV* intravenous, *PO* orally

[a] Preparing meals, shopping for groceries or clothes, using the telephone, managing money, etc.

[b] Respiratory viral nasal swab (including SARS-CoV-2), sputum cultures (bacterial, fungal, acid fast), blood cultures, urine antigen tests for legionella and pneumococcus, serum fungal markers

[c] Bathing, dressing and undressing, feeding self, toileting, taking medications

[d] Options include infliximab (5 mg/kg IV; second dose may be repeated after 14 days), mycophenolate (0.5–1 g PO every 12 h), intravenous immunoglobulin (2 g/kg over 2–5 days in divided doses), or cyclophosphamide (1–2 mg/kg/day)

General Approach to Evaluation of Suspected Drug-Induced Lung Disease

There are no universally accepted criteria for the diagnosis of drug-induced lung disease, and as treatment paradigms become more complex, identifying an individual culprit agent is increasingly challenging. Diagnosis is based on exposure, compatible clinical picture, and exclusion of other potential causes.

Patient Assessment

The most common symptoms of drug-induced lung disease include new or worsening dyspnea, nonproductive cough, fever, and sometimes weight loss. Drug-related pneumonitis may occur days, weeks, or months following therapy initiation [21]. Physical exam may be normal or may demonstrate tachypnea, resting or ambulatory hypoxemia, rales on auscultation, and, less commonly, dullness to percussion suggestive of pleural effusions [1]. Detailed drug exposure history is essential to diagnosing drug-induced lung disease. Since the development of symptoms may be considerably delayed, the offending agent may have already been discontinued. Concurrent and sequential therapies further confound accurate attribution, and synergistic toxicities must be considered [22].

Diagnostic Testing

Diagnostics should be leveraged to systematically exclude other possible causes and characterize illness severity [23]. Radiographic changes may lag symptoms by days to weeks. CT imaging is preferred over chest X-ray in detecting subtle abnormalities, with high-resolution CT imaging providing a detailed assessment of the pattern and distribution of parenchymal changes [2]. Radiographic manifestations of drug-induced lung disease are heterogeneous and nonspecific; "typical" imaging findings specific to individual agents will be discussed below. Temporal association between drug exposure and clinical presentation is key; it is prudent to compare imaging at the time of symptom onset to pre-treatment images and evaluate changes longitudinally [23]. Subclinical preexisting ILD, often underappreciated on baseline imaging, may worsen considerably with superimposed drug toxicity.

PFTs are typically abnormal in drug-induced lung disease compared to pre-treatment testing. A decrease in diffusing capacity is usually the first abnormality observed and may herald the development of symptoms or radiologic abnormalities. A reduction in lung volumes may subsequently develop [1].

The greatest utility of bronchoscopy in evaluating drug-induced lung injury is excluding other causes such as infection and progression of disease [1]. BAL can suggest drug-related causes if "bizarre" multinucleated type II pneumocytes are present, pulmonary hemorrhage is demonstrated on serial aliquots, or a lymphocytic alveolitis is seen [21]. Transbronchial biopsy may help differentiate pneumonitis from progression of malignancy but is rarely definitive [2, 21]. Typically observed histopathologic findings (e.g., usual interstitial pneumonia (UIP), nonspecific interstitial pneumonia (NSIP), organizing pneumonia (OP), diffuse alveolar damage (DAD)) are not pathognomonic for drug reactions, and some individual drugs can produce more than one pattern [24].

Assessing Severity and Principles of Management

As in radiation-related lung injuries, the CTCAE terminology helps to standardize severity gradation of drug-induced lung disease (Table 11.1) [19]. Management is guided by CTCAE grade and includes temporary or permanent drug suspension, treatment with corticosteroids, and appropriate supportive care. Prophylaxis against *Pneumocystis jirovecii* should be considered in patients receiving ≥20-mg prednisone equivalent daily for ≥4 weeks. Prophylaxis against gastritis with a proton pump inhibitor and against osteoporosis with calcium and vitamin D supplementation should be considered in those receiving long-term steroids [25].

Management of Pulmonary Complications of Systemic Therapies

Traditional Chemotherapies

Selected toxicities associated with traditional chemotherapeutic agents utilized in the treatment of lung cancer are discussed in detail below and summarized in Table 11.2.

Platinum Agents

Platinum agents are commonly used in the treatment of non-small cell lung cancer (NSCLC) and small cell lung cancer (SCLC), typically combined with an additional chemotherapeutic agent to form a "platinum doublet" [26–28]. While drugs that are combined with platinum agents pose a risk of pneumonitis, there are no reports of drug-related pneumonitis associated specifically with these drugs.

Cisplatin is associated with increased thromboembolic events, both arterial and venous. One retrospective analysis showed a 10.2% incidence of thromboembolic events in patients with small cell lung cancer, while another mixed cohort showed

Table 11.2 Chemotherapy agents and targeted therapies associated with pulmonary toxicity syndromes

Drug class (agents)	Toxicity syndromes[a]	Comments
Platinum agents (carboplatin, cisplatin)	Thromboembolism	• Specific to cisplatin; arterial and venous
Taxanes (paclitaxel, nab-paclitaxel, docetaxel)	Pneumonitis	• Higher risk with concurrent radiation
		• Fulminant, refractory cases reported
	Capillary leak	• Specific to docetaxel
Pemetrexed	Pneumonitis/ILD	• Extremely rare, higher risk in Asian populations
Gemcitabine	Dyspnea	• Typically mild, self-limited
	Pneumonitis/ILD	• Highest risk with concurrent radiation
		• Fulminant, refractory cases reported
Etoposide	Pneumonitis	• Rare, but fulminant cases reported
Topo I inhibitors (irinotecan, topotecan)	Dyspnea, cough	• Very common
	ILD	• Rare, but fulminant cases reported
Vinorelbine	Pneumonitis	• Increased risk with concurrent radiation in older patients
Alkylating agents (lurbinectedin, temozolomide)	Pneumonitis/ILD	• Unique to temozolomide
	Pneumonia	• Unique to lurbinectedin
		• May be related to associated neutropenia
	Opportunistic infections	• Unique to temozolomide
		• May be related to associated lymphopenia
Anti-VEGF (bevacizumab, ramucirumab)	Hemorrhage, hemoptysis	• Highest risk with squamous cell, thoracic radiation, central tumors
	Thromboembolism	• Predominantly arterial
	Tracheoesophageal fistulae	• Specific to bevacizumab
		• Highest risk with concurrent radiation
EGFR-TKI (afatinib, dacomitinib, crlotinib, gefitinib, mobocertinib, osimertinib)	Pneumonitis/ILD	• Highest risk with osimertinib, moboccrtinib
		• High risk in Japanese patients
	Transient, asymptomatic pulmonary opacities	• Specific to osimertinib
EGFR-mAb (amivantamab, cetuximab, necitumumab)	Pneumonitis/ILD	• No reports with necitumumab to date
	Thromboembolism	• Specific to necitumumab
ALK-TKI (alectinib, brigatinib, ceritinib, crizotinib, lorlatinib)	Pneumonitis/ILD	• Lowest risk with ceritinib, highest risk with brigatinib

(continued)

Table 11.2 (continued)

Drug class (agents)	Toxicity syndromes[a]	Comments
BRAF kinase inhibitor (dabrafenib, trametinib, vemurafenib)	Pneumonitis/ILD	• Vemurafenib associated with drug-induced and radiation recall pneumonitis
	Thromboembolism	• Specific to sabrafenib + trametinib combination
	Sarcoid-like reactions	• Specific to vemurafenib
KRAS inhibitor (sotorasib)	Pneumonitis	• Possibly higher risk following ICI use
RET (pralsetinib, selpercatinib)	Pneumonitis/ILD	• Specific to pralsetinib
	Hemorrhage, hemoptysis	• Specific to selpercatinib
MET (capmatinib, tepotinib)	Pneumonitis/ILD	• Successful challenge of one drug after toxicity from another has been reported
	Peripheral edema, pleural effusion	• Peripheral edema more common with capmatinib, pleural effusion with tepotinib

References and details can be found in the corresponding text
ILD interstitial lung disease, *VEGF* vascular endothelial growth factor, *EGFR* epidermal growth factor, *TKI* tyrosine kinase inhibitor, *mAb* monoclonal antibody, *HSR* hypersensitivity reaction, *ALK* anaplastic lymphoma kinase, *ICI* immune checkpoint inhibitor
[a] Toxicity syndromes refer to those common to all drugs in that class, unless otherwise specified in the comments

an incidence of 18.1% [29, 30]. Thromboembolism should therefore be considered in the differential diagnosis of dyspnea in this setting.

Taxanes

Paclitaxel and docetaxel are associated with pneumonitis and frequently used in advanced NSCLC and relapsed SCLC [26–28]. Rates of pneumonitis among patients with NSCLC range from 3% to 12% in those receiving concurrent radiation [31]. A phase II trial in extensive-stage SCLC (ES-SCLC) demonstrated a pneumonitis rate of 5.6% with paclitaxel monotherapy [32]. A retrospective analysis of docetaxel revealed rates up to 25% in patients with preexisting interstitial changes, though this has not been observed with other taxanes [33]. Additional risk factors associated with taxane-induced pulmonary toxicity include frequent dosing, concurrent gemcitabine administration, and concurrent radiation therapy [34–36]. Taxane pneumonitis typically presents with diffuse, bilateral ground glass opacities on CT scan within a few weeks of treatment initiation, though other imaging patterns have been described [31]. In cases of taxane pneumonitis, the offending drug should be discontinued, and treatment with systemic corticosteroids should be promptly initiated. Fulminant respiratory failure despite these measures has been reported.

Another reaction unique to docetaxel is capillary leak. This phenomenon leads to fluid retention in peripheral tissues, including pleural and peritoneal spaces. It usually occurs after several cycles of docetaxel, and pre-treatment with steroids may reduce risk or delay onset [37]. Diuretics can manage fluid retention, and thoracentesis can be considered for severely symptomatic patients.

Pemetrexed

Pemetrexed is a frequently used chemotherapy agent in the treatment of NSCLC. Though trials involving pemetrexed in the United States did not observe significant pneumonitis events, one phase II trial in Japan reported eight cases of ILD/pneumonitis (incidence 3.5%), including one fatal event [38]. Japanese post-marketing surveillance data suggest an overall incidence of 1.8% with a high proportion of high-grade events [39]. Pemetrexed should be withheld for any patient with acute-onset pulmonary symptoms and permanently discontinued if pemetrexed-related pneumonitis is strongly suspected [40]. Corticosteroids are typically administered. Re-challenge is not recommended, as fatalities have been reported [41].

Gemcitabine

Gemcitabine is used in combination with a platinum agent to treat NSCLC, especially squamous cell tumors [27]. One systematic review of gemcitabine in the treatment of multiple malignancies suggested an incidence of severe (grade ≥ 3) pulmonary toxicity from 0% to 5%, though rates were substantially higher (13.8%) in NSCLC [42]. This is complicated by frequent coadministration of taxane agents in this population [35]. Mortality may be as high as 20–37%, with risk factors including prior thoracic radiation and preexisting lung disease. One study investigating concurrent chemoradiation with gemcitabine had to be terminated early due to high rates (31.6%) of high-grade pneumonitis [43]. Symptoms are typically observed following the second cycle of treatment. Though considerable variability exists, reticulonodular interstitial infiltrates are the most common radiographic pattern seen. Pathology is heterogeneous, ranging from capillary leak to DAD [44, 45]. Once recognized, prompt initiation of corticosteroids is indicated with administration of diuretics as an additional supportive measure [42, 44]. Steroid-refractory cases have been reported [45].

Etoposide

Etoposide is typically used in combination with other chemotherapeutic agents in the treatment of NSCLC and SCLC [26–28]. Pneumonitis has rarely been reported in association with etoposide, including steroid-refractory, fatal events. Risk factors remain unknown, and rechallenge is discouraged since recurrent pneumonitis typically develops [46, 47].

Topoisomerase I Inhibitors

Topoisomerase I inhibitors are used to treat some patients with SCLC [28]. The incidence of topotecan-related ILD is unknown, though there are case reports of fatal respiratory failure [48]. Irinotecan-related ILD is rare (1.3%) but accounted for 11% of treatment-related deaths in one study [49]. Risk factors include preexisting lung disease and concurrent use of other pneumotoxic drugs, thoracic radiation, or colony-stimulating factors [50, 51]. Imaging most commonly reveals reticulonodular infiltrates, and 80% of cases occur within 16 weeks of treatment initiation [52, 53]. Most patients respond to systemic corticosteroids, but fatal steroid-refractory cases have been described.

Vinorelbine

Vinorelbine is used with cisplatin to treat advanced-stage NSCLC and relapsed ES-SCLC [26–28]. Vinorelbine-associated pneumonitis is subacute, occurs days after infusion, presents with progressive dyspnea, and rarely evolves into respiratory failure [54]. One phase II study reported an incidence of 2.5%, with imaging demonstrating either a reticulonodular pattern or diffuse ground glass opacities. There is heightened risk of pneumonitis in elderly patients receiving concurrent thoracic radiation [15]. Systemic corticosteroids are typically employed, and steroid refractory cases may improve with cyclophosphamide [55].

Alkylating Agents

Alkylating agents have recently been introduced in treating relapsed ES-SCLC [28]. Though high-grade events of pneumonia (7%), dyspnea (6%), and respiratory tract infection (5%) were reported in patients receiving lurbinectedin, there are no established pulmonary toxicities associated with this drug [56].

For temozolomide-associated pulmonary toxicity, data are largely gleaned from use in other cancers. A phase II trial in patients with recurrent or progressive brain metastases from different primary malignancies reported pneumonitis in up to 5% [57]. There are additional case reports of temozolamide-associated lung toxicity with use for glioglastoma [58, 59]. Cessation of temozolomide and trial of corticosteroids appears successful in most cases.

There is an increased risk of opportunistic infections, most notably *Pneumocystis jirovecii* pneumonia, associated with use of temozolomide, attributed to either drug-related lymphopenia or concomitant corticosteroid use [60]. As temozolomide use increases for lung cancer treatment, the rate of opportunistic infections will have to be closely observed.

Immunotherapy/Immune Checkpoint Inhibitors

ICIs include antibodies directed against the PD-1 receptor (nivolumab, pembrolizumab, cemiplimab), the PD-L1 ligand (durvalumab, atezolizumab), or the cytotoxic T-lymphocyte antigen (CTLA-4) receptor (ipilimumab), and target tumor-induced immunosuppression of T cells, restoring intrinsic antitumor responses [61, 62]. Treatment with ICIs confers risk for unique toxicities known collectively as immune-related adverse events (IRAEs) which can affect any organ. Pneumonitis and sarcoid-like reactions are the primary pulmonary toxicities of interest, though IRAEs affecting other organ systems (such as myocarditis and endocrinopathies) can present with respiratory symptoms and relevant radiographic abnormalities [63].

Pneumonitis Epidemiology and Risk Factors

Pneumonitis is a relatively rare side effect of ICIs. As is typically the case, rates in real-world practice are higher than clinical trials suggested, owing to treatment of patients excluded from clinical trials and heightened awareness of IRAEs. The incidence of pneumonitis associated with anti-PD-1/PD-L1 use is estimated at 3–5%, though some studies report rates up to 19% [62, 64, 65]. Approximately 40% of those who develop ICI pneumonitis present with grade ≥3 disease; pneumonitis is the most frequent fatal IRAE and a common reason for termination of ICI therapy [65].

ICI pneumonitis occurs more commonly in patients with NSCLC than with other cancer types [66]. Additional risk factors include female sex, poor functional status, prior thoracic radiation, combination immunotherapy, tumor infiltration with pulmonary lymphangitis, and squamous pathology [63, 65, 67]. Patients with preexisting ILD are at increased risk for both all-grade and high-grade pneumonitis compared to those without (27% vs. 10% all-grade, 15% vs. 4% grade ≥3) [68]. ILD is not an absolute contraindication to receiving ICI therapy, and pneumonitis in these patients is often manageable.

ICIs are increasingly used in combination with other treatment modalities. Dual ICI therapy with PD-1 and CTLA-4 inhibition increases pneumonitis risk (7% vs. 3–5% for monotherapy) [69]. Combining nivolumab with carboplatin/paclitaxel/bevacizumab resulted in increased rates of all-grade pneumonitis compared to chemotherapy alone (7.3% vs. 1.1%), and in a trial of nivolumab with gemcitabine/cisplatin, 10 of 12 patients discontinuing therapy did so due to pneumonitis [70, 71]. A trial evaluating concomitant durvalumab with the EGFR-TKI osimertinib was discontinued due to increased incidence of ILD (22%) [72].

As patients segue from one treatment to another, prior therapies become relevant to current clinical presentations [62]. For example, sequential use of nivolumab followed by an EGFR-TKI resulted in a 25.7% pneumonitis rate [73]. There may be a synergistic effect between ICI and the *KRAS* inhibitor sotorasib, as all three patients who died of pneumonitis in a phase II trial of sotorasib had received prior treatment with an ICI [74]. The PACIFIC trial evaluated durvalumab consolidation therapy following concurrent platinum-doublet-based chemoradiation. Reported rates did not discriminate between radiation- and drug-induced pneumonitis, but the group receiving durvalumab showed elevated rates of all-grade pneumonitis compared with chemoradiation alone (30% vs. 26%); the rate of high-grade pneumonitis was similar between the two groups (3%) [75]. This is in contrast to rates of pneumonitis observed with concurrent use of pembrolizumab with chemoradiation (~19% all-grade, 7–8% grade ≥3) [76].

Clinical Presentation and Evaluation of ICI Pneumonitis

Onset of ICI pneumonitis varies, but median time of onset is 2–3 months [77]. Higher-grade (grade ≥3) pneumonitis tends to occur earlier, while reactions developing >6 months after initiation are typically low grade [67]. Presentation may be masked or delayed if patients received corticosteroids to manage extrapulmonary ICI toxicities [70].

Symptoms of ICI pneumonitis include nonproductive cough, dyspnea, hypoxemia, fever, and chest pain [65]. Up to 33% of patients with ICI-pneumonitis are asymptomatic at the time of diagnosis [77]. Physical exam may reveal tachypnea, hypoxemia, or inspiratory rales, but is often unremarkable [78].

Evaluation with CT scan is recommended. No one radiologic feature is pathognomonic for ICI pneumonitis; however common findings include ground glass opacities or confluent areas of peripheral consolidation [77, 79]. Additional radiographic features may include increased interstitial markings with interlobular septal thickening and subpleural reticulation, centrilobular and tree-in-bud nodules, or a mixture of any of these imaging features [77]. Eighty-six percent of imaging changes occur away from the peritumoral area, so new radiographic findings near known malignant lesions are suspicious for disease progression [67].

As with all suspected drug-induced lung disease cases, steps should be taken to exclude infection as an alternative cause for symptoms and radiographic findings [25]. Bronchoscopy with BAL should be considered, when feasible, for patients with grade ≥2 pneumonitis to help exclude infection prior to initiation of immunosuppression, and may reveal lymphocytosis [64, 65]. While transbronchial biopsy is not required to diagnose ICI pneumonitis, it should be performed if there is concern for progression of disease [64].

Management of ICI Pneumonitis

Management of ICI-related pneumonitis and other IRAEs is based solely on clinical experience, as no prospective trials evaluating optimal treatment strategy have been completed [79]. Since ICI pneumonitis is the leading cause of ICI-related deaths in patients with lung cancer, multidisciplinary collaboration is strongly recommended, particularly for severe or ambiguous presentations [65, 69]. Recommendations for management of ICI pneumonitis based on the American Society of Clinical Oncology (ASCO) and National Comprehensive Cancer Network (NCCN) guidelines are summarized in Table 11.1; treatment involves drug suspension/discontinuation with initiation of corticosteroids as indicated [25, 80]. Ideally, infection should be definitively ruled out prior to initiation of immunosuppression. The role of empiric antibiotics is debated, but they are commonly administered for high-grade events [65].

Initiation of systemic corticosteroids typically results in rapid improvement in patient symptoms and oxygenation. Patients failing to improve within 48 h of corticosteroid initiation may warrant consideration of additional immunosuppression. Steroid-refractory pneumonitis constitutes 10–40% of cases and is associated with 50% 90-day all-cause mortality [77, 81, 82]. Options for therapy include infliximab, mycophenolate mofetil (MMF), intravenous immunoglobulin (IVIG), and cyclophosphamide (Table 11.1) [80].

In cases of grade 2 pneumonitis, ICI rechallenge may be considered once symptoms improve to grade 1 or better; 50–70% tolerate therapy without recurrence, while 25% develop recurrent pneumonitis [77, 83]. In the event of grade 3 or 4 toxicity, permanent discontinuation of ICI is recommended.

ICI-Related Sarcoidosis

Several reports of ICI-induced pulmonary sarcoidosis have been published, more commonly with anti-CTLA-4 therapy [69, 84]. Isolated mediastinal/hilar lymphadenopathy, often with significant PET avidity, is the most common presentation; however concurrent parenchymal subpleural micronodular opacities is also observed [69, 80]. Half of patients are asymptomatic.

This sarcoid-like reaction should be considered in patients receiving ICIs who demonstrate new lymphadenopathy. Evaluation should include bronchoscopy with endobronchial ultrasound (EBUS) to rule out disease progression [69].

Radiographic findings will often regress when treatment is discontinued. Corticosteroids or other immunomodulators can be considered for those with symptoms or progressive radiographic changes [85]. Some studies suggest that the development of sarcoid-like reactions from ICI therapy is associated with increased survival [84].

Molecularly Targeted Agents

The use of molecularly targeted agents in treating advanced NSCLC has greatly advanced in recent years. Known pulmonary and related toxicities related to these drugs are summarized in Table 11.2 and discussed by class.

VEGF

Antiangiogenic agents targeting vascular endothelial growth factor (VEGF) are used in combination with traditional chemotherapeutic agents for advanced or progressive NSCLC, regardless of specific driver mutations [26, 27].

Bevacizumab is associated with hemorrhagic complications, including hemoptysis and alveolar hemorrhage. Phase IV studies, which excluded individuals deemed high-risk for hemorrhage (squamous histology, cavitation, central tumor location), demonstrated 1% rates of grade $\geq$3 pulmonary hemorrhage and fatal hemoptysis [86–88]. Most cases of hemoptysis occur within weeks of treatment initiation. Bevacizumab should be permanently discontinued in the case of grade $\geq$3 bleeding. The management of localized bleeding may be treated bronchoscopically or endovascularly with interventional radiology, depending on resources available.

Arterial thromboembolic events have also been linked to bevacizumab use for other malignancies (incidence of grade 3–5 events ~5%). In cases of high-grade severe arterial thromboembolism, bevacizumab should be discontinued [89]. Concurrent treatment with bevacizumab and radiation is avoided due to increased risk of tracheoesophageal fistulae formation; in the event of fistula formation, management consists of placement of a covered stent [90].

Ramucirumab is second-line therapy used less commonly [27]. It is similarly associated with the risk of high-grade hemorrhage including hemoptysis (2–5%), arterial thromboembolic events (grade $\geq$3 1–2%), and infusion-related reactions [91].

EGFR

Though pneumonitis is considered low frequency (~1%), it remains the most common fatal adverse effect related to EGFR-TKI use [92, 93]. Incidence varies across studies depending on patient cohort and specific agent. Low rates ($\leq$1%) are seen with gefitinib, afatinib, erlotinib, and dacomitinib, though approximately one-third of cases of ILD from gefitinib are fatal [94–97]. Osimertinib has a higher incidence of 2.4%, and mobocertinib is the highest at 4.3% [93, 98]. Onset of pneumonitis/ILD is generally within 24–42 days following treatment initiation; fulminant, severe presentations can be seen [94].

Risk factors for EGFR-TKI-associated pneumonitis include older age, smoking, pre-existing ILD, poor functional status, recent NSCLC diagnosis, and abnormal baseline lung parenchyma on CT scan [93]. Incidence of pneumonitis appears highest in Japanese cohorts [93, 94]. As previously discussed, there is an increased risk of pneumonitis with combined use of ICIs and EGFR-TKIs, especially with osimertinib [73, 99]. This effect was not seen when an EGFR-TKI was administered before immunotherapy, suggesting that therapy order may impact risk [100, 101].

Imaging can vary from nonspecific areas of ground glass opacity to extensive consolidations and traction bronchiectasis, with the latter form having poorer prognosis; variability in presentations suggests multiple pathophysiologic mechanisms [102, 103]. Association between transient, asymptomatic pulmonary opacities, and improved survival has been observed with osimertinib but requires further study [104]. Management includes discontinuation of the offending agent and consideration of systemic corticosteroids, though some patients deteriorate despite these interventions [103]. For low-grade cases that completely resolve, trial of an alternative drug within the class can be considered [93].

Development of ILD appears to be rare with the use of the EGFR-targeting monoclonal antibody cetuximab, including those previously treated with EGFR-TKI [105]. Amivantamab potentially poses a greater risk of ILD/pneumonitis at 3.3% [106]. No reports of ILD/pneumonitis have been reported with the use of necitumumab, though this medication confers risks of arterial and venous thromboembolisms and increased risk of all-cause mortality when used for non-squamous NSCLC [107].

ALK and ROS1

In patients with *ALK*-rearranged NSCLC, the likelihood of exposure to multiple drugs targeting *ALK and ROS* is high, as almost all patients with this mutation ultimately progress on first-line crizotinib, typically with metastases to the central nervous system [108]. While pulmonary toxicity from ALK-inhibitors as a class is relatively rare, significant differences have been observed between specific agents. Incidence ranges from 1.1% with ceritinib to 7% with brigatinib, with higher rates reported in individual clinical trials [109–111]. Risk factors for ILD from ALK-tyrosine kinase inhibitors (ALK-TKIs) include older age, lower performance status, smoking, prior or concurrent ILD, and pleural effusion [111].

There is variability in presentation and severity, ranging from asymptomatic radiographic changes to severe, irreversible, and potentially fatal disease. Brigatinib appears to have two distinct presentations—one within 7 days of drug initiation associated with fulminant and often fatal ILD, and another more indolent course that presents after months of therapy [108, 109]. Crizotinib-associated pneumonitis typically occurs within 2 months of drug initiation [112]. While other imaging patterns have been described, the most common imaging abnormality is that of NSIP with bilateral ground glass opacities on CT scan [113, 114]. OP is rare among ALK-TKI reactions and principally associated with ceritinib use. In severe cases, dense consolidations and/or pleural effusions may be seen [115].

When ALK-TKI-associated pulmonary toxicity is suspected, prompt discontinuation has been associated with clinical and radiographic improvement and improved survival [113]. Steroids have been used with subsequent improvement but have not been found to have a clear impact on survival; they are still recommended in cases of severe, life-threatening reactions [116]. Once a diagnosis of drug-related ILD is established, permanent drug discontinuation is advised. The exception to this is brigatinib, which allows for consideration of rechallenge at lower doses for grade ≤ 2 reactions [109].

BRAF

As approval for *BRAF*-targeted agents is recent and the mutation somewhat rare in NSCLC, knowledge about the toxicity profile derives from treatment of metastatic melanoma [117]. In melanoma, pneumonitis is reported in up to 2.4% of patients on trametinib monotherapy and 2.2% of patients concurrently receiving dabrafenib [117, 118]. Trametinib should be held for new or progressive respiratory symptoms and permanently discontinued if pneumonitis is apparent on imaging.

Vemurafenib use is rarely associated with pneumonitis, though the possibility of radio-sensitizing properties and association with radiation recall pneumonitis has been described [12, 119]. Sarcoid-like reactions have been reported in patients with metastatic melanoma [120].

There is additionally a 4.3% risk of thromboembolic events with the combined use of dabrafenib and trametinib for NSCLC [117].

Other Newer Agents

Drugs targeting additional mutations in NSCLC are constantly emerging with limited data available to characterize toxicities. Eventual real-world experience with novel therapeutics will reveal information that cannot be gleaned from curated populations included in clinical trials. The Pneumotox database is a helpful resource to review established toxicity profiles of systemic therapies, highlighting common presentations while acknowledging pathologic diversity seen with many agents; it can also be helpful in exploring rare and recently identified toxicities that may have significant impact in clinical practice [121].

Sotorasib is *KRAS* inhibitor approved for *KRAS* G12C-mutated metastatic NSCLC. Relevant safety data from a phase I/II trial of sotorasib in NSCLC suggest a 1.6% risk of pneumonitis [74]. Broader evaluation of sotorasib in treating mixed populations of patients with *KRAS*-mutated malignancies reported three cases of pneumonitis, one of which was fatal; all three patients had received prior treatment with an ICI [122].

Selpercatinib and pralsetinib target *RET* gene rearrangements. Notable adverse events related to selpercatinib in phase I/II clinical trials involve hemorrhagic events including hemoptysis (2.3%) [123]. In the case of hemorrhagic complications, selpercatinib should be held and permanently discontinued for severe or life-threatening events. Pralsetinib has been associated with pneumonitis (4%, including 2% with grade $\geq$3) [124]. A study including both lung and thyroid *RET*-mutated cancers found pneumonitis in 10% of patients, including fatal events in 0.5% of patients [125].

Capmatinib and tepotinib target *MET* exon 14 skipping mutations or alterations. Frequent serious adverse reactions that occurred in trials of capmatinib include pleural effusion (3.6%) and ILD/pneumonitis (4.5%, including high-grade events) [126, 127]. Similar rates of pleural effusion (7%) and pneumonia (5%) are seen with tepotinib when treating lung and thyroid cancers [126]. While ILD and pneumonitis are possible with both drugs, challenge with one after toxicity from the other has been successfully attempted [128].

Summary

Lung cancer treatment guidelines continue to evolve as new targets are discovered, novel treatments are developed, and existing therapies are applied in new combinations or for expanded indications. This shifting treatment landscape requires vigilance in recognizing established toxicities and identifying new phenomena. While treatment-related toxicities are relatively rare, their clinical impact on individual patients is profound. Therefore, a well-informed discussion of potential risks and established complications should be incorporated into shared decision-making with lung cancer patients and multidisciplinary treatment teams, and monitoring strategies should be adapted based on assessment of individual vulnerabilities. Pulmonologists are essential in detecting, evaluating, and managing treatment complications when they arise, ensuring that optimal therapy can be provided to the greatest number of patients in the safest manner possible.

References

1. Limper AH. Chemotherapy-induced lung disease. Clin Chest Med. 2004,25(1).53–64.
2. Muller NL, White DA, Jiang H, Gemma A. Diagnosis and management of drug-associated interstitial lung disease. Br J Cancer. 2004;91(Suppl 2):S24–30.
3. Gaga M, Powell CA, Schraufnagel DE, Schonfeld N, Rabe K, Hill NS, et al. An official American Thoracic Society/European Respiratory Society statement: the role of the pulmonologist in the diagnosis and management of lung cancer. Am J Respir Crit Care Med. 2013;188(4):503–7.
4. Bahig H, Filion E, Vu T, Chalaoui J, Lambert L, Roberge D, et al. Severe radiation pneumonitis after lung stereotactic ablative radiation therapy in patients with interstitial lung disease. Pract Radiat Oncol. 2016;6(5):367–74.
5. Monson JM, Stark P, Reilly JJ, Sugarbaker DJ, Strauss GM, Swanson SJ, et al. Clinical radiation pneumonitis and radiographic changes after thoracic radiation therapy for lung carcinoma. Cancer. 1998;82(5):842–50.

6. Abratt RP, Morgan GW, Silvestri G, Willcox P. Pulmonary complications of radiation therapy. Clin Chest Med. 2004;25(1):167–77.
7. Barriger RB, Forquer JA, Brabham JG, Andolino DL, Shapiro RH, Henderson MA, et al. A dose-volume analysis of radiation pneumonitis in non-small cell lung cancer patients treated with stereotactic body radiation therapy. Int J Radiat Oncol Biol Phys. 2012;82(1):457–62.
8. Liu H, Zhang X, Vinogradskiy YY, Swisher SG, Komaki R, Chang JY. Predicting radiation pneumonitis after stereotactic ablative radiation therapy in patients previously treated with conventional thoracic radiation therapy. Int J Radiat Oncol Biol Phys. 2012;84(4):1017–23.
9. Bledsoe TJ, Nath SK, Decker RH. Radiation pneumonitis. Clin Chest Med. 2017;38(2):201–8.
10. Robnett TJ, Machtay M, Vines EF, McKenna MG, Algazy KM, McKenna WG. Factors predicting severe radiation pneumonitis in patients receiving definitive chemoradiation for lung cancer. Int J Radiat Oncol Biol Phys. 2000;48(1):89–94.
11. Yamaguchi S, Ohguri T, Ide S, Aoki T, Imada H, Yahara K, et al. Stereotactic body radiotherapy for lung tumors in patients with subclinical interstitial lung disease: the potential risk of extensive radiation pneumonitis. Lung Cancer. 2013;82(2):260–5.
12. Forschner A, Zips D, Schraml C, Rocken M, Iordanou E, Leiter U, et al. Radiation recall dermatitis and radiation pneumonitis during treatment with vemurafenib. Melanoma Res. 2014;24(5):512–6.
13. Cousin F, Desir C, Ben Mustapha S, Mievis C, Coucke P, Hustinx R. Incidence, risk factors, and CT characteristics of radiation recall pneumonitis induced by immune checkpoint inhibitor in lung cancer. Radiother Oncol. 2021;157:47–55.
14. Adhikari B, Dongol RM, Baral D, Hewett Y, Shah BK. Pemetrexed and interstitial lung disease. Acta Oncol. 2016;55(4):521–2.
15. Harada H, Seto T, Igawa S, Tsuya A, Wada M, Kaira K, et al. Phase I results of vinorelbine with concurrent radiotherapy in elderly patients with unresectable, locally advanced non-small-cell lung cancer: West Japan Thoracic Oncology Group (WJTOG3005-DI). Int J Radiat Oncol Biol Phys. 2012;82(5):1777–82.
16. Jia W, Gao Q, Wang M, Li J, Jing W, Yu J, et al. Overlap time is an independent risk factor of radiation pneumonitis for patients treated with simultaneous EGFR-TKI and thoracic radiotherapy. Radiat Oncol. 2021;16(1):41.
17. McDonald S, Rubin P, Phillips TL, Marks LB. Injury to the lung from cancer therapy: clinical syndromes, measurable endpoints, and potential scoring systems. Int J Radiat Oncol Biol Phys. 1995;31(5):1187–203.
18. Hanania AN, Mainwaring W, Ghebre YT, Hanania NA, Ludwig M. Radiation-induced lung injury: assessment and management. Chest. 2019;156(1):150–62.
19. Common Terminology Criteria for Adverse Events (CTCAE). 2017. Accessed 29 Aug 2022.
20. Zhang P, Yan H, Wang S, Kai J, Pi G, Peng Y, et al. Post-radiotherapy maintenance treatment with fluticasone propionate and salmeterol for lung cancer patients with grade III radiation pneumonitis: a case report. Medicine (Baltimore). 2018;97(21):e10681.
21. Flieder DB, Travis WD. Pathologic characteristics of drug-induced lung disease. Clin Chest Med. 2004;25(1):37–45.
22. Camus P. Interstitial lung disease in patients with non-small-cell lung cancer: causes, mechanisms and management. Br J Cancer. 2004;91(Suppl 2):S1–2.
23. Camus P, Fanton A, Bonniaud P, Camus C, Foucher P. Interstitial lung disease induced by drugs and radiation. Respiration. 2004;71(4):301–26.
24. Camus P, Kudoh S, Ebina M. Interstitial lung disease associated with drug therapy. Br J Cancer. 2004;91(Suppl 2):S18–23.
25. NCCN. Management of immunotherapy-related toxicities. National Comprehensive Cancer Network. v1.2022. 2022. https://www.nccn.org/professionals/physician_gls/pdf/immunotherapy.pdf.
26. Hanna NH, Schneider BJ, Temin S, Baker S Jr, Brahmer J, Ellis PM, et al. Therapy for stage IV non-small-cell lung cancer without driver alterations: ASCO and OH (CCO) Joint Guideline Update. J Clin Oncol. 2020;38(14):1608–32.

27. NCCN. Non-small cell lung cancer. National Comprehensive Cancer Network. v3.2022. 2022. https://www.nccn.org/professionals/physician_gls/pdf/nscl.pdf.
28. NCCN. Small cell lung cancer. National Comprehensive Cancer Network. v2.2022. 2021. https://www.nccn.org/professionals/physician_gls/pdf/sclc.pdf.
29. Moore RA, Adel N, Riedel E, Bhutani M, Feldman DR, Tabbara NE, et al. High incidence of thromboembolic events in patients treated with cisplatin-based chemotherapy: a large retrospective analysis. J Clin Oncol. 2011;29(25):3466–73.
30. Lee YG, Lee E, Kim I, Lee KW, Kim TM, Lee SH, et al. Cisplatin-based chemotherapy is a strong risk factor for thromboembolic events in small-cell lung cancer. Cancer Res Treat. 2015;47(4):670–5.
31. Wang GS, Yang KY, Perng RP. Life-threatening hypersensitivity pneumonitis induced by docetaxel (taxotere). Br J Cancer. 2001;85(9):1247–50.
32. Graziano SL, Herndon JE II, Socinski MA, Wang X, Watson D, Vokes E, et al. Phase II trial of weekly dose-dense paclitaxel in extensive-stage small cell lung cancer: cancer and leukemia group B study 39901. J Thorac Oncol. 2008;3(2):158–62.
33. Tamiya A, Naito T, Miura S, Morii S, Tsuya A, Nakamura Y, et al. Interstitial lung disease associated with docetaxel in patients with advanced non-small cell lung cancer. Anticancer Res. 2012;32(3):1103–6.
34. Chen YM, Shih JF, Perng RP, Tsai CM, Whang-Peng J. A randomized trial of different docetaxel schedules in non-small cell lung cancer patients who failed previous platinum-based chemotherapy. Chest. 2006;129(4):1031–8.
35. Thomas AL, Cox G, Sharma RA, Steward WP, Shields F, Jeyapalan K, et al. Gemcitabine and paclitaxel associated pneumonitis in non-small cell lung cancer: report of a phase I/II dose-escalating study. Eur J Cancer. 2000;36(18):2329–34.
36. Onishi H, Kuriyama K, Yamaguchi M, Komiyama T, Tanaka S, Araki T, et al. Concurrent two-dimensional radiotherapy and weekly docetaxel in the treatment of stage III non-small cell lung cancer: a good local response but no good survival due to radiation pneumonitis. Lung Cancer. 2003;40(1):79–84.
37. Semb KA, Aamdal S, Oian P. Capillary protein leak syndrome appears to explain fluid retention in cancer patients who receive docetaxel treatment. J Clin Oncol. 1998;16(10):3426–32.
38. Ohe Y, Ichinose Y, Nakagawa K, Tamura T, Kubota K, Yamamoto N, et al. Efficacy and safety of two doses of pemetrexed supplemented with folic acid and vitamin B12 in previously treated patients with non-small cell lung cancer. Clin Cancer Res. 2008;14(13):4206–12.
39. Tomii K, Kato T, Takahashi M, Noma S, Kobashi Y, Enatsu S, et al. Pemetrexed-related interstitial lung disease reported from post marketing surveillance (malignant pleural mesothelioma/non-small cell lung cancer). Jpn J Clin Oncol. 2017;47(4):350–6.
40. Eagle Pharmaceuticals. Pemfexy (pemetrexed) package insert. Woodcliff Lake, NJ: Eagle Pharmaceuticals; 2020.
41. Hochstrasser A, Benz G, Joerger M, Templeton A, Brutsche M, Fruh M. Interstitial pneumonitis after treatment with pemetrexed: a rare event? Chemotherapy. 2012;58(1):84–8.
42. Barlesi F, Villani P, Doddoli C, Gimenez C, Kleisbauer JP. Gemcitabine-induced severe pulmonary toxicity. Fundam Clin Pharmacol. 2004;18(1):85–91.
43. Arrieta O, Gallardo-Rincon D, Villarreal-Garza C, Michel RM, Astorga-Ramos AM, Martinez-Barrera L, et al. High frequency of radiation pneumonitis in patients with locally advanced non-small cell lung cancer treated with concurrent radiotherapy and gemcitabine after induction with gemcitabine and carboplatin. J Thorac Oncol. 2009;4(7):845–52.
44. Pavlakis N, Bell DR, Millward MJ, Levi JA. Fatal pulmonary toxicity resulting from treatment with gemcitabine. Cancer. 1997;80(2):286–91.
45. Binder D, Hubner RH, Temmesfeld-Wollbruck B, Schlattmann P. Pulmonary toxicity among cancer patients treated with a combination of docetaxel and gemcitabine: a meta-analysis of clinical trials. Cancer Chemother Pharmacol. 2011;68(6):1575–83.
46. Dajczman E, Srolovitz H, Kreisman H, Frank H. Fatal pulmonary toxicity following oral etoposide therapy. Lung Cancer. 1995;12(1–2):81–6.

47. Gurjal A, An T, Valdivieso M, Kalemkerian GP. Etoposide-induced pulmonary toxicity. Lung Cancer. 1999;26(2):109–12.
48. Maitland ML, Wilcox R, Hogarth DK, Desai AA, Caligiuri P, Abrahams C, et al. Diffuse alveolar damage after a single dose of topotecan in a patient with pulmonary fibrosis and small cell lung cancer. Lung Cancer. 2006;54(2):243–5.
49. Shiozawa T, Tadokoro J, Fujiki T, Fujino K, Kakihata K, Masatani S, et al. Risk factors for severe adverse effects and treatment-related deaths in Japanese patients treated with irinotecan-based chemotherapy: a postmarketing survey. Jpn J Clin Oncol. 2013;43(5):483–91.
50. Pfizer Injectables. Irinotecan package insert. New York, NY: Pfizer Injectables; 2014.
51. Teva Pharmaceuticals. Topotecan injection package insert. North Wales, PA: Teva Pharmaceuticals; 2014.
52. Yoshii N, Suzuki T, Nagashima M, Kon A, Kakihata K, Gemma A. Clarification of clinical features of interstitial lung disease induced by irinotecan based on postmarketing surveillance data and spontaneous reports. Anti-Cancer Drugs. 2011;22(6):563–8.
53. Madarnas Y, Webster P, Shorter AM, Bjarnason GA. Irinotecan-associated pulmonary toxicity. Anti-Cancer Drugs. 2000;11(9):709–13.
54. Tanvetyanon T, Garrity ER, Albain KS. Acute lung injury associated with vinorelbine. J Clin Oncol. 2006;24(12):1952–3.
55. Ribeiro de Oliveira Santos MB, Mergulhao P. Vinorelbine-induced acute respiratory distress syndrome treated with non-invasive ventilation and immunosuppressive therapy. Respirol Case Rep. 2018;6(7):e00349.
56. Singh S, Jaigirdar AA, Mulkey F, Cheng J, Hamed SS, Li Y, et al. FDA approval summary: lurbinectedin for the treatment of metastatic small cell lung cancer. Clin Cancer Res. 2021;27(9):2378–82.
57. Abrey LE, Olson JD, Raizer JJ, Mack M, Rodavitch A, Boutros DY, et al. A phase II trial of temozolomide for patients with recurrent or progressive brain metastases. J Neuro-Oncol. 2001;53(3):259–65.
58. Maldonado F, Limper AH, Lim KG, Aubrey MC. Temozolomide-associated organizing pneumonitis. Mayo Clin Proc. 2007;82(6):771–3.
59. Koschel D, Handzhiev S, Leucht V, Holotiuk O, Fisseler-Eckhoff A, Hoffken G. Hypersensitivity pneumonitis associated with the use of temozolomide. Eur Respir J. 2009;33(4):931–4.
60. De Vos FY, Gijtenbeek JM, Bleeker-Rovers CP, van Herpen CM. Pneumocystis jirovecii pneumonia prophylaxis during temozolomide treatment for high-grade gliomas. Crit Rev Oncol Hematol. 2013;85(3):373–82.
61. Gettinger SN, Horn L, Gandhi L, Spigel DR, Antonia SJ, Rizvi NA, et al. Overall survival and long-term safety of nivolumab (anti-programmed death 1 antibody, BMS-936558, ONO-4538) in patients with previously treated advanced non-small-cell lung cancer. J Clin Oncol. 2015;33(18):2004–12.
62. Chen TW, Razak AR, Bedard PL, Siu LL, Hansen AR. A systematic review of immune-related adverse event reporting in clinical trials of immune checkpoint inhibitors. Ann Oncol. 2015;26(9):1824–9.
63. Champiat S, Lambotte O, Barreau E, Belkhir R, Berdelou A, Carbonnel F, et al. Management of immune checkpoint blockade dysimmune toxicities: a collaborative position paper. Ann Oncol. 2016;27(4):559–74.
64. Haanen J, Carbonnel F, Robert C, Kerr KM, Peters S, Larkin J, et al. Management of toxicities from immunotherapy: ESMO Clinical Practice Guidelines for diagnosis, treatment and follow-up. Ann Oncol. 2017;28(suppl_4):iv119–iv42.
65. Reuss JE, Suresh K, Naidoo J. Checkpoint inhibitor pneumonitis: mechanisms, characteristics, management strategies, and beyond. Curr Oncol Rep. 2020;22(6):56.
66. Nishino M, Giobbie-Hurder A, Hatabu H, Ramaiya NH, Hodi FS. Incidence of programmed cell death 1 inhibitor-related pneumonitis in patients with advanced cancer: a systematic review and meta-analysis. JAMA Oncol. 2016;2(12):1607–16.

67. Suresh K, Voong KR, Shankar B, Forde PM, Ettinger DS, Marrone KA, et al. Pneumonitis in non-small cell lung cancer patients receiving immune checkpoint immunotherapy: incidence and risk factors. J Thorac Oncol. 2018;13(12):1930–9.
68. Zhang M, Fan Y, Nie L, Wang G, Sun K, Cheng Y. Clinical outcomes of immune checkpoint inhibitor therapy in patients with advanced non-small cell lung cancer and preexisting interstitial lung diseases: a systematic review and meta-analysis. Chest. 2022;161(6):1675–86.
69. Cadranel J, Canellas A, Matton L, Darrason M, Parrot A, Naccache JM, et al. Pulmonary complications of immune checkpoint inhibitors in patients with nonsmall cell lung cancer. Eur Respir Rev. 2019;28(153):190058.
70. Rizvi NA, Hellmann MD, Brahmer JR, Juergens RA, Borghaei H, Gettinger S, et al. Nivolumab in combination with platinum-based doublet chemotherapy for first-line treatment of advanced non-small-cell lung cancer. J Clin Oncol. 2016;34(25):2969–79.
71. Sugawara S, Lee JS, Kang JH, Kim HR, Inui N, Hida T, et al. Nivolumab with carboplatin, paclitaxel, and bevacizumab for first-line treatment of advanced nonsquamous non-small-cell lung cancer. Ann Oncol. 2021;32(9):1137–47.
72. Oxnard GR, Yang JC, Yu H, Kim SW, Saka H, Horn L, et al. TATTON: a multi-arm, phase Ib trial of osimertinib combined with selumetinib, savolitinib, or durvalumab in EGFR-mutant lung cancer. Ann Oncol. 2020;31(4):507–16.
73. Oshima Y, Tanimoto T, Yuji K, Tojo A. EGFR-TKI-associated interstitial pneumonitis in nivolumab-treated patients with non-small cell lung cancer. JAMA Oncol. 2018;4(8):1112–5.
74. Skoulidis F, Li BT, Dy GK, Price TJ, Falchook GS, Wolf J, et al. Sotorasib for lung cancers with KRAS p.G12C mutation. N Engl J Med. 2021;384(25):2371–81.
75. Antonia SJ, Villegas A, Daniel D, Vicente D, Murakami S, Hui R, et al. Durvalumab after chemoradiotherapy in stage III non-small-cell lung cancer. N Engl J Med. 2017;377(20):1919–29.
76. Jabbour SK, Lee KH, Frost N, Breder V, Kowalski DM, Pollock T, et al. Pembrolizumab plus concurrent chemoradiation therapy in patients with unresectable, locally advanced, stage III non-small cell lung cancer: the phase 2 KEYNOTE-799 nonrandomized trial. JAMA Oncol. 2021;7:1.
77. Naidoo J, Wang X, Woo KM, Iyriboz T, Halpenny D, Cunningham J, et al. Pneumonitis in patients treated with anti-programmed death-1/programmed death ligand 1 therapy. J Clin Oncol. 2017;35(7):709–17.
78. Michot JM, Bigenwald C, Champiat S, Collins M, Carbonnel F, Postel-Vinay S, et al. Immune-related adverse events with immune checkpoint blockade: a comprehensive review. Eur J Cancer. 2016;54:139–48.
79. Friedman CF, Proverbs-Singh TA, Postow MA. Treatment of the immune-related adverse effects of immune checkpoint inhibitors: a review. JAMA Oncol. 2016;2(10):1346–53.
80. Schneider BJ, Naidoo J, Santomasso BD, Lacchetti C, Adkins S, Anadkat M, et al. Management of immune-related adverse events in patients treated with immune checkpoint inhibitor therapy: ASCO guideline update. J Clin Oncol. 2021;39(36):4073–126.
81. Balaji A, Hsu M, Lin CT, Feliciano J, Marrone K, Brahmer JR, et al. Steroid-refractory PD-(L)1 pneumonitis: incidence, clinical features, treatment, and outcomes. J Immunother Cancer. 2021;9(1):e001731.
82. Horvat TZ, Adel NG, Dang TO, Momtaz P, Postow MA, Callahan MK, et al. Immune-related adverse events, need for systemic immunosuppression, and effects on survival and time to treatment failure in patients with melanoma treated with ipilimumab at Memorial Sloan Kettering Cancer Center. J Clin Oncol. 2015;33(28):3193–8.
83. Nishino M, Ramaiya NH, Awad MM, Sholl LM, Maattala JA, Taibi M, et al. PD-1 Inhibitor-related pneumonitis in advanced cancer patients: radiographic patterns and clinical course. Clin Cancer Res. 2016;22(24):6051–60.
84. Cabanie C, Ammari S, Hans S, Pobel C, Laparra A, Danlos FX, et al. Outcomes of patients with cancer and sarcoid-like granulomatosis associated with immune checkpoint inhibitors: a case-control study. Eur J Cancer. 2021;156:46–59.

85. Nishino M, Sholl LM, Awad MM, Hatabu H, Armand P, Hodi FS. Sarcoid-like granulomatosis of the lung related to immune-checkpoint inhibitors: distinct clinical and imaging features of a unique immune-related adverse event. Cancer Immunol Res. 2018;6(6):630–5.

86. Goto K, Endo M, Kusumoto M, Yamamoto N, Ohe Y, Shimizu A, et al. Bevacizumab for non-small-cell lung cancer: a nested case control study of risk factors for hemoptysis. Cancer Sci. 2016;107(12):1837–42.

87. Johnson DH, Fehrenbacher L, Novotny WF, Herbst RS, Nemunaitis JJ, Jablons DM, et al. Randomized phase II trial comparing bevacizumab plus carboplatin and paclitaxel with carboplatin and paclitaxel alone in previously untreated locally advanced or metastatic non-small-cell lung cancer. J Clin Oncol. 2004;22(11):2184–91.

88. Crino L, Dansin E, Garrido P, Griesinger F, Laskin J, Pavlakis N, et al. Safety and efficacy of first-line bevacizumab-based therapy in advanced non-squamous non-small-cell lung cancer (SAiL, MO19390): a phase 4 study. Lancet Oncol. 2010;11(8):733–40.

89. Genetech. Avastin (bevacizumab) package insert. South San Francisco, CA: Genetech; 2017.

90. Spigel DR, Hainsworth JD, Yardley DA, Raefsky E, Patton J, Peacock N, et al. Tracheoesophageal fistula formation in patients with lung cancer treated with chemoradiation and bevacizumab. J Clin Oncol. 2010;28(1):43–8.

91. Eli Lilly and Company. Cyramza (ramucirumab) package insert. Indianapolis, IN: Eli Lilly and Company; 2020.

92. Xie X, Wang X, Wu S, Yang H, Liu J, Chen H, et al. Fatal toxic effects related to EGFR tyrosine kinase inhibitors based on 53 cohorts with 9,569 participants. J Thorac Dis. 2020;12(8):4057–69.

93. Suh CH, Park HS, Kim KW, Pyo J, Hatabu H, Nishino M. Pneumonitis in advanced non-small-cell lung cancer patients treated with EGFR tyrosine kinase inhibitor: meta-analysis of 153 cohorts with 15,713 patients: meta-analysis of incidence and risk factors of EGFR-TKI pneumonitis in NSCLC. Lung Cancer. 2018;123:60–9.

94. Cohen MH, Williams GA, Sridhara R, Chen G, Pazdur R. FDA drug approval summary: gefitinib (ZD1839) (Iressa) tablets. Oncologist. 2003;8(4):303–6.

95. Sequist LV, Yang JC, Yamamoto N, O'Byrne K, Hirsh V, Mok T, et al. Phase III study of afatinib or cisplatin plus pemetrexed in patients with metastatic lung adenocarcinoma with EGFR mutations. J Clin Oncol. 2013;31(27):3327–34.

96. Reck M, van Zandwijk N, Gridelli C, Baliko Z, Rischin D, Allan S, et al. Erlotinib in advanced non-small cell lung cancer: efficacy and safety findings of the global phase IV Tarceva Lung Cancer Survival Treatment study. J Thorac Oncol. 2010;5(10):1616–22.

97. Pfizer Labs. Vizimpro (dacomitinib) package insert. New York, NY: Pfizer Labs; 2018.

98. Takeda Pharmaceuticals America. Exkivity (mobocertinib) package insert. Cambridge, MA: Takeda Pharmaceuticals America; 2021.

99. Uchida T, Kaira K, Yamaguchi O, Mouri A, Shiono A, Miura Y, et al. Different incidence of interstitial lung disease according to different kinds of EGFR-tyrosine kinase inhibitors administered immediately before and/or after anti-PD-1 antibodies in lung cancer. Thorac Cancer. 2019;10(4):975–9.

100. Schoenfeld AJ, Arbour KC, Rizvi H, Iqbal AN, Gadgeel SM, Girshman J, et al. Severe immune-related adverse events are common with sequential PD-(L)1 blockade and osimertinib. Ann Oncol. 2019;30(5):839–44.

101. Jia Y, Zhao S, Jiang T, Li X, Zhao C, Liu Y, et al. Impact of EGFR-TKIs combined with PD-L1 antibody on the lung tissue of EGFR-driven tumor-bearing mice. Lung Cancer. 2019;137:85–93.

102. Endo M, Johkoh T, Kimura K, Yamamoto N. Imaging of gefitinib-related interstitial lung disease: multi-institutional analysis by the West Japan Thoracic Oncology Group. Lung Cancer. 2006;52(2):135–40.

103. Yoneda KY, Shelton DK, Beckett LA, Gandara DR. Independent review of interstitial lung disease associated with death in TRIBUTE (paclitaxel and carboplatin with or without concurrent erlotinib) in advanced non-small cell lung cancer. J Thorac Oncol. 2007;2(6):537–43.

104. Lee H, Lee HY, Sun JM, Lee SH, Kim Y, Park SE, et al. Transient asymptomatic pulmonary opacities during osimertinib treatment and its clinical implication. J Thorac Oncol. 2018;13(8):1106–12.
105. Neal JW, Heist RS, Fidias P, Temel JS, Huberman M, Marcoux JP, et al. Cetuximab monotherapy in patients with advanced non-small cell lung cancer after prior epidermal growth factor receptor tyrosine kinase inhibitor therapy. J Thorac Oncol. 2010;5(11):1855–8.
106. Janssen Biotech. Rybrevant (amivantamab) package insert. Horsham Township, PA: Janssen Biotech; 2021.
107. Eli Lilly and Company. Portrazza (necitumumab) package insert. Indianapolis, IN: Eli Lilly and Company; 2015.
108. Gettinger SN, Bazhenova LA, Langer CJ, Salgia R, Gold KA, Rosell R, et al. Activity and safety of brigatinib in ALK-rearranged non-small-cell lung cancer and other malignancies: a single-arm, open-label, phase 1/2 trial. Lancet Oncol. 2016;17(12):1683–96.
109. Pellegrino B, Facchinetti F, Bordi P, Silva M, Gnetti L, Tiseo M. Lung toxicity in non-small-cell lung cancer patients exposed to ALK inhibitors: report of a peculiar case and systematic review of the literature. Clin Lung Cancer. 2018;19(2):e151–e61.
110. Au TH, Cavalieri CC, Stenehjem DD. Ceritinib: a primer for pharmacists. J Oncol Pharm Pract. 2017;23(8):602–14.
111. Gemma A, Kusumoto M, Kurihara Y, Masuda N, Banno S, Endo Y, et al. Interstitial lung disease onset and its risk factors in Japanese patients with ALK-positive NSCLC after treatment with crizotinib. J Thorac Oncol. 2019;14(4):672–82.
112. Ou SH. Crizotinib: a novel and first-in-class multitargeted tyrosine kinase inhibitor for the treatment of anaplastic lymphoma kinase rearranged non-small cell lung cancer and beyond. Drug Des Dev Ther. 2011;5:471–85.
113. Yoneda KY, Scranton JR, Cadogan MA, Tassell V, Nadanaciva S, Wilner KD, et al. Interstitial lung disease associated with crizotinib in patients with advanced non-small cell lung cancer: independent review of four PROFILE trials. Clin Lung Cancer. 2017;18(5):472–9.
114. Wu Y, Chen H, Guan J, Zhang K, Wu W, Li X, et al. Organizing pneumonia in ALK+ lung adenocarcinoma treated with ceritinib: a case report and literature review. Medicine (Baltimore). 2021;100(26):e26449.
115. Harrison PK, Boland HE, Aherne NJ, Palmieri DJ. An unusual case of lorlatinib-induced pneumonitis: a case report. Case Rep Oncol. 2022;15(1):225–30.
116. Lin L, Zhao J, Kong N, He Y, Hu J, Huang F, et al. Meta-analysis of the incidence and risks of interstitial lung disease and QTc prolongation in non-small-cell lung cancer patients treated with ALK inhibitors. Oncotarget. 2017;8(34):57379–85.
117. Chalmers A, Cannon L, Akerley W. Adverse event management in patients with BRAF V600E-mutant non-small cell lung cancer treated with dabrafenib plus trametinib. Oncologist. 2019;24(7):963–72.
118. Novartis Pharmaceuticals Corporation. Mekinist (trametinib) package insert. East Hanover, NJ: Novartis Pharmaceuticals Corporation; 2018.
119. Schmitt L, Schumann T, Loser C, Dippel E. Vemurafenib-induced pulmonary injury. Onkologie. 2013;36(11):685–6.
120. Lheure C, Kramkimel N, Franck N, Laurent-Roussel S, Carlotti A, Queant A, et al. Sarcoidosis in patients treated with vemurafenib for metastatic melanoma: a paradoxical autoimmune activation. Dermatology. 2015;231(4):378–84.
121. Camus P. The drug-induced respiratory disease website. v2.2. 2022. https://www.pneumotox.com/drug/index/.
122. Nakajima EC, Drezner N, Li X, Mishra-Kalyani PS, Liu Y, Zhao H, et al. FDA approval summary: sotorasib for KRAS G12C-mutated metastatic NSCLC. Clin Cancer Res. 2022;28(8):1482–6.
123. Lilly. Retevmo (selpercatinib) package insert. Indianapolis, IN: Lilly; 2020.

124. Gainor JF, Curigliano G, Kim DW, Lee DH, Besse B, Baik CS, et al. Pralsetinib for RET fusion-positive non-small-cell lung cancer (ARROW): a multi-cohort, open-label, phase 1/2 study. Lancet Oncol. 2021;22(7):959–69.
125. Kim J, Bradford D, Larkins E, Pai-Scherf LH, Chatterjee S, Mishra-Kalyani PS, et al. FDA approval summary: pralsetinib for the treatment of lung and thyroid cancers with RET gene mutations or fusions. Clin Cancer Res. 2021;27(20):5452–6.
126. Mathieu LN, Larkins E, Akinboro O, Roy P, Amatya AK, Fiero MH, et al. FDA approval summary: capmatinib and tepotinib for the treatment of metastatic NSCLC harboring MET exon 14 skipping mutations or alterations. Clin Cancer Res. 2022;28(2):249–54.
127. Wolf J, Seto T, Han JY, Reguart N, Garon EB, Groen HJM, et al. Capmatinib in MET exon 14-mutated or MET-amplified non-small-cell lung cancer. N Engl J Med. 2020;383(10):944–57.
128. Hashiguchi MH, Sato T, Yamamoto H, Watanabe R, Kagyo J, Domoto H, et al. Successful tepotinib challenge after capmatinib-induced interstitial lung disease in a patient with lung adenocarcinoma harboring MET exon 14 skipping mutation: case report. JTO Clin Res Rep. 2022;3(2):100271.

Chapter 12
Multidisciplinary Approach to Lung Cancer Care

Thomas Bilfinger, Lee Ann Santore, and Barbara Nemesure

Introduction

Although multidisciplinary cancer care has been recommended by cancer organizations, governments, and healthcare organizations since 1995 [1, 2], this date is by no means the start of the movement to establish multidisciplinary models in cancer care. A growing literature has documented the potential benefits of these approaches in the general population over the past two decades [1], while premiere cancer institutions have long used integrated models for specialized cancer care proclaiming superior results. In modern times improved diagnosis and treatment result in >50% cancer survival in developed countries with the best approaching 60%. Multidisciplinary care is central to the declared goal of achieving 70% survival by 2035 [3]. Screening, prompt diagnosis, and expeditious treatment followed by tight

T. Bilfinger (✉)
Renaissance School of Medicine, Stony Brook University, Stony Brook, NY, USA

Stony Brook Chest Clinic, Stony Brook University Hospital, Stony Brook, NY, USA

Department of Surgery, Stony Brook University, Stony Brook, NY, USA
e-mail: thomas.bilfinger@stonybrookmedicine.edu

L. A. Santore
Renaissance School of Medicine, Stony Brook University, Stony Brook, NY, USA
e-mail: lee.santore@stonybrookmedicine.edu

B. Nemesure
Renaissance School of Medicine, Stony Brook University, Stony Brook, NY, USA

Stony Brook Chest Clinic, Stony Brook University Hospital, Stony Brook, NY, USA

Department of Family, Population and Preventive, Medicine, Stony Brook University, Stony Brook, NY, USA
e-mail: barbara.nemesure@stonybrookmedicine.edu

C. MacRosty, M. P. Rivera (eds.), *Lung Cancer*, Respiratory Medicine,
https://doi.org/10.1007/978-3-031-38412-7_12

surveillance are the cornerstones of any effort to decrease the cancer burden and improve survival outcomes.

Most (46%) cases of non-small cell lung cancer (NSCLC) present in advanced stages [4] and carcinoma of the lung have the highest mortality rate of all cancer types [5]. Despite these grave statistics, lung cancer was not among the first cancer disciplines to introduce multidisciplinary models of care into practice. With advances in screening, diagnostics, and treatments that have emerged over the past two decades, a wider array of therapeutic options are now available to address this complex disease. Guidelines for optimal care of patients with NSCLC have been developed by a number of organizations, typically relying on participation from providers in different specialties. Many patients do not fit neatly into a set of schemes and therefore require individualized care plans [6]. Newer treatment modalities with immune checkpoint inhibitors, targeted therapies, new and advanced radiation techniques, and surgical advances have widened the armamentarium but have also complicated the options [7, 8]. In concert with the increase in treatment options, an increase in the number of complex cases has been observed. This together with experience from other cancers, particularly breast cancer, has led to recommendations for multidisciplinary care for patients with lung cancer.

The benefit of a multidisciplinary approach is most evident for patients with stage III NSCLC [9–11], but benefit has been demonstrated for earlier stage patients as well [12]. As a result of comorbidities, patients often do not fall neatly into pro-tocol driven algorithms. Precisely these algorithms have been used as argument against multidisciplinary care due to added cost, particularly in patients with stages I and II disease, where clear guidelines are available. Several studies however showed that adherence to guidelines is more likely to occur if a multidisciplinary team review took place [13, 14]. At present, multidisciplinary care as part of lung cancer management has been recommended in a number of guidelines in the USA [15, 16], the UK [17], Australia [18], and France [19], among others and is a man-date for accreditation.

A Framework for a Multidisciplinary Lung Cancer Program: The Front Desk Experience

Lung cancer care is becoming increasingly complex requiring high-level care coor-dination in a timely fashion. The framework for action on interprofessional educa-tion and collaborative practice published by the World Health Organization in 2010 [20] concluded that interprofessional/interdisciplinary teamwork is essential for high-quality cancer care in an increasingly complex medical environment. Today, many hospitals are promoting patient centered care where the patient is involved in their care and decision-making. From a patient's perspective, the expectation is that the healthcare system includes input on his or her specific disease from a multidis-ciplinary panel of expert providers representing all disciplines associated with his or

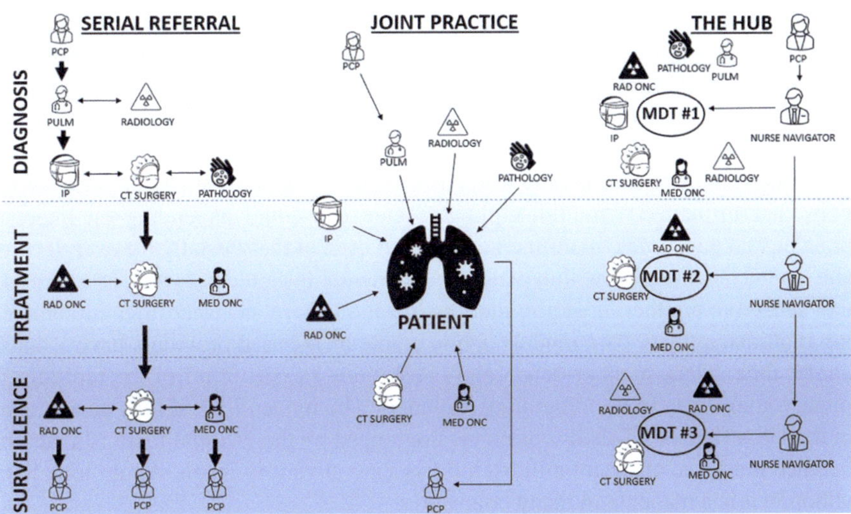

Fig. 12.1 The four distinct phases of care as described by Moody et al. [21]

her disease. Care should be timely with a clearly identifiable leader who transmits information to the patient and guides him or her through the process. Lung cancer care varies among institutions, systems, and countries according to infrastructure, available resources, quality standards, and operating procedures [9]. Three main forms of care (Fig. 12.1) can be identified within what is considered a multidisciplinary approach: (1) a serial referral model; (2) a continuous joint practice model; or (3) a hub, joint decision-making model.

The following are putative benefits of multidisciplinary lung cancer care:

- Improved consistency, continuity, coordination and cost-effectiveness of care.
- Improved clinical outcomes.
- Increased recruitment into clinical trials.
- Improved communication between cancer care providers.
- Increased satisfaction and psychological well-being of patients.
- Educational opportunities for health professionals.
- Opportunities to collect relevant data.
- Increased job satisfaction and psychological well-being of team members.

with the added expectation to resolve or improve the following:

- Nonuniform access to cancer care.
- Disjoint referral systems.
- Large variation in frequency of individual treatments used, patient survival, and cancer treatment caseloads of individual physicians.

Accepting for a moment what some have called lofty and more theoretical goals (after all, lung cancer care over the last two decades has achieved a 53% improvement in 5 year survival even with low implementation of multidisciplinary care)

[22], it becomes immediately clear that the devil is in the details. Below we describe what "multidisciplinary" may mean from a patient's perspective, but how this may look from a physician's perspective is often overlooked, particularly in the context of cancer care. Only oncologists and radiation oncologists are involved exclusively in cancer care. For all other disciplines that may be involved in care of patients with lung cancer, cancer care is only a fraction of their practice. Hence the wide variations that formalized "multidisciplinary" care can entail depending on interest, practice makeup, time commitment, perceived need of the specialty for overall care, and healthcare structure within which it is rendered. It should not come as a surprise that academic or other large provider organizations have an easier time implementing multidisciplinary care models, while community-based providers have a much harder time. Thus, most criticism and questioning of part or all of the multidisciplinary goals stem from community providers who render 70% of lung cancer care in the USA [23, 24]. This discussion is not helped by the fact that there is a lack of detailed guidance of what multidisciplinary care at various levels should look like, although it is a mandate in many countries.

The Serial Referral Model

This is the traditional system that is well established, particularly in the USA. The patient is seen by a general practitioner (not necessarily a physician) and has imaging ordered for various reasons. The report is returned as abnormal and he/she then refers the patient to a specialist. Subsequently, a series of referrals occur until a diagnosis is established, leading to a new series of referrals if cancer is found. There are numerous reasons this model is suboptimal including (but not limited to) long waiting times between appointments, easy deviation and lack of continuity for practitioners who work in isolation, less adherence to guidelines, increased costs, and less use of allied health professionals where feasible. So why is this model still in existence? The major advantage from a provider's perspective is that at any given time it is clear who is in charge. Responsibility for the patient is handed off from practitioner to practitioner, and billing episodes can easily be captured with ICD codes. This model is far from ideal from a patient's perspective where authorizations from his/her insurance must be obtained for every step, copayments must be rendered for every visit, and results must be obtained individually from every specialist involved. From a "system" perspective, however, this structure is still better than an "integrated" model where the patient does not know who is in charge, appointments are not coordinated, and bills may be difficult to reconcile.

The Joint Practice Model

The fundamental thought governing this model is that the patient, when he/she comes to clinic, remains in a single location and that multiple disciplines have patient interactions in a coordinated fashion: one stop shopping [25]. From a patient's perspective, this model is optimal and has been recognized by many professional organizations as the goal of lung cancer care [26]. Setting up such a clinic is a logistical challenge as the patient's needs change as he/she goes from diagnosis to treatment to surveillance. How does a clinic day like that look? Who sees the patient first? Perhaps a care coordinator who becomes the patient's advocate and at the end summarizes and condenses what happened that day, or the oncologist because it is likely an advanced stage cancer, or anyone who has time to see the patient because that is what is most efficient for the clinic and the physicians? What about in the next room and who starts there? How many care coordinators are required? Is coordination/sequence desirable or important, i.e., is the patient more or less confused, more or less satisfied with such an approach? How does such a clinic look behind the scenes: are all providers made familiar with the case beforehand, or when? Does a debriefing after clinic take place as a conference, as a written summary, led by whom? This model is very difficult to implement, and its success relies on strong coordination, typically by a group of allied health professionals, nurse practitioners, and/or cancer nurse specialists and a team of physicians who submit to the coordination protocols. Another challenging (behind the scenes) issue is billing. For systems that employ all providers, a solution to this is easier than for systems where different departments bill separately or for individual practices. To this date lung cancer care is not bundled, and there are strong objections to its implementation in a RVU-driven environment.

The Hub, Joint Decision-Making Model

This model is based on joint decision-making hubs where all participants and stakeholders come together to develop a patient focused plan using guidelines and best practices. There are several variations each with a slightly different focus in the application of this model. These "hubs" are sometimes referred to as tumor boards, multidisciplinary team (MDT) case reviews, MDT cancer conferences, etc. The goal of all these "hubs" is to facilitate a dialogue and subsequent ongoing collaboration to arrive at an evidence-based treatment plan for the patient and provide feedback on outcomes [27]. These hubs can serve many purposes: They can consist of a conference where all new cases are presented with the goal of establishing the most expeditious way to reach a diagnosis. The next purpose would be to determine the best means of treatment for a given patient based on guidelines and individual comorbidities. A third purpose is a quality control check if the patient is responding to the treatment prescribed and, if not, to evaluate if modifications to the treatment plan need to be made, and whether long-term surveillance requires new interventions. All of these aspects can be addressed during separate conferences which do not necessarily have to take place with equal frequency or can be combined to minimize the number of meetings. While the frequency and structure of these interdisciplinary discussions differ somewhat, the consensus from the literature is that they all contribute to a modern high-quality approach to lung cancer care [28].

Figure 12.1 illustrates various models of multidisciplinary care for patients with lung cancer.

Challenges

The recruitment of interested physicians appears easier among medical providers belonging to an organization/healthcare system. Private practitioners looking for maximum efficiency and reimbursement opportunities may be less inclined to participate in a system that is designed to optimize the patient's (and not the physician's) experience. Often private practice specialists are necessary for the care of these patients and hence pose organizational challenges. The assembled team needs to commit to regular meetings and to referring prospective patients to multidisciplinary discussions. Service duties, night coverage, Operating times, etc. all can significantly impact MDT conference attendance and MDT clinic attendance. These competing responsibilities have resulted in poor MDT attendance which subsequently leads to insufficient case preparation and inadequate clinical information, as well as unequal contribution to MDT discussions. This vicious cycle has been shown to negatively impact quality of care [29, 30]. Poor leadership, insufficient teamwork, and time pressures are recognized barriers to the effective operation of successful MDTs. Ideally, an established physician (from any specialty of the team) is named MDT chair. In addition to providing clinical expertise, the chair should assume the role of ensuring diversity, equal expression of all opinions, and a culture of respect and collaboration. The program should also include an MDT lead who can be the same person as the chair though this is not required. An advanced practice nurse with excellent organizational skills is often a good selection for the lead position to keep the meeting on track, document the proceedings, make the necessary appointments, and assure that the information is transmitted in an understandable form to the patient. Since communication is the cornerstone of success, some programs in Europe have introduced an entire curriculum in thoracic oncology to impart the skills required to share information effectively and ensure standardization of multidisciplinary thoracic oncology care practices. Graduates of these programs, regardless of their specialty background, are taught how to properly lead an MDT [31].

To optimize benefit, it is advisable to establish and agree upon standard operating procedures for all team members. This can be a challenge as members may have different perceptions of their role. Particular attention is needed to address the question of who is legally responsible for the patient's care and who will guide/interface with the patient and the referring physician. These questions should be answered from the start and documented to avoid any issues that could potentially arise. To that end, dedicated communication skills training has been advocated.

Among many things we have learned from the COVID-19 pandemic is that being in one room is no longer a prerequisite for a meeting. Although from a team bonding perspective, direct human interactions appear preferable, it has actually been shown that attendance at virtual MDT meetings is higher than in-person meetings. Reliance on technology can be a challenge when setting up an MDT conference as the quality of discussion is highly impacted by the information technology quality, especially with team members calling in. These aspects are multiplied in an MDT clinic where multiple specialties depend on access to imaging, electronic medical records, and lab data.

Organizational challenges are often a primary hurdle that may hamper the implementation of an MDT program. As a first step, financial questions must be addressed. Hospital administration needs to be convinced of the program's value with a compelling business plan, typically involving the preparation of a market share analysis of the of the lung cancer multidisciplinary program. Current data, including historic and current institutional clinic volumes, procedures, and operations should be listed. Estimates of growth of these metrics with respect to hospital operating margins as well as upfront costs, anticipated revenue, and marketing strategies are likewise encouraged. The next step is to get commitments from participating physicians as well as their clinical supervisors. This is particularly important if an MDT clinic (and not just a conference) is being planned. The clinic and conference require participation of at least one member of each specialty, taking into account vacations, service and call obligations, etc. This may require negotiations with division chiefs and administration regarding hours and compensation. A multidisciplinary clinic and conference require resources from all stakeholders and should be negotiated early. The use of conference rooms with available technology where imaging and pathology slides can be displayed are a minimum requirement. Most experts on the subject highly recommend hiring a full-time multidisciplinary clinic coordinator who serves as a dedicated and consistent point of contact for in-house and outside referrals. This person additionally serves as a liaison for referring physicians and for patients and families. Given the multiple responsibilities of this role, a program may require more than one coordinator for this position. It is important that this person(s) is dedicated to the clinic and not to individual services. A primary responsibility of the coordinator is to create and monitor the clinic's schedule/flow, and therefore institutional commitment is necessary for these key personnel. MDT coordinators command competitive salaries and cannot be framed as individual cost-centers. Advanced practice providers such as nurse practitioners, for example, with excellent communication skills, are particularly well suited for these positions.

After hiring the program coordinator, a plan to specify scheduling logistics is imperative. Prior established clinic times, conference schedules, individual team member clinic times, and available space all need to be taken into consideration. Conflicts have to be acknowledged and handled promptly. All members and their supervisors have to be willing to compromise since not every team member can expect to see patients without interruption all day, and their supervisors cannot expect uninterrupted RVU production. Space holders for urgent and unforeseen cases are necessary. This likely will require negotiations with the institutional administration. An experienced coordinator can alleviate many of these stresses by being able to foresee what team members are necessary on the basis of his/her knowledge of the case and plan accordingly. This requires a meeting with the schedulers and constant communication with the front desk. The earlier a clinic schedule can be made, the happier team members tend to be [32].

Further, thought should be given for the allotment of time and space to support services such as social work, tobacco cessation treatment, financial counseling, registered dietician consults, genetic counseling, palliative care, pre-op testing, and family/patient education. These supporting disciplines may be offered as "on-call" options, as needed.

With a strong financial business plan describing an anticipated increased revenue stream, an institution may be willing to consider the establishment of a multidisciplinary lung cancer clinic. This comes at a considerable up-front investment, however. Thus, it is imperative that the revenue stream and justification be simplified as much as possible.

In many organizations/institutions, team members are affiliated with different departments, each with its own billing structure, authorization requirements, need for co-payment, participation in different insurance plans, etc. This may pose challenges regarding how billing and payments are handled. From a patient's perspective, having to return to the front desk after each physician encounter for another co-payment and re-registration with re-entry of the same information into yet another billing system is not desirable. From an institutional perspective, this is a challenging issue that even long-established cancer centers have difficulties with because to date there exist no pathways for bundled cancer care and certainly not for lung cancer care.

Pilot projects, particularly in ENT with demonstration of feasibility, but otherwise equivocal results have been described [33]. Since issues related to complicated billing and insurance structures are known to negatively impact patient satisfaction, the program should address these matters before the first clinic day and at regular intervals (weekly) thereafter. These details deserve the attention of a senior administrator who can adjudicate the various interests of stakeholders and oversee the financial health of such a clinic. Solutions to these issues are scarce; however, there are publications describing overall savings of a multidisciplinary approach for lung cancer. For example, Voong et al. describe a 23% ($5839) savings in the pretreatment diagnostic phase alone with a multidisciplinary lung cancer clinic approach at John Hopkins [34]. In another US publication, a comparison between patients who were presented at an MDT conference versus not in a propensity matched population revealed a savings of $3001 per case in the MDT group which was statistically significant ($p < 0.0001$) [35].

Systems with a national payer have an easier time calculating overall cost savings of a multidisciplinary lung cancer clinic. For instance, a Canadian study of 428 patients (78 traditional vs. 350 MDT patients) over a 22-month period showed savings of CAD 48,389, including CAD 24,167 direct out-of-pocket patient expenses

[36]. Studies from England and the Netherlands show a similar trend [37]. The dilemma is that MDT clinics are expensive and add >$500 per case. That expense is carried by the provider, while the overall healthcare system saves [38].

It is easy to put together on paper a list of team members for an MDT conference: Many publications advocate for a pulmonologist and /or an interventional pulmonologist, thoracic oncologist, pathologist, dedicated chest radiologist, nuclear medicine physician, radiation oncologist, and thoracic surgeon and increasingly a palliative care physician to be regular attendees. They are complimented by a coordinator, allied health providers, and administrative specialists. From a practical perspective, a case can be divided into three phases: diagnostic phase, treatment phase, and surveillance phase. Each one of these phases requires input from different specialties. While in healthcare systems, predominantly in Europe, with dominant public payers, the flow and particularly the entry point are easily regulated; this is not the case in the USA. The pulmonologist is not the sole entry point: Thoracic surgery, interventional pulmonology, radiation oncology, or oncology can all be entry points for new patients. Presumably all patients need a diagnosis first, with the gold standard being a tissue diagnosis, followed by preliminary staging. The diagnostic phase is likely the most time-consuming aspect. If during this period of uncertainty for the patient additional angst is created by not knowing who is in charge of this phase, the result is an unhappy patient. The patient has to have the impression that he/she has a navigator in the system advocating for an expeditious optimal workup and who provides personal feedback of results and plans. A patient portal on the EMR is helpful but insufficient for that purpose. Again, who this person is to the patient and who is legally responsible for the patient, two separate items, need to be clarified from the beginning and documented during the MDT conference. The initial team composition may now change as the patient enters the next phase: treatment. The oncologist, radiation oncologist, or the thoracic surgeon or a combination may now be the dominant team members which should be clearly communicated to the patient. The case may likely have to be represented at MDT conference, and the change in the team should be documented and communicated to the patient. Finally, the surveillance phase has recommendations in the cancer guidelines but is often erratically handled as it is most of the time carried out by the dominant treating specialty. Each specialty and their professional organizations have different guidelines and often the patient is discharged from an MDT clinic into the care of a general practitioner. It has repeatedly been shown that long-term survival and adherence to national cancer guidelines seem better for patients who remain cared for by an MDT clinic.

Multidisciplinary Lung Cancer Care: Are There Knowledge Gaps?

Existing cancer policy and national plans make it clear that multidisciplinary care as concept is here to stay with a minimal requirement of an MDT conference. While there are everyday additions to the number of publications in favor of multidisciplinary care, a smaller but not less thoughtful number of publications asks for a critical examination of that groundswell of enthusiasm [24]. Publications on the subject often use the term "multidisciplinary care" interchangeably for MDT meetings and MDT clinics. The terms are often used without providing a definition and distinguishing features of the programs [39]. This suggests that the data to base decisions on is suboptimal. While it is difficult to argue with the theoretical and potential benefits of a multidisciplinary lung cancer care model, its real-world implementation, even in well-resourced countries, remains low. Identification of overt and covert barriers which vary in different care environments is essential for success. Most publications about multidisciplinary lung cancer care originate from academic centers; however, more than 70% of lung cancers are treated outside of such institutions in the USA [23], and the reports from those centers [40] show inconsistent high-quality evidence of benefit. Many existing reports looking at the benefit of MDT care are either retrospective, single institutional, containing non-contemporaneously collected data or no comparison group at all. They describe timeliness of care delivery, use of certain therapies but lack precise description of the "multidisciplinary" care provided. Conclusions range from no benefit to great benefit. It has been said that multidisciplinary care models disrupt established practice patterns, physician interactions, referral patterns, and infrastructure of care. Physician autonomy is challenged when a system with mutual performance monitoring is introduced where none existet. In addition, demand for manpower and infrastructure without overcoming fundamental issues of scarcity of highly specialized providers and personnel, presents a challenge, especially in post-pandemic times. Pulmonologists make more money in ICU care, not in outpatient clinics; oncologists make money administering chemotherapy, while surgeons want to operate and not spend hours in conferences or clinics. Pathologists and radiologists derive little benefit from in-person clinical interactions. The point of this harsh assessment is to demonstrate the absence of data on the true cost of MDT care (let's just start with one MDT conference/weekly) in a RVU-driven world. Existing cost analysis leave that aspect out and tend to concentrate on patient and overall savings [36, 41], but depending on altruism and belief seems a shaky starting point for a new program. Against this backdrop it seems reasonable to ask a few fundamental questions that may be answered differently for any given program based on specific environments, resources, populations, and size.

1. What should a multidisciplinary lung cancer care model look like in this particular circumstance? Is it a case discussion (tumor board), should it have a quality assurance function, or is a multidisciplinary clinic the goal?

2. What are the critical minimal components of a successful multidisciplinary care program? Which specialists are absolutely necessary and what is the most effective way for them to interact?
3. Which patients benefit from multidisciplinary care the most—everyone, or just those with complex cases not falling cleanly into the guidelines?
4. What are the signs of functional versus dysfunctional multidisciplinary programs?
5. How do we benchmark effective multidisciplinary programs? What do we measure?
6. What stops anyone from using the term "multidisciplinary" without delivering any tangible benefit?

Data for multidisciplinary lung cancer care is somewhat limited, so it may be worthwhile thinking about how to improve on the existing data. A randomized study is unlikely to be considered ethical in many countries where multidisciplinary care is already considered the standard of care. Team science principles of closed-loop communications, shared mental models, mutual trust, mutual performance monitoring, and backup behavior are new to medical thinking and are difficult to quantify given confounders such as socioeconomic status, geographic location, cultural factors, and access to resources. A quick answer is unlikely, and any answer will depend as much on the evolution of the healthcare industry and medical economics as on evidence-based policy decisions [42].

Where aspects of "multidisciplinary care" in lung cancer seem the least controversial is in the fact that MDT management shows good concordance with improved adherence to guidelines [43] and increased overall treatment rates [44]. Conditions for acquiring quality data on the effect of MDT care seem most promising in (state mandated) registries such as the Dutch Lung Cancer Audit. This two-decade-old registry reports on treatment and quality outcomes including participation in MDTs [45]. For example, it describes in a country with a mandatory MDT policy that 95% of patients receiving radiation and 97% of patients receiving surgery were discussed which represented an increase over time. The idea of using registries for high-quality data is not new: The Society of Thoracic Surgeons (voluntary) database on adult cardiac surgery for example has delivered high-quality data for decades which is currently being used for national policy and reimbursement decisions and has a voluntary participation in the high 90% of all US CT surgeons.

Evidence Supporting Multidisciplinary Care Teams

Reducing Delays in Diagnosis and Staging

Minimizing the time between initial symptom presentation or screening abnormality and cytologic diagnosis is vital to ensuring optimal patient outcomes [46] and, thus, is a primary goal of the MDT. Delays in diagnosis can occur between each step

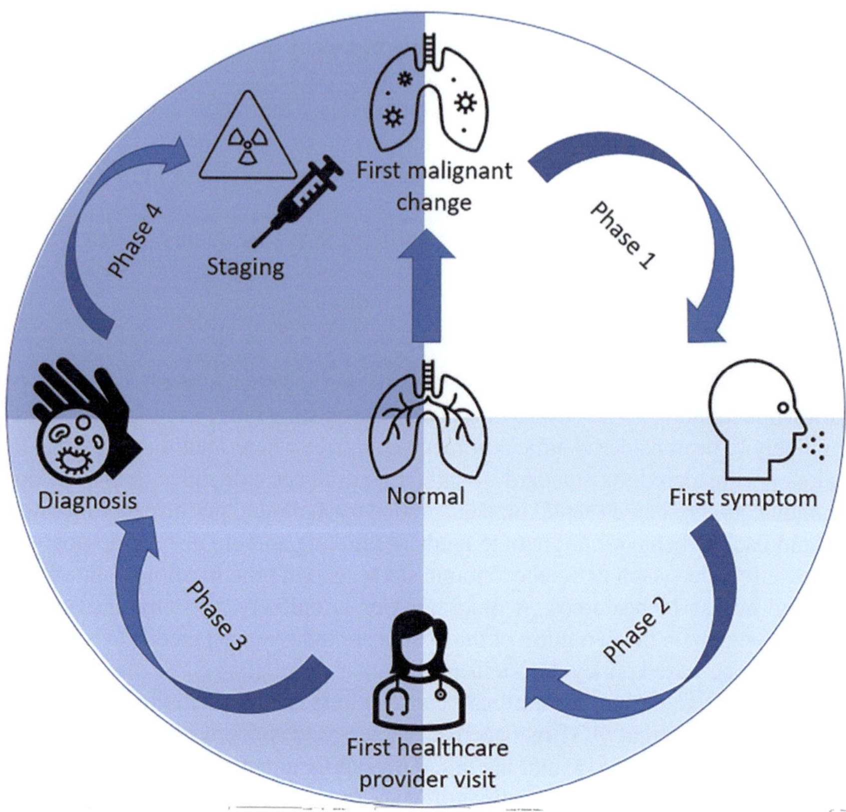

Fig. 12.2 The three main forms of multidisciplinary care. *PCP* primary care provider, *Pulm* pulmonologist, *IP* interventional pulmonology, *CT* cardiothoracic, *Rad Onc* radiation oncology, *Med Onc* medical oncology, *MDT* multidisciplinary team meeting

in the diagnostic process: from the patient's first symptomatic presentation, to their abnormal imaging result, to their referral to see a specialist, to their actual visit with the specialist, to their diagnostic test, to additional diagnostic tests, to the time they are informed of their biopsy result [47]. These timeframes have been further described as four distinct phases of care (Fig. 12.2), with phase I describing the time between the malignant change and symptom presentation, phase II describing the time between symptom presentation and first healthcare provider visit, phase III describing the time between first healthcare provider visit and diagnosis, and phase IV describing the time between diagnosis and staging [21]. Within these four phases of care, the MDT has the ability to improve phase III and phase IV [48].

Phase III and phase IV focus on diagnosis. Many patients with lung cancer face delays in care surrounding the diagnostic procedure itself including administrative, procedural, diagnostic, and staging-related issues. Administrative delays include difficulty scheduling, obtaining insurance approval, and obtaining prior authorizations. Procedural delays include the need for imaging prior to certain procedures and the need for adequate patient recovery time between staged or multiple procedures. Diagnostic delays include indeterminate cytology results due to sampling procedures that have inadequate yield, contain only normal tissue that is suggestive of the proceduralist missing the intended biopsy site, or result in cytologic atypia [49]. Finally, staging delays can occur when administrative, procedural, or diagnostic challenges occur in a staging procedure, as well as when staging itself requires a multiple procedures such as mediastinoscopy, endobronchial ultrasound-guided transbronchial needle aspiration of lymph nodes, pleural fluid aspiration, etc. [50]. The diagnostic phase may be the most multidisciplinary aspect of a lung cancer diagnosis, with challenges central to administrators, radiologists, interventional pulmonologists, thoracic surgeons, and pathologists, and thus, should be improved by the incorporation of an MDT.

A review of lung cancer staging in the multidisciplinary team setting examined just this [51] and found access to a multidisciplinary team lead to greater availability, more timely, and more accurate sampling procedures for both diagnosis and staging in patients with suspected lung cancer [51]. Patients who are discussed at an MDT meeting are also more likely to undergo mediastinoscopy and receive complete preoperative mediastinal staging [10, 43, 52]. A retrospective observational cohort study of patients treated by an MDT over a 7-year period found that patients treated by the MDT had significant reductions in the length of their phase III care when compared to the national benchmark [48]. This reduction was driven by decreases in time between positron emission tomography (PET) scan and diagnostic sampling procedures, with the MDT having a median of 13 days compared to the national benchmark of 28 days [48]. This reduction in delays in diagnosis and staging may lead to patients being diagnosed at earlier stages. A retrospective observational cohort study of a multispecialty private practice group found that implementation of an MDT resulted in an increase in the proportion of early stage (stage I or stage II) and a decrease in the proportion of late stage (stage III and stage IV) lung cancers diagnosed within the first 2 years of implementation of the MDT [53].

MDT implementation has also been associated with significant improvements in phase IV care [48]. One study found that their MDT had a median of 9 and 13 days between diagnosis and chemotherapy or radiation oncology consults, respectively, compared to the national benchmark of 24–34 days [48].

Treatment Utilization

Lung cancer treatment is rapidly evolving due to recent advances in neoadjuvant and adjuvant therapies, immunotherapy, and targeted therapies [54]. Patients with tumors that were once considered inoperable may now find themselves surgical candidates after neoadjuvant therapy [55], and patients who previously would have only followed up postoperatively with imaging and/or chemotherapy may now undergo advanced targeted adjuvant therapies [56, 57]. The role of the surgeon in caring for lung cancer patients is also rapidly evolving, as surgeons must now plan for diagnostic procedures that enable appropriate biomarker screening, plan surgeries that are minimally invasive, and allow for rapid recovery so as not to delay receipt of adjuvant therapy, and guide patient expectations in terms of the importance of receiving adjuvant therapy when appropriate [54]. It is more important than ever that surgeons be familiar with different mutations in non-small cell lung cancer as guidelines regarding which biomarkers to screen for are lacking [54]. In this setting, collaboration with other medical specialties through an MDT is paramount [58].

Patients with lung cancer who are discussed at an MDT meeting are more likely to receive treatment in general, and more likely to receive curative treatment [12, 13, 58–61]. While being discussed at an MDT meeting does not increase the odds of undergoing surgical treatment overall [43], it does increase the likelihood of receiving surgical treatment for patients with stage I and stage II non-small cell lung cancer [62, 63], as well as for patients seen at regional centers associated with tertiary care centers with thoracic surgery departments via the MDT [64], Patients discussed at an MDT meeting are also more likely to receive both palliative and curative radiation therapy than patients who are not [65]. Discussion at an MDT meeting is associated with increased utilization of chemotherapy [43, 65]; however, this increase has only been demonstrated in neoadjuvant chemotherapy [43], as opposed to adjuvant chemotherapy [66]. While it is expected that due to the complexity of immunotherapy and targeted therapy, the MDT's facilitation of collaboration between medical oncology, thoracic surgery, pathology, and even geneticists will be vital to increasing utilization of these treatment modalities [54]; research providing empirical evidence on this topic is currently lacking [58].

Patient-Reported Outcomes

There is strong quality evidence with conflicting conclusions that MDTs improve patient-reported outcomes [58, 67]. A randomized control trial of 103 patients undergoing radiation therapy with a 5-year estimated survival of less than 50% found that patients randomized to the MDT had significantly improved patient-reported quality of life compared to baseline, while patients in the control arm experienced a decline in patient reported quality of life compared to their baseline [68]. A second randomized control trial found that patients randomized to treatment by an MDT had worse quality of life compared to patients who received normal standard of care, however, was limited by the fact that a larger proportion of patients in the MDT arm were receiving chemotherapy and may have experienced more treatment-related side effect that impacted quality of life [69]. Current literature thus suggests that patients receiving care from an MDT may have worse overall quality of life compared to patients who do not receive care from an MDT secondary to receipt of more rigorous treatment, but treatment from an MDT may improve patient quality of life compared to baseline.

Improving Patient Survival

The impact of an MDT on survival in patients with lung cancer is unclear [58]. A review of the literature evaluating MDT care on patient outcomes between 2000 and 2019 identified 15 studies assessing the impact of the MDT on lung cancer survival [58]. Of these 15 studies [58], 10 found significant improvements in survival [13, 52, 60–62, 70–73], 1 found nonsignificant trends toward improvement in survival [10], and 4 found no difference in survival between patients treated by an MDT and patients who were treated in other settings [65, 66, 69, 74].

Evidence suggesting MDTs improve survival in patients with lung cancer comes largely from retrospective analyses [58]. A study of a heterogenous and robust sample of 4271 lung cancer patients diagnosed between 2002 and 2016 at a single tertiary academic center in the USA found increased survival in the 1956 patients treated by an MDT compared to the 2315 patients who were not treated by an MDT [62]. Similarly, a study of 388 non-small cell lung cancer patients with nonmetastatic disease treated between 2008 and 2014 at a single tertiary academic center in the USA found improved median survival in patients treated by an MDT [70].

While these studies highlight improvements in survival among patients with early-stage disease, MDTs have also demonstrated improved survival in patients with later-stage disease. Two studies of patients with inoperable stage III or stage IV non-small cell lung cancer found improved survival in patients treated by an MDT compared to those who were not [60, 72]. Other studies found the improvements in survival seen by MDT patients were consistent across all stages of lung cancer [11, 62] or across all stages except stage IIIB [73].

Similar patterns of improved survival occur internationally. A retrospective Australian study of 386 MDT patients and 207 non-MDT patients diagnosed with cancer between 2009 and 2012 found that presentation at an MDT meeting prior to receiving treatment resulted in decreased mortality [13]. Another Australian study of 1197 lung cancer patients found improved survival in patients treated by an MDT 1, 2, and 7 5-year post-treatment [73]. A retrospective study of 841 patients identified on a state cancer registry in Australia in 2003 found that survival was significantly improved for patients discussed at an MDT meeting and that this improvement in survival was independent of prognostic factors [61]. In Italy, a retrospective study of patients with non-small cell lung cancer managed with surgery between 2008 and 2015 found significant improvements in 1-year survival in patients seen by an MDT compared to patients treated prior to initiation of the MDT [52]. A large and more heterogenous retrospective study of 32,569 patients with newly diagnosed non-small cell lung cancer identified from a national cancer registry in Taiwan between 2005 and 2011 found improved 2-year survival in patients treated by an MDT and identified the use of an MDT as an independent predictor of survival [11].

These improvements in survival have also been demonstrated in older patient populations. A retrospective study of 542 patients aged over 70 and with non-small cell lung registered in a radiation oncology department in Southeast Scotland between 1995 and 2000 found increased 1-year survival in patients treated by an MDT compared to those who were not [71].

These studies are limited by their retrospective nature [11, 13, 52, 60–62, 70–73], homogenous sample [60, 70, 71], lack of a comparison group [70], and time effect in studies with a comparison non-MDT group treated years prior to the MDT group [11, 52, 58, 62, 71, 72, 75].

The strongest evidence against the use of MDTs improving patient survival may come from a randomized control trial that enrolled 88 patients with suspected lung cancer at 3 different clinics in the UK between 1998 and 2001 [69]. With 45 patients randomized to an MDT meeting and 43 patients to receiving conventional treatment, no significant differences were found in overall survival between these groups or in survival of a subset of patients who did go on to receive radical treatment [69]. While this study has the benefit of being a randomized control trial, it is limited by a small homogenous sample size and by a high proportion of enrolled patients who were not diagnosed with lung cancer [58, 69]. Other evidence against MDTs improving survival in patients with lung cancer include retrospective analyses of patients registered at Veterans Affairs (VA) centers [66, 74]. Both a study of 24,616 patients with small cell and non-small cell lung cancer [66] and a smaller study of 345 patients with NSCLC [74] reported no differences in survival regardless of presentation at an MDT meeting [66]. Both studies are limited by their homogenous sample, limited enrollment of women, and retrospective nature [58, 66, 74]. This pattern of results has also been demonstrated internationally, as an Australian study of patients with non-small cell lung cancer treated between 2005 and 2008 also found no significant differences in survival between patients discussed at MDT meeting and those who were not [65]. Advances in treatment options for lung cancer have changed significantly since these studies were published and results may not be directly applicable in today's landscape of lung cancer care.

More recent studies have demonstrated improvements in survival for patients treated by MDTs. A retrospective study of 9628 patients identified in the Victorian Lung Cancer Registry between 2011 and 2020 found patients discussed at an MDT meeting had a 25% lower risk of mortality compared to patients who were not presented at an MDT meeting [76]. This improvement in survival has been driven by increases in survival among patients with stage III and stage IV lung cancer. A retrospective study of patients treated at a VA center between 2013 and 2016 found the use of an MDT was independent prognostic factor in patients with stage III non-small cell lung cancer [77]. Another retrospective study of 300 patients treated at a single institution found that treatment by an MDT improved overall survival and cancer-specific survival in patients with stage III and stage IV lung cancer [78]. In the setting of the COVID-19 pandemic, MDTs may have minimized worsening survival outcomes in patients with lung cancer [79]. However, these improvements in survival associated with patients being treated by MDTs may be confounded by MDTs being offered more often at academic institutions as opposed to community centers and academic center being better equipped to offer novel treatment methods [75, 80]. Although it appears MDTs may improve survival in lung cancer, a randomized control trial of a large heterogeneous sample is needed to truly determine

MDT's impact [58, 75]. Although MDT's effect on survival in lung cancer is currently unclear, rapid advancements in immunotherapy, chemotherapy, and surgical treatment modalities may reveal greater effects on survival in the future [67].

Disparities in the Receipt of Multidisciplinary Care

Despite the aforementioned evidence in support of MDTs, not all patients have access to care from an MDT. A recent study of the Surveillance, Epidemiology and End Results (SEER) database analyzing trends in MDT prevalence in Medicare beneficiaries with surgically respectable breast, colorectal, or lung cancer over a 10-year period found that patient, surgeon, neighborhood, and healthcare organization factors significantly impede access to MDT [81]. Furthermore, patients who were Black, had comorbidities, had dual Medicare and Medicaid coverage, lived in rural areas, or lived in areas with higher proportions of black or Hispanic residents were less likely to receive care from an MDT than patients who did not have these factors [81]. Development of an MDT in under-resourced health systems, however, may not lead to the same benefits seen at more well-funded institutions. For example, in one study, the implementation of an MDT lead to improvements in diagnosis, but failed to meet goals related to time between diagnosis and treatment due to the amount of patients successfully identified to have lung cancer by the MDT overwhelming the practice's radiation oncology services [53]. Research around reducing barriers to access to MDT lung cancer care is essential to reduce these inequities and bring MDT care to underrepresented patients and under-resourced areas.

Conclusion

Multidisciplinary lung cancer care is here to stay; it is a national mandate, and in many states is part of accreditation for cancer care. "Multidisciplinary" means different things to different stakeholders. At present there is no categorization of what encompasses "multidisciplinary" care for lung cancer. In the near future, it behooves national and international cancer organizations to come up with comprehensive definitions of what constitutes different categories of multidisciplinary care in detail. In the meantime, each provider at the institutional level should define, best in writing, what multidisciplinary lung cancer care locally entails. Based on that local definition goals can be set, allowing for verification. Periodic review of outcome measures, objectives, programmatic needs, and patient and provider satisfaction is essential. At present it has to be acknowledged that data favoring multidisciplinary care is enthusiastic but not beyond scrutiny. Randomized studies to resolve this knowledge gap are not likely to take place when multidisciplinary care is standard of care. The added costs, hidden and real, and the future developments of the healthcare market, policies, and economic outlook will be as influential as is the current enthusiasm for implementation of what is thought to be a logical and good idea.

References

1. Borras JM, Albreht T, Audisio R, Briers E, Casali P, Esperou H, et al. Policy statement on multidisciplinary cancer care. Eur J Cancer. 2014;50(3):475–80.
2. Selby P, Gillis C, Haward R. Benefits from specialised cancer care. Lancet. 1996;348(9023):313–8.
3. Lawler M, Banks I, Law K, Albreht T, Armand J-P, Barbacid M, et al. The European cancer patient's bill of rights, update and implementation 2016. ESMO Open. 2016;1(6):e000127.
4. Fitzmaurice C, Allen C, Barber RM, Barregard L, Bhutta ZA, Brenner H, et al. Global, regional, and national cancer incidence, mortality, years of life lost, years lived with disability, and disability-adjusted life-years for 32 cancer groups, 1990 to 2015: a systematic analysis for the global burden of disease study. JAMA Oncol. 2017;3(4):524–48.
5. Siegel RL, Miller KD, Jemal A. Cancer statistics, 2018. CA Cancer J Clin. 2018;68(1):7–30.
6. Howington JA, Blum MG, Chang AC, Balekian AA, Murthy SC. Treatment of stage I and II non-small cell lung cancer: diagnosis and management of lung cancer: American College of Chest Physicians evidence-based clinical practice guidelines. Chest. 2013;143(5):e278S–313S.
7. Duma N, Santana-Davila R, Molina JR, editors. Non–small cell lung cancer: epidemiology, screening, diagnosis, and treatment. Mayo Clinic proceedings. Amsterdam: Elsevier; 2019.
8. Kris MG, Johnson BE, Berry LD, Kwiatkowski DJ, Iafrate AJ, Wistuba II, et al. Using multiplexed assays of oncogenic drivers in lung cancers to select targeted drugs. JAMA. 2014;311(19):1998–2006.
9. Blum TG, Rich A, Baldwin D, Beckett P, De Ruysscher D, Faivre-Finn C, et al. The European initiative for quality management in lung cancer care. Eur Respir Soc. 2014;43:1254.
10. Friedman EL, Kruklitis RJ, Patson BJ, Sopka DM, Weiss MJ. Effectiveness of a thoracic multidisciplinary clinic in the treatment of stage III non-small-cell lung cancer. J Multidiscip Healthc. 2016;9:267.
11. Pan C-C, Kung P-T, Wang Y-H, Chang Y-C, Wang S-T, Tsai W-C. Effects of multidisciplinary team care on the survival of patients with different stages of non-small cell lung cancer: a national cohort study. PLoS One. 2015;10(5):e0126547.
12. Stevens W, Stevens G, Kolbe J, Cox B. Management of stages I and II non-small-cell lung cancer in a New Zealand study: divergence from international practice and recommendations. Intern Med J. 2008;38(10):758–68.
13. Rogers MJ, Matheson L, Garrard B, Maher B, Cowdery S, Luo W, et al. Comparison of outcomes for cancer patients discussed and not discussed at a multidisciplinary meeting. Public Health. 2017;149:74–80.
14. Vinod SK, Sidhom MA, Delaney GP. Do multidisciplinary meetings follow guideline-based care? J Oncol Pract. 2010;6(6):276–81.
15. American Society of Clinical Oncology, European Society for Medical Oncology. ASCO-ESMO consensus statement on quality cancer care. Ann Oncol. 2006;17(7):1063–4.
16. Network NCCN. Non-small cell lung cancer (version 2.2023). J Natl Compr Canc Netw. 2023;21(4):340–50.
17. NIfHaC E Lung cancer: diagnosis and management. NICE Clinical Guideline 2011. Nice.org,uk/guidance/ng122/evidence/full-guideline-april2011-6722113501.
18. Australian Cancer Network Colorectal Cancer Guidelines Revision Committee. Clinical practice guidelines for the prevention, diagnosis and management of lung cancer. The Cancer Council Australia and Australian Cancer Network, National Health and Medical Research Council Canberra. 2004. Cancer.org.au/health-professionals/clinical-practice-guidelines/lung-cancer.

19. Leo F, Venissac N, Poudenx M, Otto J, Mouroux J. Multidisciplinary management of lung cancer: how to test its efficacy? J Thorac Oncol. 2007;2(1):69–72.
20. World Health Organization. Framework for action on interprofessional education & collaborative practice; 2010.
21. Moody A, Muers M, Forman D. Delays in managing lung cancer. BMJ Publishing London; 2004. p. 1–3.
22. American Cancer Society. Key statistics for lung cancer. 2019. https://www.cancer.org/cancer/lung-cancer.html.
23. Little AG, Gay EG, Gaspar LE, Stewart AK. National survey of non-small cell lung cancer in the United States: epidemiology, pathology and patterns of care. Lung Cancer. 2007;57(3):253–60.
24. Osarogiagbon RU. Making the evidentiary case for universal multidisciplinary thoracic oncologic care. Clin Lung Cancer. 2018;19(4):294–300.
25. Kedia SK, Ward KD, Digney SA, Jackson BM, Nellum AL, McHugh L, et al. 'One-stop shop': lung cancer patients' and caregivers' perceptions of multidisciplinary care in a community healthcare setting. Transl Lung Cancer Res. 2015;4(4):456.
26. Gaga M, Powell CA, Schraufnagel DE, Schönfeld N, Rabe K, Hill NS, et al. An official American Thoracic Society/European Respiratory Society statement: the role of the pulmonologist in the diagnosis and management of lung cancer. Am J Respir Crit Care Med. 2013;188(4):503–7.
27. Denton E, Conron M. Improving outcomes in lung cancer: the value of the multidisciplinary health care team. J Multidiscip Healthc. 2016;9:137.
28. Osarogiagbon RU, Phelps G, McFarlane J, Bankole O. Causes and consequences of deviation from multidisciplinary care in thoracic oncology. J Thorac Oncol. 2011;6(3):510–6.
29. Lamb BW, Sevdalis N, Arora S, Pinto A, Vincent C, Green JS. Teamwork and team decision-making at multidisciplinary cancer conferences: barriers, facilitators, and opportunities for improvement. World J Surg. 2011;35(9):1970–6.
30. Rosell L, Alexandersson N, Hagberg O, Nilbert M. Benefits, barriers and opinions on multidisciplinary team meetings: a survey in Swedish cancer care. BMC Health Serv Res. 2018;18(1):1–10.
31. Gamarra F, Noël J-L, Brunelli A, Dingemans A-MC, Felip E, Gaga M, et al. Thoracic oncology HERMES: European curriculum recommendations for training in thoracic oncology. Breathe. 2016;12(3):249–55.
32. Meguid C, Ryan CE, Edil BH, Schulick RD, Gajdos C, Boniface M, et al. Establishing a framework for building multidisciplinary programs. J Multidiscip Healthc. 2015;8:519.
33. Spinks T, Guzman A, Beadle BM, Lee S, Jones D, Walters R, et al. Development and feasibility of bundled payments for the multidisciplinary treatment of head and neck cancer: a pilot program. J Oncol Pract. 2018;14(2):e103–e12.
34. Voong KR, Liang OS, Dugan P, Torto D, Padula WV, Senter JP, et al. Thoracic oncology multidisciplinary clinic reduces unnecessary health care expenditure used in the workup of patients with non–small-cell lung cancer. Clin Lung Cancer. 2019;20(4):e430–e41.
35. Freeman RK, Ascioti AJ, Dake M, Mahidhara RS. The effects of a multidisciplinary care conference on the quality and cost of care for lung cancer patients. Ann Thorac Surg. 2015;100(5):1834–8.
36. Stone CJ, Johnson AP, Robinson D, Katyukha A, Egan R, Linton S, et al. Health resource and cost savings achieved in a multidisciplinary lung cancer clinic. Curr Oncol. 2021;28(3):1681–95.
37. van der Linden N, Bongers M, Coupé V, Smit E, Groen H, Welling A, et al. Costs of non-small cell lung cancer in The Netherlands. Lung Cancer. 2016;91:79–88.
38. Munro A. Multidisciplinary team meetings in cancer care: an idea whose time has gone? Clin Oncol. 2015;27(12):728–31.
39. Quality AfHR. Working for quality annual report; 2011. www.ahrq.gov/qual/qrdr10.htm.
40. Osarogiagbon RU, Freeman RK, Krasna MJ. Implementing effective and sustainable multidisciplinary clinical thoracic oncology programs. Transl Lung Cancer Res. 2015;4(4):448.
41. Rankin NM, Fradgley EA, Barnes DJ. Implementation of lung cancer multidisciplinary teams: a review of evidence-practice gaps. Transl Lung Cancer Res. 2020;9(4):1667.

42. Iyer NG, Chua ML. Multidisciplinary team meetings—challenges of implementation science. Nat Rev Clin Oncol. 2019;16(4):205–6.
43. Freeman RK, Van Woerkom JM, Vyverberg A, Ascioti AJ. The effect of a multidisciplinary thoracic malignancy conference on the treatment of patients with lung cancer. Eur J Cardiothorac Surg. 2010;38(1):1–5.
44. Wang J, Kuo YF, Freeman J, Goodwin JS. Increasing access to medical oncology consultation in older patients with stage II-IIIA non-small-cell lung cancer. Med Oncol. 2008;25(2):125–32.
45. Liu H, Song Y. MDT is still important in the treatment of early stage lung cancer. J Thorac Dis. 2018;10(Suppl 33):S3984.
46. Mackillop WJ. Killing time: the consequences of delays in radiotherapy. Radiother Oncol. 2007;84(1):1–4.
47. Vidaver RM, Shershneva MB, Hetzel SJ, Holden TR, Campbell TC. Typical time to treatment of patients with lung cancer in a multisite, US-based study. J Oncol Pract. 2016;12(6):e643–e53.
48. Albano D, Bilfinger T, Feraca M, Kuperberg S, Nemesure B. A multidisciplinary lung cancer program: does it reduce delay between diagnosis and treatment? Lung. 2020;198(6):967–72.
49. Albano D, Santore LA, Bilfinger T, Feraca M, Novotny S, Nemesure B. Clinical implications of "atypia" on biopsy: possible precursor to lung cancer? Curr Oncol. 2021;28(4):2516–22.
50. Liam CK, Andarini S, Lee P, Ho JCM, Chau NQ, Tscheikuna J. Lung cancer staging now and in the future. Respirology. 2015;20(4):526–34.
51. Liam C-K, Liam Y-S, Poh M-E, Wong C-K. Accuracy of lung cancer staging in the multidisciplinary team setting. Transl Lung Cancer Res. 2020;9(4):1654.
52. Tamburini N, Maniscalco P, Mazzara S, Maietti E, Santini A, Calia N, et al. Multidisciplinary management improves survival at 1 year after surgical treatment for non-small-cell lung cancer: a propensity score-matched study. Eur J Cardiothorac Surg. 2018;53(6):1199–204.
53. LeMense GP, Waller EA, Campbell C, Bowen T. Development and outcomes of a comprehensive multidisciplinary incidental lung nodule and lung cancer screening program. BMC Pulm Med. 2020;20(1):1–8.
54. Donington JS, Gitlitz B, Lim E, Opitz I, Kim YT, Altorki N. Integration of new systemic adjuvant therapies for non-small cell lung cancer: role of the surgeon. Ann Thorac Surg. 2023;115:1544.
55. Forde PM, Spicer J, Lu S, Provencio M, Mitsudomi T, Awad MM, et al. Neoadjuvant nivolumab plus chemotherapy in resectable lung cancer. N Engl J Med. 2022;386:1973.
56. Felip E, Altorki N, Zhou C, Csőszi T, Vynnychenko I, Goloborodko O, et al. Adjuvant atezolizumab after adjuvant chemotherapy in resected stage IB–IIIA non-small-cell lung cancer (IMpower010): a randomised, multicentre, open-label, phase 3 trial. Lancet. 2021;398(10308):1344–57.
57. Paz-Ares L, O'Brien M, Mauer M, Dafni U, Oselin K, Havel L, et al. VP3-2022: Pembrolizumab (pembro) versus placebo for early-stage non-small cell lung cancer (NSCLC) following complete resection and adjuvant chemotherapy (chemo) when indicated: randomized, triple-blind, phase III EORTC-1416-LCG/ETOP 8-15–PEARLS/KEYNOTE-091 study. Ann Oncol. 2022;33(4):451–3.
58. Heinke MY, Vinod SK. A review on the impact of lung cancer multidisciplinary care on patient outcomes. Transl Lung Cancer Res. 2020;9(4):1639.
59. Bjegovich-Weidman M, Haid M, Kumar S, Huibregtse C, McDonald J, Krishnan S. Establishing a community-based lung cancer multidisciplinary clinic as part of a large integrated health care system: aurora health care. J Oncol Pract. 2010;6(6):e27–30.
60. Bydder S, Nowak A, Marion K, Phillips M, Atun R. The impact of case discussion at a multidisciplinary team meeting on the treatment and survival of patients with inoperable non-small cell lung cancer. Intern Med J. 2009;39(12):838–41.
61. Mitchell PL, Thursfield VJ, Ball DL, Richardson GE, Irving LB, Torn-Broers Y, et al. Lung cancer in Victoria: are we making progress? Med J Aust. 2013;199(10):674–9.
62. Bilfinger TV, Albano D, Perwaiz M, Keresztes R, Nemesure B. Survival outcomes among lung cancer patients treated using a multidisciplinary team approach. Clin Lung Cancer. 2018;19(4):346–51.

63. Kehl KL, Landrum MB, Kahn KL, Gray SW, Chen AB, Keating NL. Tumor board participation among physicians caring for patients with lung or colorectal cancer. J Oncol Pract. 2015;11(3):e267–e78.
64. Davison A, Eraut C, Haque A, Doffman S, Tanqueray A, Trask C, et al. Telemedicine for multidisciplinary lung cancer meetings. J Telemed Telecare. 2004;10(3):140–3.
65. Boxer MM, Vinod SK, Shafiq J, Duggan KJ. Do multidisciplinary team meetings make a difference in the management of lung cancer? Cancer. 2011;117(22):5112–20.
66. Keating NL, Landrum MB, Lamont EB, Bozeman SR, Shulman LN, McNeil BJ. Tumor boards and the quality of cancer care. J Natl Cancer Inst. 2013;105(2):113–21.
67. Batra U, Munshi A, Kabra V, Momi G. Relevance of multi-disciplinary team approach in diagnosis and management of Stage III NSCLC. Indian J Cancer. 2022;59(Suppl 1):S46.
68. Rummans TA, Clark MM, Sloan JA, Frost MH, Bostwick JM, Atherton PJ, et al. Impacting quality of life for patients with advanced cancer with a structured multidisciplinary intervention: a randomized controlled trial. J Clin Oncol. 2006;24(4):635–42.
69. Murray P, O'Brien M, Sayer R, Cooke N, Knowles G, Miller A, et al. The pathway study: results of a pilot feasibility study in patients suspected of having lung carcinoma investigated in a conventional chest clinic setting compared to a centralised two-stop pathway. Lung Cancer. 2003;42(3):283–90.
70. Senter J, Hooker C, Lang M, Voong K, Hales R. Thoracic multidisciplinary clinic improves survival in patients with lung cancer. Int J Radiat Oncol Biol Phys. 2016;96(2):S134.
71. Price A, Kerr G, Gregor A, Ironside J, Little F. The impact of multidisciplinary teams and site specialisation on the use of radiotherapy in elderly people with non-small cell lung cancer (NSCLC). Radiother Oncol. 2002;64(Suppl 1):80.
72. Forrest L, McMillan D, McArdle C, Dunlop D. An evaluation of the impact of a multidisciplinary team, in a single centre, on treatment and survival in patients with inoperable non-small-cell lung cancer. Br J Cancer. 2005;93(9):977–8.
73. Stone E, Rankin N, Kerr S, Fong K, Currow DC, Phillips J, et al. Does presentation at multidisciplinary team meetings improve lung cancer survival? Findings from a consecutive cohort study. Lung Cancer. 2018;124:199–204.
74. Riedel RF, Wang X, McCormack M, Toloza E, Montana GS, Schreiber G, et al. Impact of a multidisciplinary thoracic oncology clinic on the timeliness of care. J Thorac Oncol. 2006;1(7):692–6.
75. Bertolaccini L, Mohamed S, Bardoni C, Lo Iacono G, Mazzella A, Guarize J, et al. The Interdisciplinary Management of Lung Cancer in the European community. J Clin Med. 2022;11(15):4326.
76. Lin T, Pham J, Paul E, Conron M, Wright G, Ball D, et al. Impacts of lung cancer multidisciplinary meeting presentation: drivers and outcomes from a population registry retrospective cohort study. Lung Cancer. 2022;163:69–76.
77. Hung H-Y, Tseng Y-H, Chao H-S, Chiu C-H, Hsu W-H, Hsu H-S, et al. Multidisciplinary team discussion results in survival benefit for patients with stage III non-small-cell lung cancer. PLoS One. 2020;15(10):e0236503.
78. Gaudioso C, Sykes A, Whalen PE, Attwood KM, Masika MM, Demmy TL, et al. Impact of a thoracic multidisciplinary conference on lung cancer outcomes. Ann Thorac Surg. 2022;113(2):392–8.
79. Round T, L'Esperance V, Bayly J, Brain K, Dallas L, Edwards JG, et al. COVID-19 and the multidisciplinary care of patients with lung cancer: an evidence-based review and commentary. Br J Cancer. 2021;125(5):629–40.
80. Popat S, Navani N, Kerr KM, Smit EF, Batchelor TJP, Van Schil P, et al. Navigating diagnostic and treatment decisions in non-small cell lung cancer: expert commentary on the multidisciplinary team approach. Oncologist. 2020;26(2):e306–e15.
81. Sanchez JI, Doose M, Zeruto C, Chollette V, Gasca N, Verhoeven D, et al. Multilevel factors associated with inequities in multidisciplinary cancer consultation. Health Serv Res. 2022;57:222.

Chapter 13
Physiologic and Patient-Centered Considerations in Lung Cancer Care

Duc M. Ha

Introduction

The goals of lung cancer treatment are to achieve a cure where possible and/or control tumor burden, improve symptoms, and enhance health-related quality of life (HRQL), depending on the stage of disease, patients' fitness to tolerate the recommended therapies, and their personal values and preferences [1]. Curative intent therapy of lung cancer usually includes surgical treatment, with anatomic lung resection (e.g., lobectomy) being the guideline-recommended approach for appropriately selected patients [2]. However, surgical treatment is accompanied by a risk of perioperative morbidity and mortality, with 1–5% of patients having major complications including death [3]. This mortality risk can be even higher (e.g., 10–15%) depending on the patients' fitness, surgical approach, extent of resection, surgical expertise, hospital volume, and other factors [2, 4, 5]. In addition, following lobectomy, patients typically lose 10–15% of lung function (i.e., forced expiratory volume in 1 s, FEV_1; diffusion capacity of the lungs for carbon monoxide, DL_{CO}) [6, 7] or 3% per segment of lung resected [8], which can contribute to gas-exchange and other physiologic impairments. Also, many patients experience increased dyspnea and symptom burden, decrements in functional exercise capacity, and/or decreased HRQL [9–12]. Therefore, there is a need for risk assessment to weigh the probabilities of harms against benefits in the management of patients with lung cancer being considered for curative intent therapy [13, 14].

The primary goal of the physiologic evaluation of patients with lung cancer being considered for surgical treatment is to identify those with increased risk for

D. M. Ha (✉)
Section of Pulmonary and Critical Care, Rocky Mountain Regional Veterans
Affairs Medical Center, Aurora, CO, USA

Division of Pulmonary Sciences and Critical Care Medicine, University of Colorado
Anschutz Medical Campus, Aurora, CO, USA
e-mail: duc.ha@va.gov; duc.ha@cuanschutz.edu

C. MacRosty, M. P. Rivera (eds.), *Lung Cancer*, Respiratory Medicine,
https://doi.org/10.1007/978-3-031-38412-7_13

277

perioperative complications and long-term disability using the least invasive tests possible, the results of which are used in informed decision-making and patient counseling regarding the treatment options and their associated risks [13]. In addition, identifying patients with an elevated surgical risk provides an opportunity for interventions to reduce the risk of perioperative complications and long-term disability associated with treatment [13]. This chapter will summarize the physiological bases and supporting evidence for these evaluations. In addition, it will discuss other (physiologic and non-physiologic) measures and considerations that may guide decision-making for clinicians caring for patients with lung cancer being considered for curative intent therapy.

Pulmonary Function Testing

The physiologic evaluation of patients with lung cancer being considered for curative intent therapy starts with pulmonary function testing to measure forced expiratory volume in 1 second (FEV_1) and diffusion capacity of the lungs for carbon monoxide (DL_{CO}). Reduced FEV_1 and DL_{CO} have been associated with increased respiratory morbidity and mortality among patients undergoing lung cancer resection surgery [15, 16], including in those undergoing open thoracotomy [17], video-assisted [18], and robotically assisted thoracoscopic surgery [19]. While the thresholds used to determine risk can vary, a preoperative FEV_1 of <60% predicted has been associated with perioperative mortality and respiratory morbidity [20], with approximately 20% of patients experiencing adverse respiratory outcomes [17]. In addition, a reduced DL_{CO} is an important predictor of surgical outcomes—approximately 40% of patients with preoperative $DL_{CO} < 60\%$ can have perioperative respiratory morbidity [21]. This morbidity risk also exists in patients without spirometric airflow limitation [22, 23].

The predicted postoperative lung function ($ppoFEV_1$ and $ppoDL_{CO}$) is considered more useful than the measured values because it accounts for the quantity of lung tissue that would be resected. The $ppoFEV_1$ and $ppoDL_{CO}$ values can be calculated using the anatomic or perfusion method. In the anatomic method, the ppo values are calculated as a fraction of the number of segments that would be removed with the planned surgery [8]:

$$ppoFEV_1 \left(or\ ppoDL_{CO} \right) = preoperative\ FEV_1 \left(or\ DL_{CO} \right) predicted$$
$$\times \left(1 - planned\ number\ of\ lung\ segments\ to\ be\ resected \div 19 \right)$$

For instance, in a patient with preoperative FEV_1 70% predicted being considered for right upper lobectomy, the $ppoFEV_1$ would equal 70% × (1 − 3 ÷ 19), or 59%.

A limitation of the anatomic approach is the underlying assumption that all lung segments participate in gas-exchange equally, which may be highly inaccurate in some patients (e.g., in those with significant bullous emphysema). The perfusion method uses quantitative radionuclide perfusion scanning to evaluate perfusion in the lung that would be resected to more accurately calculate the ppo values. This method is also known as a split-function study. In this method, the ppo values are calculated as a fraction of perfused lung that would be removed [24]:

$$\mathrm{ppoFEV_1\left(or\,ppoDL_{CO}\right)=preoperative\,FEV_1\left(or\,DL_{CO}\right)predicted}$$
$$\times\left(1-\mathrm{fraction\ of\ perfusion\ for\ the\ lung\ planned\ to\ be\ resected}\right)$$

For instance, for a patient with preoperative FEV_1 70% predicted being considered for right pneumonectomy and quantitative radionuclide perfusion demonstrating 60% perfusion on the right lung, the $ppoFEV_1$ would equal 70% × (1 − 0.60), or 28%. The anatomic method is usually recommended for patients being considered for lobectomy and the perfusion method for those being considered for pneumonectomy [13].

Exercise Testing

Cardiopulmonary Exercise Testing

In patients with impaired lung function, exercise testing to evaluate functional or peak exercise capacity can better delineate surgical risk. In exercising individuals, the physiologic responses to meet the metabolic demands of contracting skeletal muscles include changes in ventilation, cardiac output, pulmonary, and systemic blood flow, with a goal to ultimately preserve cellular oxygenation and acid-base homeostasis. Assessment of exercise capacity traditionally relies on cardiopulmonary exercise testing (CPET) to measure oxygen consumption (VO_2), reflecting the body's ability to take in, transport, and use oxygen to produce adenosine triphosphate during exercise. In healthy individuals, VO_2 increases with increasing exercise intensity and reaches a plateau, at which point increasing exercise intensity no longer leads to increased VO_2 due to the limited oxidative capacity of skeletal muscles and/or cardiac output (maximal VO_2, or VO_{2max}). A normal VO_{2max} usually excludes significant pulmonary, cardiovascular, hematologic, neuropsychological, and skeletal muscle disease. Therefore, VO_{2max} is often regarded as the accepted standard measure of cardiopulmonary fitness. In individuals who do not reach VO_{2max} during CPET, typically due to prohibitive symptoms, the term VO_{2peak} is often used to indicate the highest VO_2 reached.

In patients with lung cancer, VO_2 may be low due to the effects of advanced age, comorbid cardiopulmonary or other conditions, and/or cancer. Among the largest studies, the cancer and leukemia group B performed a prospective, multi-institutional study to investigate the use of VO_{2peak} in predicting surgical risk among patients with known or suspected resectable non-small cell lung cancer (NSCLC) [25]. This study used an algorithmic approach in which patients with $ppoFEV_1$ < 33% underwent

CPET and found that, among 346 participants, those with VO_{2peak} < 15 ml/min/kg (or <65% predicted) were more likely to experience a poor surgical outcome of respiratory failure or death [25]. A systematic review of 14 studies including 955 patients also showed that preoperative VO_{2max} was lower (by an average of 3 ml/kg/min, or 8% predicted) among those who developed clinically relevant complications after curative lung resection [26]. Consequently, the measurement of VO_2 is recommended by the American College of Chest Physicians (ACCP) [13], British Thoracic Society (BTS) [27], and European Respiratory Society/European Society of Thoracic Surgery (ERS/ESTS) [28] clinical practice guidelines for patients with impaired lung function being considered for lung cancer resection surgery [29]. Differences in recommendations vary between societies and are discussed later in this chapter.

Simple Field Exercise Tests

Despite its predictive usefulness however, VO_2 measurement with CPET requires a high degree of equipment and technological expertise, with often complex interpretation strategies [30]. Further, many lung cancer patients are not able to perform CPET due to significant comorbidities. For instance, one study identified that approximately 20% of patients undergoing evaluation for lung cancer resection surgery are unable to perform CPET due to musculoskeletal disease, neurologic impairment, peripheral vascular disease, or psychiatric illness [31]. As such, low-technology and simple field exercise tests have been used to complement CPET [29]. These simple field exercise tests include the stair climbing test (SCT), incremental shuttle walk test (ISWT), and 6-minute walk test (6MWT).

A study of 640 lung cancer patients undergoing lobectomy or pneumonectomy identified that those who climbed to SCT heights <12 m, compared to those who climbed >22 m, had 2.5- and 13-fold higher odds of having perioperative cardiopulmonary complications and mortality, respectively [32]. The SCT height has also been shown to correlate well ($r = 0.70$) with VO_{2peak}, with SCT height >22 m having a positive predictive value of 86% for VO_{2peak} > 15 ml/kg/min [33]. A systematic review of six studies also showed that while there were high variations in the cutoffs of SCT height used (range 2.4–12.0 m), a pooled height of <10 m was associated with 2.3-fold increased odds of postoperative morbidity following lung cancer resection surgery, with positive and negative predictive values 62% and 75%, respectively [34]. Indeed, the height reached during the SCT is recommended by the ACCP to risk stratify patients being considered for lung cancer resection surgery [13]. However, a significant limitation of the SCT is the absence of standardization, including of test duration, instructions for speed of ascend, number of steps per flight, height per step, and test termination criteria [13].

The ISWT and 6MWT are simple field exercise tests with established standards for performance and interpretation in patients with chronic lung disease [35–37]. In the ISWT, patients are instructed to walk back and forth between two cones set 9 m apart, with increasing speed externally paced by a series of pre-recorded auditory signals [36]. The test terminates when patients indicate not being able to continue (e.g., due to exhaustion) or by the assessor (e.g., deemed unfit or unsafe to continue) or until the maximum test duration of 20 min is reached [36]. The primary measure is total distance walked [37]. In a study of 125 patients with potentially operable lung cancer, the ISWT distance was found to correlate moderately well ($r = 0.67$) with VO_{2peak}, with all 55 of those who achieved ISWT distance >400 m having $VO_{2peak} \geq 15$ ml/kg/min [38]. A retrospective study of 101 patients undergoing lung cancer resection surgery identified that ISWT distance cutoffs of <400 m and <250 m were associated with 3.0- and 2.5-fold increased odds of postoperative cardiopulmonary complications in univariable analyses, respectively, with ISWT distance <400 m (but not <250 m) being associated with a 4.3-fold increased odds of postoperative cardiopulmonary complications in multivariable analyses [39]. A systemic review identified three studies involving 236 patients found that while this one study described an association between the ISWT distance and perioperative complications, the other two studies found no association [40]. Albeit, given the degree of correlation between the ISWT distance and VO_2, the ISWT is recommended by the ACCP [13] and BTS [27] to risk stratify patients being considered for lung cancer resection surgery.

The 6MWT is a self-paced test in which patients are instructed to walk as far as possible, back and forth along a flat 30-m corridor, for 6 min [35]. The test terminates after 6 min or if patients are unable to continue (e.g., due to symptoms or safety concerns). The primary measure is distance walked. In patients with lung cancer, 2 systematic reviews identified 6 studies involving 681 patients, all of which showed associations between the 6MWT distance (or % predicted) and perioperative morbidity or mortality following lung cancer resection surgery [29, 40]. In addition, three studies by other investigators involving 1,100 patients showed similar findings [41–43]. Except for one older study, all more recent studies used 6MWT distance thresholds <400–500 m to indicate elevated surgical risk, with no study reporting additional exercise testing used beyond the 6MWT to determine risk and treatment selection [41–47]. The perioperative mortality rates for all these studies were <1% [41–47].

Among the prospective observational studies, 1 enrolled 416 participants undergoing lobectomy and identified that, among those with moderately reduced ppo lung function (i.e., $ppoFEV_1$ or $ppoDL_{CO} < 60\%$ and both >30%), participants with 6MWT distance <400 m, compared to $\geq$400 m, had approximately eightfold increased odds of having cardiopulmonary complications; however only a small number of 14 participants were allocated to this "moderate-risk and short-distance" group, with perioperative mortality <1% and not analyzed separately [42]. Another similar prospective cohort study of 224 participants also identified that those with 6MWT distance <400 m, compared to $\geq$400 m, had 2.4-fold increased hazards of death at 5 years following lobectomy; however, this threshold did not provide additional prognostic value beyond the Eastern Cooperative Oncology Group performance status [44].

Physiologically, due to its self-paced nature, the 6MWT is traditionally considered a sub-maximal test and used to measure functional capacity [35]. A study of 20 patients with stage I–IIIB lung cancer, 35% of whom had comorbid chronic obstructive pulmonary disease (COPD), identified that the 6MWT distance correlated poorly ($r = 0.24$) with VO_{2peak} [48]. However, in patients with chronic lung disease, performance on the 6MWT is known to elicit a VO_{2peak} response similar to that during CPET [36], with the 6MWT distance demonstrating high correlation ($r = 0.59$–0.93) with VO_{2peak} [37]. As such, the European Respiratory Society/American Thoracic Society supports the use of the 6MWT to test functional exercise capacity of patients with chronic lung disease (e.g., those with impaired lung function) [36, 37]. Given that simple field exercise tests are typically indicated in patients with impaired FEV_1 and DL_{CO} and ppo values, the 6MWT distance has both construct and predictive validity in the physiologic evaluation of patients being considered for lung cancer resection surgery. In addition, another study of 62 patients with lung cancer following curative intent therapy identified that the 6MWT distance correlated moderately well ($r = 0.45$) with HRQL [49], supporting its use to assess and predict other outcomes following curative lung resection.

Additional Physiologic and Other Measures

Adjunct Physiologic Measures

In addition to measuring or estimating VO_2, exercise testing can elicit other physiologic responses that can be used to predict perioperative outcomes in patients undergoing lung cancer resection surgery [29]. For instance, the relationship between minute ventilation (VE) and carbon dioxide production (VCO_2) obtained up to peak exercise intensity during CPET, expressed as a linear regression line (ventilatory efficiency slope), has been shown to be associated with perioperative outcomes [50]. A VE/VCO_2 slope > 35 has been associated with 3- and 12-fold increased odds of respiratory complications and mortality, respectively [51]. In addition, oxygen desaturation (>4% decrease during the SCT) has been shown to be associated a twofold increased odds of perioperative respiratory complications [52]. Impaired heart rate recovery (≤ 12 beats/min following the 6MWT)—a measure thought to reflect impaired parasympathetic nervous system function [53]—has been shown to be associated with a five-fold increased odds of perioperative cardiopulmonary complications following lung cancer resection surgery [54]. However, the use of these adjunct physiologic measures to guide clinical decision making is not well-established [13, 29].

Other Measures

In addition to pulmonary function and exercise testing, other measures can be used to predict perioperative outcomes. A state of increased vulnerability to stressors is referred to as frailty, conceptualized as "physical" (and manifested by muscle weakness, low energy level, slowed motor performance, low physical activity, and unintentional weight loss [55]) or "cumulative deficit" (resulting from an accumulation of medical conditions, functional, psychological, cognitive declines, and nonspecific health issues that include poor nutrition, over time [56, 57]). A study of the US National Inpatient Sample database identified that frailty, assessed by ICD-9 diagnoses clustered around malnutrition or catabolic illness, incontinence, weight loss, social support needs, difficulty walking, and falls, was prevalent in 4% of adults who underwent anatomic lung resections [58]. This study identified that frailty was associated with 5.0- and 3.5-fold increased odds of postoperative non-home discharge and mortality, respectively [58]. However, another retrospective, single-institutional study of 193 patients identified that preoperative patient-reported frailty, prevalent in 7% of patients, was not associated with surgical complications [59]. In this study, frailty was assessed by self-reported weight loss, fatigue, physical inactivity, poor grip strength (awareness of the presence of muscle weakness), and (awareness of) slow walking speed [59]. Another retrospective, single-institutional study of 552 patients with stage I–IIIA lung cancer, 44% of whom underwent surgical treatment, also identified significant associations of pre-diagnosis patient-reported physical inactivity with post-diagnosis acute health care utilization and overall survival [60]; however, postoperative complications were not assessed in this study [60]. A systematic review of 16 studies involving 4,183 lung cancer patients identified that 45% are frail, with frailty being associated with three-fold increased hazards of death [61]. However, there was significant heterogeneity in the prevalence of frailty (e.g., range 0–80% among males assessed by the Fried frailty index), with only one study focusing on patients undergoing surgical treatment [61].

Sarcopenia, or the age-related loss of muscle mass and strength or physical function [62], has also been associated with perioperative complications. In a retrospective study of 328 patients undergoing curative lung resection, sarcopenia, assessed by a psoas muscle mass index on computed tomography and prevalent in 56% of patients, was associated with postoperative complications [63]. However, another similar retrospective study of 391 patients showed no association between sarcopenia and postoperative complications [64]. A systematic review of 23 studies focusing on patients with stage I–III NSCLC and surgical treatment identified that pretreatment nutritional status, conceptualized by multiple measures that include sarcopenia, functional or biochemical (e.g., serum albumin) tests, anthropometric characteristics (e.g., body-mass index), and nutrition risk indices, showed significant associations of poor pretreatment nutritional status with posttreatment complications and mortality [65]. However, this study also identified a need for (and easy-to-use) pretreatment nutritional assessments that accurately identify patients who are at risk for treatment complications [65]. Other radiographic assessments include emphysema (e.g., by quantitative computed tomography) [66, 67] and pulmonary hypertension (e.g., pulmonary artery-to-ascending-aorta size ratio) [68] also show promise, however with limited studies.

Practical Challenges and Considerations

Variations in Guideline Recommendations

The ACCP, BTS, and ERS/ESTS clinical practice guidelines endorse the use of algorithms to risk stratify patients being considered for lung cancer resection surgery [13, 27, 28], with the indications and thresholds used to guide testing and clinical decision-making varying between them [29]. For instance, the ACCP recommends that patients with ppoFEV$_1$ or ppoDL$_{CO}$ 30–60% to undergo SCT or ISWT and subsequently CPET if performance on the SCT or ISWT is impaired— i.e., SCT height <22 m, or ISWT <400 m [13]. In such patients, lung cancer resection surgery is generally not recommended if VO$_{2peak}$ is <10 ml/kg/min (or <35% predicted), due to concerns of excessive/prohibitive operative risk [13]. In contrast, the ERS/ESTS recommends that all patients with FEV$_1$ or DL$_{CO}$ < 80% predicted undergo CPET and does not endorse the use of any simple field exercise testing for risk stratification, with a similar VO$_{2peak}$ threshold used to indicate excessive/prohibitive operative risk [28]. The BTS, on the other hand, recommends that patients with ppoFEV$_1$ or ppoDL$_{CO}$ ≤ 40% undergo ISWT or CPET, with ISWT distance <400 m or VO$_{2peak}$ < 15 ml/kg/min indicating excessive and prohibitive risk [27] (Table 13.1).

Table 13.1 Summary of clinical guidelines on the physiologic evaluation for lung cancer resection surgery

Clinical question	ACCP guideline [13]	BTS guideline [27]	ERS/ESTS guideline [28]
Whom to test and which test	ppoFEV$_1$ or ppoDL$_{CO}$ 30–60%: SCT or ISWT	ppoFEV$_1$ or ppoDL$_{CO}$ ≤ 40%: ISWT or CPET	FEV$_1$ or DL$_{CO}$ < 80% predicted: CPET
	ppoFEV$_1$ or ppoDL$_{CO}$ < 30%: CPET		
Functional cutoff indicating elevated surgical risk	SCT height < 22 m or ISWT distance <400 m and/or VO$_{2peak}$ < 20 ml/kg/min (or <75% predicted)	ISWT distance <400 m or VO$_{2peak}$ < 15 ml/kg/min	VO$_{2peak}$ < 20 ml/kg/min (or <75% predicted)
Anatomic resection generally not recommended (i.e., "prohibitive risk")	VO$_{2peak}$ < 10 ml/kg/min (or <35% predicted)		VO$_{2peak}$ < 10 ml/kg/min (or <35% predicted)

ACCP American College of Chest Physicians, *BTS* British Thoracic Society, *CPET* cardiopulmonary exercise testing, *DL$_{CO}$* diffusion capacity of the lung for carbon monoxide, *ERS/ESTS* European Respiratory Society/European Society of Thoracic Surgery, *FEV$_1$* forced expiratory volume in 1 second, *ISWT* incremental shuttle walk test, *ppo* predicted postoperative, *SCT* stair climbing test, *VO$_{2peak}$* peak oxygen consumption

Defining Risk and Acceptable Thresholds

Due to the historically poor prognosis associated with lung cancer, a high surgical mortality risk has been accepted for the potential benefit of a cure. For instance, the ACCP defines high (and prohibitive) surgical risk as >10%, moderate 1–10%, and low risk as <1% chance of perioperative mortality following lung cancer resection surgery. However, advances in therapeutic techniques, including video-assisted thoracoscopic surgery and stereotactic body radiotherapy (SBRT), have improved survival rates for patients with early-stage lung cancer [69]. Concerns have been raised for patients deemed at "moderate" surgical risk as defined by guideline-recommended algorithms, with perioperative mortality rates of 8–9% following bi-lobectomy or pneumonectomy reported in one study [70]. The American Society of Clinical Oncology guideline recommends no more than a 5% perioperative mortality risk for patients being considered for surgical treatment of stage III NSCLC [71]. Moreover, there is not a well-accepted/validated definition of poor (and nonfatal) composite surgical outcomes, with some studies including clinical events of unclear significance (e.g., atelectasis with or without therapeutic bronchoscopy) and possibly not related to cardiopulmonary function and/or fitness (e.g., intrathoracic or extrathoracic bleeding). As such, concerns have been raised regarding the significance of the surgical outcomes commonly evaluated to date [72].

Real-World Challenges

Despite the available physiologic predictors and associated algorithms, real-world challenges exist. Many patients with lung cancer are older and with significant comorbidities that render them unable to perform exercise testing, including simple field exercise testing such as the SCT [31, 73]. The inability to perform the indicated exercise test has been associated with worse perioperative outcomes [31, 73]. In addition, while VO_{2peak} is a well-accepted physiologic predictor of perioperative morbidity and mortality, CPET has limited availability and the SCT height, despite its construct and predictive validity, does not have accepted standards for testing performance and interpretation. A 2021 survey of a panel of thoracic surgeons, pulmonologists, and radiation oncologist suggested that the five most important risk factors considered in practice when assessing surgical risk for lung cancer resection surgery are: the use of home oxygen, frailty, ppo lung function (i.e., $ppoFEV_1$; $ppoDL_{CO}$), and functional status [74]. CPET and simple field exercise test were ranked 13th and tenth, respectively, out of the 16 risk factors considered [74].

Patient-Centered Care

In addition to physiologic measures and associated algorithms, a patient-centered approach can further guide clinical decision making for patients with lung cancer being considered for curative intent therapy [14, 29]. A cross-sectional study of 114 patients with early-stage lung cancer at 4–6 months following surgical resection or SBRT showed high (about 50%) discordance between preferred and actual treatment received, with more patients valuing independence and HRQL as "most important" compared to traditionally accepted clinical outcomes of survival or cancer recurrence [75]. This study also identified that an overwhelming majority (about 80%) of patients were willing to accept no more than a 2% chance of perioperative death for one additional year of life [75]. Another cross-sectional study of 660 lung cancer patients identified that ≥90% ranked quality of life, maintaining independence, and ability to perform normal activities as "very important" or "important," regardless of disease stage (metastatic or not) or status (disease-free or not) [76]. Longitudinal studies have also shown that within 1 year following curative intent therapy of lung cancer, many patients experience increased dyspnea and symptom burden, impaired functional exercise capacity, and decreased HRQL [9–12]. A meta-synthesis of qualitative studies also showed that following surgical treatment, lung cancer patients "long to get back on track with their lives," feeling that they are in "a pendulum between needing support and wanting independence," and "burdened with postoperative symptoms" [77]. A systematic review of qualitative and quantitative studies specifically identified that many lung cancer patients experience significant dyspnea, fatigue, sleep difficulties, and worrying about limitations on activities of daily life, losing independence, and physical disability [78]. Therefore, patient-centered care, particularly to incorporate patient preferences, values, and patient-centered outcomes such as HRQL and disability can guide decision-making [1, 13, 79]. A standard set of patient-centered outcomes has been proposed in lung cancer, to include patient-reported domains of HRQL (e.g., fatigue, dyspnea, and cough), in addition to complications during or within 6 months of treatment, and survival [80].

Moreover, shared decision-making is an essential component of patient-centered care [81]. The use of decision aids to facilitate shared decision-making has been shown to improve patient satisfaction, value agreement, and knowledge and decrease conflict and anxiety among patients undergoing elective surgery [82, 83]. In lung cancer, shared decision-making is recommended to facilitate decision making on screening [84, 85] and can be effective [86]. In patients with lung cancer being considered for curative intent therapy, shared decision-making has been shown to be suboptimal [87, 88]. The use of decision aids to facilitate shared decision-making with patients being considered for diagnostic procedures [89, 90] and lung cancer treatment [91] has been explored.

Additional Considerations

Mitigating Risk

A component of risk evaluation also includes identification of strategies to mitigate risk. Given that low exercise capacity is associated with poor perioperative surgical outcomes, exercise training to improve exercise capacity has been attempted to reduce surgical risk. For instance, a randomized controlled trial (RCT) of 151 participants with operable lung cancer, 38% of whom had comorbid COPD, demonstrated that those in the high-intensity interval exercise training, compared to usual care group, had significant improvements in VO_{2peak} and 6MWT distance [92]. Also, a subsequent systematic review and meta-analysis of RCTs identified 791 participants in 14 studies showed that compared to usual care, preoperative exercise training reduced overall, and clinically relevant postoperative complications [93]. The estimates of the effect of exercise training on mortality was imprecise (and statistically nonsignificant), with exercise training possibly improving exercise capacity, lung function, HRQL, although the clinical significance of these changes was unclear [93]. The preoperative exercise training program durations identified in this systematic review ranged 1–8 weeks [93].

In the posttreatment phase, a RCT of 61 participants who underwent surgical treatment, 30% of whom had comorbid COPD, demonstrated that compared to usual care, participants allocated to a 20-week high-intensity endurance and strength exercise training program, starting approximately 1 month posttreatment, experienced improvements in VO_{2peak}, leg muscle strength, total muscle mass, and HRQL [94]. A subsequent systematic review and meta-analysis of eight RCTs involving 450 participants within 12 months of lung cancer resection surgery showed that exercise training improves exercise capacity and leg muscle strength, and possibly physical HRQL and dyspnea control [95]. Exercise training programs evaluated in this phase ranged 4–20 weeks [95]. Therefore, exercise training or rehabilitation programs can mitigate the risk of perioperative surgical complications and possibly improve HRQL posttreatment. Indeed, pulmonary rehabilitation is recommended for lung cancer patients with impaired lung function and exercise capacity in the pre- or postoperative settings [13].

Smoking cessation can also positively impact outcomes. A prospective study of 517 current smokers with stage I–IIIA NSCLC, followed for an average of 7 years, identified that, compared to those who continued smoking postdiagnosis, those who had quit had an adjusted median overall survival time of 22 months longer; their 5-year overall and progression-free survival rates were also significantly higher: 61% vs. 49% and 54% vs. 44%, respectively [96]. In this study, smoking cessation was associated with approximately 30% decreased hazard of all-cause mortality, cancer-specific mortality, and disease progression, regardless of stage [96]. Moreover, smoking cessation prior to surgical treatment has been associated with lower rates of surgical complications, although this relationship has not been consistently identified across studies [97–99]. Albeit, given its potential benefits, smoking cessation is recommended to mitigate surgical risk for patients with lung cancer being considered for surgical treatment [13].

Care Team Characteristics

Care team and hospital characteristics have been associated with outcomes in lung cancer. Surgical outcomes can depend on expertise (i.e., better with thoracic compared to general surgery) [100] and surgeon or hospital volume (i.e., better with higher volumes compared to low) [101, 102], with guideline recommendations to have lung cancer resection surgery performed by thoracic surgeons in high volume centers (e.g., $\geq$20–25 cases/year) [2, 28]. In addition, involvement of multidisciplinary teams has been associated with better timeliness to treatment, treatment selection, adherence to clinical guideline recommendations, and lower health care costs and expenditures [103–107]. The ACCP recommends that multidisciplinary teams for patients being considered for lung cancer resection surgery include thoracic surgeons, radiation oncologists, medical oncologists, and pulmonologists [1, 13]. However, approximately 30% of lung cancer resection surgery cases are performed by general surgeons [2], with significant real-world disparities in outcomes with regard to medical center characteristics (better with specialized/complex compared to nonspecialized/affiliate centers [108]), access to care (e.g., better in urban compared to rural areas [109]), and geography (by state and county levels in the USA [110, 111]). Therefore, considerations with regard to team- and center-level characteristics, as well as access to care, can guide clinical decision-making with patients with lung cancer being considered for curative intent therapy.

A Consolidated Approach

The patient's ability to survive surgical treatment is a principal consideration in the physiologic assessment for curative intent therapy of lung cancer. Traditionally, due to the absence of effective alternative treatment options, relatively high risks have been taken to achieve the potential benefit of a cure. As such, older studies of physiologic evaluation for curative lung cancer resection reported much higher rates of surgical mortality (e.g., 20%) [16, 112]. Advances in surgical and radiation techniques have allowed for safer, better-tolerated, and effective treatment modalities, with survival rates significantly improving for patients diagnosed with early-stage lung cancer [69]. Additional outcome measures, such as HRQL and disability, should be considered in clinical decision-making [3, 79].

Therefore, a consolidated physiologic and patient-centered approach may better guide treatment selection for patients with lung cancer being considered for curative intent therapy, with important considerations [3, 13, 14, 29]:

1. Physiologic measures and associated algorithms that incorporate pulmonary function testing and exercise capacity assessments can, to a reasonable extent, predict patients' ability to tolerate the necessary stresses induced by curative lung resection, particularly on the cardiopulmonary system. The ability of direct or indirect measures of VO_{2peak} with exercise testing (either with CPET or simple field exercise tests) to predict surgical outcomes is fairly well established in patients with impaired lung function. However, given the imprecise nature of risk assessments, including thresholds used and unclear acceptance of the clinical outcomes traditionally considered, no single variable or algorithm involving physiologic measures should be used in decision-making.
2. While perioperative mortality is an important and well-accepted outcome to assess surgical risk, the available literature and supporting evidence highlights the importance of patient-centered care, including the incorporation of patient-centered outcomes such as HRQL and disability, as well as eliciting patients' preferences and values in shared decision-making.
3. Clinical decision-making, especially regarding binary decisions (e.g., surgery or no surgery), is complex and multifaceted and should be made in a multidisciplinary approach, with access to care taken into account.

With these considerations, patients with $ppoFEV_1$ and $ppoDL_{CO} > 60\%$ can be considered low risk for perioperative morbidity and mortality for lung cancer resection surgery [13]. Patients with marginal $ppoFEV_1$ and/or $ppoDL_{CO}$ 30–60% and acceptable performance on exercise testing can also be considered low risk. The decision to pursue exercise testing should consider patients' ability to undergo the indicated test, testing availability, and interpretation to guide decision-making. Acceptable performance on simple field exercise tests can be defined as SCT height > 22 m, ISWT distance >400 m, or 6MWT distance >400–500 m. Poor performance on exercise testing that indicates high (and usually prohibitive) surgical risk includes $VO_{2peak} < 10$ ml/kg/min (or <35% predicted) on CPET, or if not available, the higher distance thresholds on simple field exercise tests (i.e., SCT height <22 m, ISWT distance <400 m, or 6MWT distance <500 m). Strategies to mitigate surgical risk in the preoperative setting, particularly for patients deemed at "moderate" risk, should include exercise training programs to reduce perioperative complications, especially if such programs are accessible. Patients with $ppoFEV_1$ or $ppoDL_{CO} < 30\%$, particularly with poor performance on exercise testing, can be considered high risk and offered nonsurgical treatment or sub-lobar resection. A perioperative mortality risk >5% can be used as a threshold to indicate high and prohibitive risk [71]. For all patients, a patient-centered approach with a goal of informed shared decision-making and optimal treatment selection should be pursued. This patient-centered approach should incorporate patient preferences, values, and considerations of patient-centered outcomes such as HRQL, disability, and team- and center-level characteristics (Fig. 13.1).

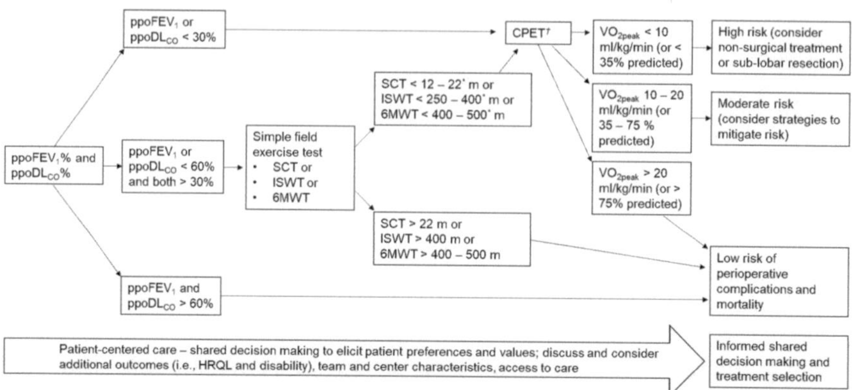

Fig. 13.1 A consolidated approach to the evaluation of patients being considered for lung cancer resection surgery. *Consider using the higher distance or height cutoff to suggest high surgical risk if CPET is not available. †Consider using simple field exercise testing (i.e., 6MWT, ISWT, or SCT) if CPET is not available (and higher distance or height cutoffs to suggest high surgical risk). *6MWT* 6-minute walk test, *CPET* cardiopulmonary exercise testing, DL_{CO} diffusion capacity of the lungs for carbon monoxide, FEV_1 forced expiratory volume in 1 s, *HRQL* health-related quality of life, *ISWT* incremental shuttle walk test, *ppo* predicted postoperative, *SCT* stair-climbing test, VO_{2peak} peak oxygen consumption

References

1. Ost DE, Jim Yeung SC, Tanoue LT, Gould MK. Clinical and organizational factors in the initial evaluation of patients with lung cancer: diagnosis and management of lung cancer, 3rd ed: American College of Chest Physicians evidence-based clinical practice guidelines. Chest. 2013;143(5 Suppl):e121S–e41S.
2. Howington JA, Blum MG, Chang AC, Balekian AA, Murthy SC. Treatment of stage I and II non-small cell lung cancer: diagnosis and management of lung cancer, 3rd ed: American College of Chest Physicians evidence-based clinical practice guidelines. Chest. 2013;143(5 Suppl):e278S–313S.
3. Donington J, Ferguson M, Mazzone P, Handy J Jr, Schuchert M, Fernando H, et al. American College of Chest Physicians and Society of Thoracic Surgeons consensus statement for evaluation and management for high-risk patients with stage I non-small cell lung cancer. Chest. 2012;142(6):1620–35.
4. Tabutin M, Couraud S, Guibert B, Mulsant P, Souquet PJ, Tronc F. Completion pneumonectomy in patients with cancer: postoperative survival and mortality factors. J Thorac Oncol. 2012;7(10):1556–62.
5. Thibout Y, Guibert B, Bossard N, Tronc F, Tiffet O, de la Roche E, et al. Is pneumonectomy after induction chemotherapy for non-small cell lung cancer a reasonable procedure? A multicenter retrospective study of 228 cases. J Thorac Oncol. 2009;4(12):1496–503.
6. Win T, Groves AM, Ritchie AJ, Wells FC, Cafferty F, Laroche CM. The effect of lung resection on pulmonary function and exercise capacity in lung cancer patients. Respir Care. 2007;52(6):720–6.
7. Bolliger CT, Jordan P, Soler M, Stulz P, Tamm M, Wyser C, et al. Pulmonary function and exercise capacity after lung resection. Eur Respir J. 1996;9(3):415–21.
8. Zeiher BG, Gross TJ, Kern JA, Lanza LA, Peterson MW. Predicting postoperative pulmonary function in patients undergoing lung resection. Chest. 1995;108(1):68–72.

9. Ha D, Ries AL, Lippman SM, Fuster MM. Effects of curative-intent lung cancer therapy on functional exercise capacity and patient-reported outcomes. Supportive Care Cancer. 2020;28(10):4707–20.
10. Nugent SM, Golden SE, Hooker ER, Sullivan DR, Thomas CR Jr, Deffebach ME, et al. Longitudinal health-related quality of life among individuals considering treatment for stage I non-small-cell lung cancer. Ann Am Thorac Soc. 2020;17(8):988–97.
11. Granger CL, McDonald CF, Irving L, Clark RA, Gough K, Murnane A, et al. Low physical activity levels and functional decline in individuals with lung cancer. Lung Cancer (Amsterdam, Netherlands). 2014;83(2):292–9.
12. Pompili C, Rogers Z, Absolom K, Holch P, Clayton B, Callister M, et al. Quality of life after VATS lung resection and SABR for early-stage non-small cell lung cancer: a longitudinal study. Lung Cancer. 2021;162:71–8.
13. Brunelli A, Kim AW, Berger KI, Addrizzo-Harris DJ. Physiologic evaluation of the patient with lung cancer being considered for resectional surgery: diagnosis and management of lung cancer, 3rd ed: American College of Chest Physicians Evidence-Based Clinical Practice Guidelines. Chest. 2013;143(5 Suppl):e166S–90S.
14. Choi H, Mazzone P. Preoperative evaluation of the patient with lung cancer being considered for lung resection. Curr Opin Anaesthesiol. 2015;28(1):18–25.
15. Markos J, Mullan BP, Hillman DR, Musk AW, Antico VF, Lovegrove FT, et al. Preoperative assessment as a predictor of mortality and morbidity after lung resection. Am Rev Respir Dis. 1989;139(4):902–10.
16. Pierce RJ, Copland JM, Sharpe K, Barter CE. Preoperative risk evaluation for lung cancer resection: predicted postoperative product as a predictor of surgical mortality. Am J Respir Crit Care Med. 1994;150(4):947–55.
17. Berry MF, Villamizar-Ortiz NR, Tong BC, Burfeind WR Jr, Harpole DH, D'Amico TA, et al. Pulmonary function tests do not predict pulmonary complications after thoracoscopic lobectomy. Ann Thorac Surg. 2010;89(4):1044–51; discussion 1051–2.
18. Zhang R, Lee SM, Wigfield C, Vigneswaran WT, Ferguson MK. Lung function predicts pulmonary complications regardless of the surgical approach. Ann Thorac Surg. 2015;99(5):1761–7.
19. Cao C, Louie BE, Melfi F, Veronesi G, Razzak R, Romano G, et al. Impact of pulmonary function on pulmonary complications after robotic-assisted thoracoscopic lobectomy. Eur J Cardiothorac Surg. 2020;57(2):338–42.
20. Licker MJ, Widikker I, Robert J, Frey JG, Spiliopoulos A, Ellenberger C, et al. Operative mortality and respiratory complications after lung resection for cancer: impact of chronic obstructive pulmonary disease and time trends. Ann Thorac Surg. 2006;81(5):1830–7.
21. Ferguson MK, Little L, Rizzo L, Popovich KJ, Glonek GF, Leff A, et al. Diffusing capacity predicts morbidity and mortality after pulmonary resection. J Thorac Cardiovasc Surg. 1988;96(6):894–900.
22. Brunelli A, Refai MA, Salati M, Sabbatini A, Morgan-Hughes NJ, Rocco G. Carbon monoxide lung diffusion capacity improves risk stratification in patients without airflow limitation: evidence for systematic measurement before lung resection. Eur J Cardiothorac Surg. 2006;29(4):567–70.
23. Ferguson MK, Vigneswaran WT. Diffusing capacity predicts morbidity after lung resection in patients without obstructive lung disease. Ann Thorac Surg. 2008;85(4):1158–64; discussion 1164–5.
24. Olsen GN, Block AJ, Tobias JA. Prediction of postpneumonectomy pulmonary function using quantitative macroaggregate lung scanning. Chest. 1974;66(1):13–6.
25. Loewen GM, Watson D, Kohman L, Herndon JE 2nd, Shennib H, Kernstine K, et al. Preoperative exercise Vo2 measurement for lung resection candidates: results of Cancer and Leukemia Group B Protocol 9238. J Thorac Oncol. 2007;2(7):619–25.
26. Benzo R, Kelley GA, Recchi L, Hofman A, Sciurba F. Complications of lung resection and exercise capacity: a meta-analysis. Respir Med. 2007;101(8):1790–7.

27. Lim E, Baldwin D, Beckles M, Duffy J, Entwisle J, Faivre-Finn C, et al. Guidelines on the radical management of patients with lung cancer. Thorax. 2010;65(Suppl 3):iii1–27.
28. Brunelli A, Charloux A, Bolliger CT, Rocco G, Sculier JP, Varela G, et al. ERS/ESTS clinical guidelines on fitness for radical therapy in lung cancer patients (surgery and chemoradiotherapy). Eur Respir J. 2009;34(1):17–41.
29. Ha D, Mazzone PJ, Ries AL, Malhotra A, Fuster M. The utility of exercise testing in patients with lung cancer. J Thorac Oncol. 2016;11(9):1397–410.
30. American Thoracic Society, American College of Chest Physicians. ATS/ACCP statement on cardiopulmonary exercise testing. Am J Respir Crit Care Med. 2003;167(2):211–77.
31. Epstein SK, Faling LJ, Daly BD, Celli BR. Inability to perform bicycle ergometry predicts increased morbidity and mortality after lung resection. Chest. 1995;107(2):311–6.
32. Brunelli A, Refai M, Xiume F, Salati M, Sciarra V, Socci L, et al. Performance at symptom-limited stair-climbing test is associated with increased cardiopulmonary complications, mortality, and costs after major lung resection. Ann Thorac Surg. 2008;86(1):240–7; discussion 247–8.
33. Brunelli A, Xiumé F, Refai M, Salati M, Di Nunzio L, Pompili C, et al. Peak oxygen consumption measured during the stair-climbing test in lung resection candidates. Respiration. 2010;80(3):207–11.
34. Boujibar F, Gillibert A, Gravier FE, Gillot T, Bonnevie T, Cuvelier A, et al. Performance at stair-climbing test is associated with postoperative complications after lung resection: a systematic review and meta-analysis. Thorax. 2020;75(9):791–7.
35. ATS Committee on Proficiency Standards for Clinical Pulmonary Function Laboratories. ATS statement: guidelines for the six-minute walk test. Am J Respir Crit Care Med. 2002;166(1):111–7.
36. Holland AE, Spruit MA, Troosters T, Puhan MA, Pepin V, Saey D, et al. An official European Respiratory Society/American Thoracic Society technical standard: field walking tests in chronic respiratory disease. Eur Respir J. 2014;44(6):1428–46.
37. Singh SJ, Puhan MA, Andrianopoulos V, Hernandes NA, Mitchell KE, Hill CJ, et al. An official systematic review of the European Respiratory Society/American Thoracic Society: measurement properties of field walking tests in chronic respiratory disease. Eur Respir J. 2014;44(6):1447–78.
38. Win T, Jackson A, Groves AM, Sharples LD, Charman SC, Laroche CM. Comparison of shuttle walk with measured peak oxygen consumption in patients with operable lung cancer. Thorax. 2006;61(1):57–60.
39. Fennelly J, Potter L, Pompili C, Brunelli A. Performance in the shuttle walk test is associated with cardiopulmonary complications after lung resections. J Thorac Dis. 2017;9(3):789–95.
40. Voorn MJJ, Franssen RFW, Verlinden J, Bootsma GP, de Ruysscher DK, Bongers BC, et al. Associations between pretreatment physical performance tests and treatment complications in patients with non-small cell lung cancer: a systematic review. Crit Rev Oncol Hematol. 2021;158:103207.
41. Hattori K, Matsuda T, Takagi Y, Nagaya M, Inoue T, Nishida Y, et al. Preoperative six-minute walk distance is associated with pneumonia after lung resection. Interact Cardiovasc Thorac Surg. 2018;26(2):277–83.
42. Lee H, Kim HK, Kang D, Kong S, Lee JK, Lee G, et al. Prognostic value of 6-min walk test to predict postoperative cardiopulmonary complications in patients with non-small cell lung cancer. Chest. 2020;157(6):1665–73.
43. Wesolowski S, Orlowski TM, Kram M. The 6-min walk test in the functional evaluation of patients with lung cancer qualified for lobectomy. Interact Cardiovasc Thorac Surg. 2020;30(4):559–64.
44. Hamada K, Irie M, Fujino Y, Hyodo M, Hanagiri T. Prognostic value of preoperative exercise capacity in patients undergoing thoracoscopic lobectomy for non-small cell lung cancer. Lung Cancer (Amsterdam, Netherlands). 2019;128:47–52.

45. Marjanski T, Badocha M, Wnuk D, Dziedzic R, Ostrowski M, Sawicka W, et al. Result of the 6-min walk test is an independent prognostic factor of surgically treated non-small-cell lung cancer. Interact Cardiovasc Thorac Surg. 2019;28(3):368–74.
46. Marjanski T, Wnuk D, Bosakowski D, Szmuda T, Sawicka W, Rzyman W. Patients who do not reach a distance of 500 m during the 6-min walk test have an increased risk of postoperative complications and prolonged hospital stay after lobectomy. Eur J Cardiothorac Surg. 2015;47(5):e213–9.
47. Irie M, Nakanishi R, Yasuda M, Fujino Y, Hamada K, Hyodo M. Risk factors for short-term outcomes after thoracoscopic lobectomy for lung cancer. Eur Respir J. 2016;48(2):495–503.
48. Granger CL, Denehy L, Parry SM, Martin J, Dimitriadis T, Sorohan M, et al. Which field walking test should be used to assess functional exercise capacity in lung cancer? An observational study. BMC Pulm Med. 2015;15:89.
49. Ha D, Ries AL, Mazzone PJ, Lippman SM, Fuster MM. Exercise capacity and cancer-specific quality of life following curative intent treatment of stage I-IIIA lung cancer. Support Care Cancer. 2018;26(7):2459–69.
50. Brunelli A. Ventilatory efficiency slope: an additional prognosticator after lung cancer surgery. Eur J Cardiothorac Surg. 2016;50(4):780–1.
51. Brunelli A, Belardinelli R, Pompili C, Xiumé F, Refai M, Salati M, et al. Minute ventilation-to-carbon dioxide output (VE/VCO2) slope is the strongest predictor of respiratory complications and death after pulmonary resection. Ann Thorac Surg. 2012;93(6):1802–6.
52. Brunelli A, Refai M, Xiume F, Salati M, Marasco R, Sciarra V, et al. Oxygen desaturation during maximal stair-climbing test and postoperative complications after major lung resections. Eur J Cardiothorac Surg. 2008;33(1):77–82.
53. Ha D, Fuster M, Ries AL, Wagner PD, Mazzone PJ. Heart rate recovery as a preoperative test of perioperative complication risk. Ann Thorac Surg. 2015;100(5):1954–62.
54. Ha D, Choi H, Zell K, Raymond DP, Stephans K, Wang XF, et al. Association of impaired heart rate recovery with cardiopulmonary complications after lung cancer resection surgery. J Thorac Cardiovasc Surg. 2015;149(4):1168–73.e3.
55. Fried LP, Tangen CM, Walston J, Newman AB, Hirsch C, Gottdiener J, et al. Frailty in older adults: evidence for a phenotype. J Gerontol A Biol Sci Med Sci. 2001;56(3):M146–56.
56. Mitnitski AB, Mogilner AJ, Rockwood K. Accumulation of deficits as a proxy measure of aging. ScientificWorldJournal. 2001;1:323–36.
57. Walston J, Bandeen-Roche K, Buta B, Bergman H, Gill TM, Morley JE, et al. Moving frailty toward clinical practice: NIA intramural frailty science symposium summary. J Am Geriatr Soc. 2019;67(8):1559–64.
58. Karunungan KL, Hadaya J, Tran Z, Sanaiha Y, Mandelbaum A, Revels SL, et al. Frailty is independently associated with worse outcomes after elective anatomic lung resection. Ann Thorac Surg. 2021;112(5):1639–46.
59. Kaneda H, Nakano T, Murakawa T. The predictive value of preoperative risk assessments and frailty for surgical complications in lung cancer patients. Surg Today. 2021;51(1):86–93.
60. Ha DM, Zeng C, Chan ED, Gray M, Mazzone PJ, Samet JM, et al. Association of exercise behavior with overall survival in stage I-IIIA lung cancer. Ann Am Thorac Soc. 2021;18(6):1034–42.
61. Komici K, Bencivenga L, Navani N, D'Agnano V, Guerra G, Bianco A, et al. Frailty in patients with lung cancer: a systematic review and meta-analysis. Chest. 2022;162:485.
62. Batsis JA, Villareal DT. Sarcopenic obesity in older adults: aetiology, epidemiology and treatment strategies. Nat Rev Endocrinol. 2018;14(9):513–37.
63. Nakamura R, Inage Y, Tobita R, Yoneyama S, Numata T, Ota K, et al. Sarcopenia in resected NSCLC: effect on postoperative outcomes. J Thorac Oncol. 2018;13(7):895–903.
64. Shinohara S, Otsuki R, Kobayashi K, Sugaya M, Matsuo M, Nakagawa M. Impact of sarcopenia on surgical outcomes in non-small cell lung cancer. Ann Surg Oncol. 2020;27(7):2427–35.
65. Voorn MJJ, Beukers K, Trepels CMM, Bootsma GP, Bongers BC, Janssen-Heijnen MLG. Associations between pretreatment nutritional assessments and treatment

complications in patients with stage I-III non-small cell lung cancer: a systematic review. Clin Nutr ESPEN. 2022;47:152–62.
66. Sato S, Nakamura M, Shimizu Y, Goto T, Koike T, Ishikawa H, et al. The impact of emphysema on surgical outcomes of early-stage lung cancer: a retrospective study. BMC Pulm Med. 2019;19(1):73.
67. Yasuura Y, Maniwa T, Mori K, Miyata N, Mizuno K, Shimizu R, et al. Quantitative computed tomography for predicting cardiopulmonary complications after lobectomy for lung cancer in patients with chronic obstructive pulmonary disease. Gen Thorac Cardiovasc Surg. 2019;67(8):697–703.
68. Asakura K, Mitsuboshi S, Tsuji M, Sakamaki H, Otake S, Matsuda S, et al. Pulmonary arterial enlargement predicts cardiopulmonary complications after pulmonary resection for lung cancer: a retrospective cohort study. J Cardiothorac Surg. 2015;10:113.
69. Siegel RL, Miller KD, Fuchs HE, Jemal A. Cancer statistics, 2021. CA Cancer J Clin. 2021;71(1):7–33.
70. Gooseman MR, Falcoz PE, Decaluwe H, Szanto Z, Brunelli A. Morbidity and mortality of lung resection candidates defined by the American College of Chest Physicians as 'moderate risk': an analysis from the European Society of Thoracic Surgeons database. Eur J Cardiothorac Surg. 2021;60(1):91–7.
71. Daly ME, Singh N, Ismaila N, Antonoff MB, Arenberg DA, Bradley J, et al. Management of stage III non-small-cell lung cancer: ASCO guideline. J Clin Oncol. 2022;40(12):1356–84.
72. Lim E, Beckles M, Warburton C, Baldwin D. Cardiopulmonary exercise testing for the selection of patients undergoing surgery for lung cancer: friend or foe? Thorax. 2010;65(10):847–9.
73. Brunelli A, Sabbatini A, Xiume F, Borri A, Salati M, Marasco RD, et al. Inability to perform maximal stair climbing test before lung resection: a propensity score analysis on early outcome. Eur J Cardiothorac Surg. 2005;27(3):367–72.
74. Pennathur A, Brunelli A, Criner GJ, Keshavarz H, Mazzone P, Walsh G, et al. Definition and assessment of high risk in patients considered for lobectomy for stage I non-small cell lung cancer: The American Association for Thoracic Surgery expert panel consensus document. J Thorac Cardiovasc Surg. 2021;162(6):1605–18.e6.
75. Sullivan DR, Eden KB, Dieckmann NF, Golden SE, Vranas KC, Nugent SM, et al. Understanding patients' values and preferences regarding early stage lung cancer treatment decision making. Lung Cancer. 2019;131:47–57.
76. Gralla RJ, Hollen PJ, Msaouel P, Davis BV, Petersen J. An evidence-based determination of issues affecting quality of life and patient-reported outcomes in lung cancer: results of a survey of 660 patients. J Thorac Oncol. 2014;9(9):1243–8.
77. Salander P, Lilliehorn S. To carry on as before: a meta-synthesis of qualitative studies in lung cancer. Lung Cancer (Amsterdam, Netherlands). 2016;99:88–93.
78. Maguire R, Papadopoulou C, Kotronoulas G, Simpson MF, McPhelim J, Irvine L. A systematic review of supportive care needs of people living with lung cancer. Eur J Oncol Nurs. 2013;17(4):449–64.
79. Colt HG, Murgu SD, Korst RJ, Slatore CG, Unger M, Quadrelli S. Follow-up and surveillance of the patient with lung cancer after curative-intent therapy: diagnosis and management of lung cancer, 3rd ed: American College of Chest Physicians evidence-based clinical practice guidelines. Chest. 2013;143(5 Suppl):e437S–54S.
80. Mak KS, van Bommel AC, Stowell C, Abrahm JL, Baker M, Baldotto CS, et al. Defining a standard set of patient-centred outcomes for lung cancer. Eur Respir J. 2016;48(3):852–60.
81. Barry MJ, Edgman-Levitan S. Shared decision making--pinnacle of patient-centered care. N Engl J Med. 2012;366(9):780–1.
82. Niburski K, Guadagno E, Abbasgholizadeh-Rahimi S, Poenaru D. Shared decision making in surgery: a meta-analysis of existing literature. Patient. 2020;13(6):667–81.
83. Niburski K, Guadagno E, Mohtashami S, Poenaru D. Shared decision making in surgery: a scoping review of the literature. Health Expect. 2020;23(5):1241–9.

84. Krist AH, Davidson KW, Mangione CM, Barry MJ, Cabana M, Caughey AB, et al. Screening for lung cancer: US Preventive Services Task Force recommendation statement. JAMA. 2021;325(10):962–70.
85. Mazzone PJ, Silvestri GA, Souter LH, Caverly TJ, Kanne JP, Katki HA, et al. Screening for lung cancer: CHEST guideline and expert panel report. Chest. 2021;160:e427.
86. Volk RJ, Lowenstein LM, Leal VB, Escoto KH, Cantor SB, Munden RF, et al. Effect of a patient decision aid on lung cancer screening decision-making by persons who smoke: a randomized clinical trial. JAMA Netw Open. 2020;3(1):e1920362.
87. De Roo AC, Vitous CA, Rivard SJ, Bamdad MC, Jafri SM, Byrnes ME, et al. High-risk surgery among older adults: not-quite shared decision-making. Surgery. 2021;170(3):756–63.
88. Golden SE, Thomas CR Jr, Moghanaki D, Slatore CG. Dumping the information bucket: a qualitative study of clinicians caring for patients with early stage non-small cell lung cancer. Patient Educ Couns. 2017;100(5):861–70.
89. Olling K, Stie M, Winther B, Steffensen KD. The impact of a patient decision aid on shared decision-making behaviour in oncology care and pulmonary medicine-a field study based on real-life observations. J Eval Clin Pract. 2019;25(6):1121–30.
90. Søndergaard SR, Madsen PH, Hilberg O, Jensen KM, Olling K, Steffensen KD. A prospective cohort study of shared decision making in lung cancer diagnostics: impact of using a patient decision aid. Patient Educ Couns. 2019;102(11):1961–8.
91. Spronk I, Meijers MC, Heins MJ, Francke AL, Elwyn G, van Lindert A, et al. Availability and effectiveness of decision aids for supporting shared decision making in patients with advanced colorectal and lung cancer: results from a systematic review. Eur J Cancer Care (Engl). 2019;28(3):e13079.
92. Licker M, Karenovics W, Diaper J, Fresard I, Triponez F, Ellenberger C, et al. Short-term preoperative high-intensity interval training in patients awaiting lung cancer surgery: a randomized controlled trial. J Thorac Oncol. 2017;12(2):323–33.
93. Gravier FE, Smondack P, Prieur G, Medrinal C, Combret Y, Muir JF, et al. Effects of exercise training in people with non-small cell lung cancer before lung resection: a systematic review and meta-analysis. Thorax. 2022;77(5):486–96.
94. Edvardsen E, Skjonsberg OH, Holme I, Nordsletten L, Borchsenius F, Anderssen SA. High-intensity training following lung cancer surgery: a randomised controlled trial. Thorax. 2015;70(3):244–50.
95. Cavalheri V, Burtin C, Formico VR, Nonoyama ML, Jenkins S, Spruit MA, et al. Exercise training undertaken by people within 12 months of lung resection for non-small cell lung cancer. Cochrane Database Syst Rev. 2019;6:CD009955.
96. Sheikh M, Mukeriya A, Shangina O, Brennan P, Zaridze D. Postdiagnosis smoking cessation and reduced risk for lung cancer progression and mortality : a prospective cohort study. Ann Intern Med. 2021;174(9):1232–9.
97. Lugg ST, Tikka T, Agostini PJ, Kerr A, Adams K, Kalkat MS, et al. Smoking and timing of cessation on postoperative pulmonary complications after curative-intent lung cancer surgery. J Cardiothorac Surg. 2017;12(1):52.
98. Mason DP, Subramanian S, Nowicki ER, Grab JD, Murthy SC, Rice TW, et al. Impact of smoking cessation before resection of lung cancer: a Society of Thoracic Surgeons General Thoracic Surgery Database study. Ann Thorac Surg. 2009;88(2):362–70; discussion 370–1.
99. Takenaka T, Shoji F, Tagawa T, Kinoshita F, Haratake N, Edagawa M, et al. Does short-term cessation of smoking before lung resections reduce the risk of complications? J Thorac Dis. 2020;12(12):7127–34.
100. von Meyenfeldt EM, Gooiker GA, van Gijn W, Post PN, van de Velde CJ, Tollenaar RA, et al. The relationship between volume or surgeon specialty and outcome in the surgical treatment of lung cancer: a systematic review and meta-analysis. J Thorac Oncol. 2012;7(7):1170–8.
101. Birkmeyer JD, Stukel TA, Siewers AE, Goodney PP, Wennberg DE, Lucas FL. Surgeon volume and operative mortality in the United States. N Engl J Med. 2003;349(22):2117–27.

102. Birkmeyer JD, Siewers AE, Finlayson EV, Stukel TA, Lucas FL, Batista I, et al. Hospital volume and surgical mortality in the United States. N Engl J Med. 2002;346(15):1128–37.
103. Boxer MM, Vinod SK, Shafiq J, Duggan KJ. Do multidisciplinary team meetings make a difference in the management of lung cancer? Cancer. 2011;117(22):5112–20.
104. Coory M, Gkolia P, Yang IA, Bowman RV, Fong KM. Systematic review of multidisciplinary teams in the management of lung cancer. Lung Cancer. 2008;60(1):14–21.
105. Freeman RK, Ascioti AJ, Dake M, Mahidhara RS. The effects of a multidisciplinary care conference on the quality and cost of care for lung cancer patients. Ann Thorac Surg. 2015;100(5):1834–8; discussion 1838.
106. Freeman RK, Van Woerkom JM, Vyverberg A, Ascioti AJ. The effect of a multidisciplinary thoracic malignancy conference on the treatment of patients with lung cancer. Eur J Cardiothorac Surg. 2010;38(1):1–5.
107. Voong KR, Liang OS, Dugan P, Torto D, Padula WV, Senter JP, et al. Thoracic oncology multidisciplinary clinic reduces unnecessary health care expenditure used in the workup of patients with non-small-cell lung cancer. Clin Lung Cancer. 2019;20(4):e430–e41.
108. Boffa DJ, Mallin K, Herrin J, Resio B, Salazar MC, Palis B, et al. Survival after cancer treatment at top-ranked US cancer hospitals vs affiliates of top-ranked cancer hospitals. JAMA Netw Open. 2020;3(5):e203942.
109. Nicoli CD, Sprague BL, Anker CJ, Lester-Coll NH. Association of rurality with survival and guidelines-concordant management in early-stage non-small cell lung cancer. Am J Clin Oncol. 2019;42(7):607–14.
110. Sineshaw HM, Sahar L, Osarogiagbon RU, Flanders WD, Yabroff KR, Jemal A. County-level variations in receipt of surgery for early-stage non-small cell lung cancer in the United States. Chest. 2020;157(1):212–22.
111. Sineshaw HM, Wu XC, Flanders WD, Osarogiagbon RU, Jemal A. Variations in receipt of curative-intent surgery for early-stage non-small cell lung cancer (NSCLC) by state. J Thorac Oncol. 2016;11(6):880–9.
112. Holden DA, Rice TW, Stelmach K, Meeker DP. Exercise testing, 6-min walk, and stair climb in the evaluation of patients at high risk for pulmonary resection. Chest. 1992;102(6):1774–9.

Index

A

Acute radiation pneumonitis, 232
Adenocarcinoma in situ (AIS), 114
Adenocarcinomas, 180
Adjuvant chemotherapy, 268
Administrative delays, 266
Advanced imaging modalities, 214
Affordable Care Act, 27
ALK-tyrosine kinase inhibitors (ALK-TKIs), 245
Alkylating agents, 240, 241
American Academy of Family Physicians (AAFP), 27
American College of Chest Physicians (ACCP), 106, 114, 127, 280
American College of Chest Physicians Quality Improvement Registry, Evaluation, And Education (AQuIRE) registry, 112
American College of Radiology (ACR), 30
American Joint Committee on Cancer (AJCC) tumor, 147
American Society of Clinical Oncology (ASCO), 125, 243, 285
2018 American Thoracic Society (ATS), 56, 62, 219, 282
Amivantamab, 245
Anaplastic lymphoma kinase (*ALK*) gene, 171
Anatomic lung resection, 277
Anatomic method, 278, 279
Anterior mediastinoscopy, 110
Anti-angiogenic biologic agents, 166, 168
Anti-CTLA-4 antibody ipilimumab, 177

Anti-EGFR therapy, 158
Anti-LAG3 antibody relatlimab, 181
Anti-PD1/PD-L1 inhibitors, 174
Arterial thromboembolic events, 244
Asbestos, 15, 16, 73
Atezolizumab, 176
2018 Australasian Malignant Pleural Effusion (AMPLE-2) Trial, 220
Australian study, 269
Automated radiomics, 76
Azathioprine, 233

B

Behavioral interventions, 55
Behavioral Risk Factor Surveillance System (BRFS) data, 39–40
Bevacizumab, 166, 174, 231, 244
Bilobectomy, 128
Biomarkers, 87–88, 268
Biopsy, 85
Blastomycosis, 74
Blood tests, 40
BRAF inhibitors, 231
BRAF-targeted agents, 246
Breast cancer screening, 36
Brief motivational interventions, 55
Brigatinib, 245
Brims' decision tree, 212
British Thoracic Society (BTS), 31, 280
Brock models, 82
Bronchoalveolar lavage (BAL), 230
Bronchoscopy, 85, 128, 233, 242
Bupropion sustained release (S.R.), 61

C
Calcium, 236
Canadian study, 262
Cancer and Leukemia Group B (CALGB)
    30407 trial, 157
Cancer and Leukemia Group B (CALGB)
    30610, 192
Cancer Intervention and Surveillance
    Modeling Network (CISNET), 26
Capmatinib, 247
Carbon dioxide production (VCO_2), 282
Cardiopulmonary comorbidities, 230
Cardiopulmonary exercise testing (CPET),
    127, 279
CASPIAN study, 196
Cellulitis, 220
Centers for Medicare and Medicaid Services
    (CMS), 27, 37
Centers for Medicare and Medicaid Services
    National Coverage
    Determination, 51
Centralized programs, 38
Cerebellar degeneration, 187
Chamberlain procedure, 110
Charleston Comorbidity Index (CCI), 188
CheckMate9LA, 177
CheckMate017, 175
CheckMate057, 175
CheckMate227, 178, 180
Chemical pleurodesis, 218
Chemoimmunotherapy, 174, 176, 178, 179
Chemotherapy, 173, 237–238, 242, 268, 271
Chest radiographs (CXR), 75
Chest radiotherapy, 191, 200
Chronic obstructive pulmonary disease
    (COPD), 281–282
Chronic respiratory failure, 233
Cigarette smoking, 39, 49, 73
Circulating tumor DNA (ctDNA), 215
Cisplatin, 236
Clinical decision making, 289
Clinical staging, cTNM, 98
Clinician-level barriers, 37
Closed-loop communications, 265
Combination immunotherapy, 241
Combination immunotherapy-
    chemoradiotherapy, 155, 157
Combined EBUS/EUS, 106
Common Terminology Criteria for Adverse
    Events (CTCAE) scale, 233
Computed tomographic (CT) chest imaging,
    104, 235

Concurrent chemoradiation (CCRT), 149
Consolidative radiotherapy, 199
Constitutional symptoms, 187
Contrast-enhanced computed tomography
    (CT), 214
Conventional computed tomography (CT)
    imaging, 230
Conventional transbronchial needle aspiration
    (TBNA) of lymph nodes, 106
Conventional treatment, 270
CONVERT study, 192
Corticosteroids, 239, 243
Cough, 230
Counseling and interventions, 40
COVID-19 pandemic, 41, 261
Crizotinib-associated pneumonitis, 245
Cryoablation, 127
Cumulative deficit, 283
Curative intent therapy, 286
Curative lung resection, 283
Cyclophosphamide, 243
Cyclophosphamide, doxorubicin, and
    vincristine (CAV), 198
Cytotoxic T-lymphocyte associated protein-4
    (CTLA-4) inhibitor, 196, 241

D
Danish LCS Trial (DLCST), 28
Decentralized programs, 39
Department of Health and Human Services
    Healthy People 2030 goals, 36
Dermatomyositis, 187
Diagnostic delays, 267
Diagnostic testing, 235, 236, 267, 286
Diffusion impairments, 230
Digital tomosynthesis augmentation, 115
Disparities, 136
Diuretics, 239
DNA miscoding, 51
Doublet regimens, 173
Drainage frequency, 220
Drug-related pneumonitis, 235
Dual anti-CTLA-4 plus anti-PD1/PD-L1
    immunotherapy, 181
Dual immune blockade, 178
Dual immunotherapy, 177, 178
Durvalumab, 196
Dutch-Belgian Randomized Lung Cancer
    Screening Trial, 28
Dutch Lung Cancer Audit, 265
Dyspnea, 230

E

EAGLES trial, 61

Early Pleurodesis via IPC with Talc for Malignant Effusion (EPIToME) observational trial, 221

Early-stage lung cancer
determination of operability, 127
extent of lung resection, 127, 128
preoperative work up, 128, 129
presentation, 124
radiotherapy techniques, 137
staging schema, 124
surgical approach, 129–131
surgical techniques, 131, 133–135, 137
treatment options for, 125–127

Eastern Cooperative Oncology Group Performance Status (ECOG-PS), 212

EGFR-TKI osimertinib, 241

Electronic cigarettes, 9, 10, 62

Electronic health records (EHR), 36

Emphysema, 283

Endobronchial ultrasound (EBUS), 106–108, 243

Endobronchial ultrasound-guided lymph node aspiration (EBUS-TBNA), 107, 108

Endobronchial ultrasound scope, 107

Endobronchial ultrasound using the EBUS scope (EUS-B), 109

Endoscopic ultrasound (EUS), 106, 108

Endosonography versus mediastinoscopy, 111

Epidermal growth factor receptor (EGFR), 166, 170, 180, 244, 245

Epidermal growth factor receptor-tyrosine kinase inhibitors, 231

Etoposide, 196, 239

European Respiratory Society (ERS) statement, 221, 280, 282

European Society for Medical Oncology (ESMO), 106

European Society of Thoracic Surgeons (ESTS), 106, 280

Exercise testing
cardiopulmonary exercise testing, 279
simple field exercise tests, 280–282
training programs, 287

Extended cervical mediastinoscopy, 111

Extensive-stage SCLC (ES-SCLC), 238

Extrathoracic evaluations, 74

Extrinsic obstruction, 220

F

Fagerstrom test for nicotine dependence (FTND), 53

18F-flurodeoxyglucose (FDG), 129

Fibrosis, 232

Financial business plan, 262

5As Model for Behavior Change, 54

Fleischner Society guidelines, 81

Flexible EBUS scope with a 21-gauge needle, 107

Flow cytometry, 215

G

Gemcitabine, 231, 239

General anesthesia (GA), 108

Geographic location, 265

German LCS Intervention (LUSI), 28

Glioglastoma, 240

H

Hamartomas, 77

Healthcare providers, 55

Healthcare systems, 263

Health-related quality of life (HRQOL), 136, 277

Help with Oncologic Mediastinal Evaluation for Radiation (HOMER) prediction model, 113

Help with the assessment of Adenopathy in Lung cancer (HAL) prediction model, 112, 113

Hilar exposure, 132

Human epidermal growth factor receptor 2, 172

Hybrid program, 38

I

ICD-9 diagnoses, 283

Immune checkpoint inhibitors (ICIs), 148, 231, 241, 242

Immune-related adverse events (IRAEs), 241

Immunosuppression, 242

Immunotherapy, 241, 271

IMpower131, 176, 196

IMpower150, 176

Incremental shuttle walk test (ISWT), 280

Indwelling pleural catheter (IPC), 219

Infliximab, 243

INSIGNA trial, 179

International Association for the Study of
Lung Cancer (IASLC), 33, 101
International Early Lung Cancer Action
Program (I-ELCAP), 31, 82
International Lung Screening Trial, 35
Interstitial lung disease (ILD), 231
Intrathoracic metastases (M1a), 101
Intravenous immunoglobulin (IVIG), 243
Invasive biopsy, 83
Invasive mediastinal staging, 106
Invasive staging with tissue biopsy, 105, 106
Italian Lung Cancer Screening Trial
(ITALUNG), 39

J
Joint practice model, 259

K
KEYNOTE trials, 179, 180
Kiersten rat sarcoma virus (*KRAS*), 168
KRAS G12C, 172
KRAS inhibitor sotorasib, 242

L
Lambert-Eaton myasthenic syndrome
(LEMS), 187
Large cell neuroendocrine carcinoma
(LCNEC), 166, 168, 169
Laser ablation, 127
LENT score, 212
LGBTQ+ community, 50
Lobectomy, 131, 132, 134, 135
Low-dose computed tomography (LDCT) lung
cancer screening, 71
Lung cancer, 213
care, 257
evidence for screening, 27–30
familial risk factors, 15
global incidence of, 1
history of screening, 25–27
incidence and mortality of, 1
influential factors of
age, 2
sex, 2
socioeconomic factors, 5
tobacco use, 4
low dose CT screening exam
technique, 30–31
nonsmoking-related risk factors
diet and supplements, 12

race, 12
sex, 11, 12
weight, 13
occupational and environmental factors
asbestos, 15, 16
environmental pollution, 16, 17
radon, 16
radiation therapy, 14
resection surgery, 284, 285, 289, 290
screening interpretation, 31
smoking-related risk factors
cannabis smoking, 9
cigarette smoking, 5–7, 9, 10
never-smoking, 10, 11
secondhand smoke, 7–9
smoking cessation, 10
stage grouping, 102, 148
treatment, 231
2021 USPSTF LCS Recommendations, 30
with multiple lesions, 102, 103
Lung cancer screening (LCS) programs, 38
Lung Reporting and Data System
(Lu-RADS), 82
Lurbinectedin, 197
Lymphadenopathy, 104
Lymph node staging, 85
Lymph node station, 101
Lymph nodes accessibility, 112
Lymphocyte-activation gene 3 (LAG-3), 181
Lymphocytic alveolitis, 236

M
Magnetic resonance imaging (MRI), 188, 214
Malignant airway obstruction, 213–214
Malignant pleural effusion (MPE), 110
clinical presentation, 213
definitive pleural intervention, 218, 219
epidemiology, 211–213
imaging, 214
loculated/septated MPE, 222, 223
management, 216
nonexpandable lung, 222
pathophysiology, 213, 214
pleural biopsy, 216
pleural fluid analysis, 214, 215
surgical management, 217, 222
therapeutic thoracentesis, 218
Median OS, 180
Mediastinal lymph nodes assessment, 135
Medicaid, 37
Medical oncologists, 230
Medical thoracoscopy, 216

Medicare, 37, 271
Melanoma, 246
Metastatic disease on imaging, 110
Metronomic chemotherapy, 197
Microscopic injury, 232
Minimally invasive adenocarcinomas
    (MIA), 114
Minute ventilation (VE), 282
Molecularly targeted agents
    ALK & ROS1, 245, 246
    BRAF-targeted agents, 246
    EGFR, 244, 245
    vascular endothelial growth factor, 244
    VEGF, 244
Motivational interviewing (MI), 54
Multicentric Italian Lung Detection
    (MILD), 28
Multidisciplinary care, 258, 264–266
Multidisciplinary lung cancer program,
    230, 257
    diagnosis and staging, 265, 267
    disparities in receipt of, 271
    hub, joint decision-making model,
        259, 260
    joint practice model, 259
    patient survival, 269, 271
    patient-reported outcomes, 268
    serial referral model, 258
    treatment utilization, 267, 268
Multidisciplinary team (MDT), 147, 263
Multifocal adenocarcinoma, 103
Multiple extrathoracic metastases
    (M1c), 101
Musculoskeletal disease, 280
Mutual performance monitoring, 265
Mutual trust, 265
Mycophenolate mofetil (MMF), 243

N
National Cancer Database, 130
National Cancer Institute Common
    Terminology Criteria for Adverse
    Events (CTCAE) grading
    scale, 234
National Commission on Cancer Network
    (NCCN) guidelines, 41, 106, 125,
    149, 243
National Institutes of Health and National
    Cancer Institute, 52
National Lung Screening Trial (NLST), 26,
    27, 37, 72
National Radiology Data Registry, 37

Navigational bronchoscopy, with or without
    radial ultrasound and fluoroscopic
    guidance, 115
Nederlands-Leuvens Longkanker Screenings
    Onderzoek (NELSON) study, 29, 77
Neoadjuvant chemotherapy, 149, 151,
    152, 268
Neurohormonal alterations, 62
Neurologic impairment, 280
Nicotine, 52
Nicotinic acetylcholine receptors (nAChR)
    binding, 61
Nicotine addiction, 52, 53
Nicotine inhaler, 60
Nicotine replacement therapy, 60
Nicotinic acetylcholine receptors
    (nAChRs), 52
Nodule contour, 76
Nodule size, 31
Nonexpandable lung, 222
Noninvasive staging, 104, 105
Non-mucinous adenocarcinomas, 114
Non-small cell lung cancer (NSCLC), 97,
    236, 256
    defined, 147
    first-line therapy
        actionable mutations, 169–172
        adenocarcinoma vs. squamous cell
            carcinoma, 167, 168
        histology, 166
        large cell neuroendocrine carcinoma
            (LCNEC), 168, 169
        sarcomatoid carcinoma, 167, 169
    immunotherapy for
        combination immunotherapy-
            chemoradiotherapy, 155, 157
        neoadjuvant setting, 154, 155
    neoadjuvant chemotherapy, 151, 152
    nonsurgical treatment, 152–154
    principles of management, 149
    surgery plus adjuvant therapy, 150, 151
    treatment strategies for, 148, 149, 166
Nonsurgical treatment, 152–154

O
Occupational exposures, 74
Organizational challenges, 261
Organizational skills, 260
Osimertinib, 244
Overall survival (OS), 166
Overdiagnosis, 34
Oxygen desaturation, 282

P
PACIFIC trial, 156
Palliative medicine specialists, 230
Particle-based therapy, 194, 195
Pathological staging, pTNM, 98
Pathologic lymphadenopathy, 104
Patient assessment, 235
Patient-centered approach, 286, 288, 289
Patient-centered care, 286
Patient-centered outcomes, 286
Patient level barriers, 39
Patient-related factors, 149
Patient satisfaction, 262
Patients' fitness, 277
PD-L1 expression, 179
PD-L1 tumor proportion score (TPS), 175
Pembrolizumab, 198
Pemetrexed, 168, 231, 239
Perioperative mortality, 289
Peripheral vascular disease, 280
PET-based imaging, 193
Pharmacotherapy, 56, 60
Phase III randomized controlled trial
        (RCT), 169
Physiologic responses, 279
Pilot projects, 262
Platinum agents, 236
Pleuoroscopy, 110
Pleural effusions, 235
Pleural fluid analysis, 214
Pleural fluid cytology, 215
Pleural fluid markers, 212
Pleural space, 220
Pneumocystis jirovecii, 236, 240
Pneumonitis, 241
Pneumotox database, 246
Polyaromatic hydrocarbons (PAHs), 50
POSEIDON, 177
Positron emission tomography (PET),
        40, 84, 267
Posterolateral thoracotomy, 130
Postoperative cardiopulmonary
        complications, 281
Postoperative radiotherapy, 126, 190
Pralsetinib, 246, 247
Predicted postoperative lung function, 278
Private practitioners, 260
Programmed death ligand-1 (PD-L1)
        inhibitor, 196
Prophylactic cranial irradiation
        (PCI), 200–202
Prostate, Lung, Colon, and Ovarian (PLCO)
        trial, 26

Proton-based therapy, 195
Proton pump inhibitor, 236
Proton therapy, 194
Psychiatric illness, 280
Pulmonary embolism, 230
Pulmonary function tests (PFTs), 230, 278
Pulmonary hypertension, 283
Pulmonary lymphangitis, 241
Pulmonary nodules, 71, 81
    causes and characteristics of, 73
    clinical and pulmonary risk factors for, 74
    diagnostic evaluations, 72
    etiology, 72
    evaluation, 73, 75
    imaging, 75–77, 79, 81, 82
    pulmonary biomarkers, 85, 89
    risk assessment on diagnostic
        evaluation, 84
    risk stratification models, 82, 85
Pulmonary toxicity syndromes, 237–238
Pulmonologists, 230

Q
Qualitative studies, 286
Quality of life (QoL), 130
Quitlines (800-QUIT-NOW), 56

R
Radiation fibrosis, 232
Radiation oncologists, 230
Radiation pneumonitis, 233
Radiation recall pneumonitis, 231
Radiation therapy, 14
    diagnostic testing, 235, 236
    epidemiology, risk factors, and risk
        reduction, 231
    patient assessment, 235
    radiation-induced lung injury, 232
    radiation-related pulmonary toxicity, 233
    severity and principles of management, 236
    suspected radiation-induced lung injury,
        232, 233
Radiogenomics approaches, 76
Radiographic abnormalities, 230
Radiographic features, 242
Radiologic abnormalities, 235
Radiologists, 230
Radiotherapy techniques, 137
Radon, 16
Ramucirumab, 166, 244
Randomized controlled trial (RCT), 287

Randomized LDCT trials, 34
2017 Randomized Trial of Pleural Fluid
        Drainage Frequency in Patients with
        Malignant Pleural Effusions Trial
        (ASAP Trial), 220
Rapid On-Site cytologic Evaluation
        (ROSE), 108
Reliable Change Index (RCI), 203
Resectable cN2, 149
Retrospective analysis, 238
Retrospective study, 281
Right upper lobectomy, 132
Robotic-assisted thoracic surgery (RATS), 129
Robotic systems, 115

S
Sarcomatoid carcinoma, 167, 169
Sarcopenia, 283
SCALE Collaboration, 52
Segmentectomy, 133
Selpercatinib, 246, 247
Semi-solid nodules, 81
Shared decision making (SDM), 37, 38, 286
Shared mental models, 265
Single agent immunotherapy, 174, 180
Single checkpoint inhibitor, 177, 179
Single extrathoracic metastasis (M1b), 101
Six-minute walk test (6MWT), 280
Sleeve lobectomy, 135
Sleeve resections, 134
Small cell lung cancer (SCLC), 236
    extensive stage disease
        initial systemic treatment, 195, 196
        oligometastatic SCLC, 199, 200
        palliative, attenuated dose radiotherapy
            in ED-SCLC, 200
        prophylactic cranial irradiation
            (PCI), 200–203
        systemic treatment for relapsed
            disease, 196–199
        thoracic radiation considerations, 199
    particle-based therapy, 194, 195
    radiation treatment, 192, 194
    staging and diagnosis, 187–189
    surgical considerations, 190
    systemic treatment considerations,
        189, 190
    thoracic radiation, 190–192
Smoking cessation, 287
Society of Thoracic Radiology clinical
        practice guidelines, 219
Society of Thoracic Surgeons (STS), 219, 265

Socioeconomic status, 265
Solid pulmonary nodules (SPN), 77
Sotorasib, 246
South West Oncology Group (SWOG) S0023
        trial, 158
Squamous cell carcinoma (SCIS), 114
Squamous pathology, 241
Staging
    clinical *vs.* pathologic stage, 98
    combination of EUS and EBUS, 109
    conventional TBNA, 107
    EBUS-TBNA, 107, 108
    elastin stains, 113
    EUS, 108
    5-year survival percentages, 102
    invasive, 105, 106
    metastatic disease, 110
    N (nodal) component, 100
    nodal metastases, 115
    noninvasive, 104, 105
    peripheral pulmonary nodules with
        complication rates, 115
    proposed approach, 102
    significance, 97
    T (tumor) component, or tumor size, 99
    TNM, 98–102
Stage IIIA adenocarcinoma, 232
Stair climbing test (SCT), 280
Standard cervical mediastinoscopy, 110
Standard-of-care treatment, 200
Stereotactic body radiotherapy (SBRT),
        137–139, 231, 285
Steroid-refractory pneumonitis, 243
Subclinical disease, 231
Subsolid pulmonary nodules, 80
Supraclavicular lymph node involvement, 188
Surgical treatment, 271, 277
Surveillance, Epidemiology, and End Results
        (SEER) registry, 34, 271
Symptomatic fluid reaccumulation, 220
Synchronous primaries, 102
Syndrome of inappropriate diuretic hormone
        (SIADH), 187
Systemic steroids, 233
System-level barriers, 36

T
Talc pleurodesis, 221
Taxane, 231, 238, 239
T descriptor, 99, 116
Temozolomide, 198, 240
Therapeutic approaches, 147

Therapeutic Intervention in Malignant
	Effusion (TIME-2) trial, 221
Thermal ablation, 127
Thoracentesis, 188
Thoracic radiotherapy, 189–191, 232
Thoracic surgeons, 230
Thoracic ultrasonography, 219
Thromboembolism, 238
Time to first cigarette (TTFC), 53
Tobacco prevalence and treatment
	bupropion sustained release (S.R.), 61
	comprehensive tobacco history and
		examination, 55
	counseling, 55, 56
	development of lung cancer, 50, 51
	disparities in, 50
	5As Model for Behavior Change, 54
	lung cancer care, 52
	lung cancer screening, 51
	motivational interviewing (MI), 54
	nicotine addiction, 52, 53
	nicotine replacement therapy, 60
	ongoing research, 52
	pharmacotherapy, 56, 60
	relapse prevention, 62
	self-awareness and proactive work, 53
	varenicline, 61
Tobacco prevention, 6, 49
Topoisomerase I inhibitors, 231, 240
Topotecan, 197
Traction bronchiectasis, 232
Traditional chemotherapeutic agents, 231
	alkylating agents, 240, 241
	etoposide, 239
	gemcitabine, 239
	pemetrexed, 239
	platinum agents, 236
	taxanes, 238, 239
	topoisomerase I inhibitors, 240
	vinorelbine, 240
Trametinib, 246
Transbronchial biopsy, 236, 242
Transcervical extended mediastinal
	lymphadenectomy (TEMLA), 111
Transthoracic needle aspiration (TTNA) of
	lung nodules, 110
Treatment complications, 283

Treatment modalities, 268
Tremelimumab, 178
Tumor-derived vascular endothelial growth
	factor (VEGF), 213
Tumor infiltration, 241
Tumor necrosis factor (TNF), 213
Tumor, nodes, and metastases (TNM)
	classification system, 98
Tyrosine kinase inhibitor (TKI) therapy, 157

U
UK Lung Cancer Screening Trial (UKLS), 28
United States, 165, 174
United States Preventive Services Task Force
	(USPSTF), 26, 54, 62, 82
Upper lobe location, 77
US National Inpatient Sample database, 283

V
Validated Pulmonary Nodule Risk
	Calculators, 83
Varenicline, 61
Vemurafenib, 246
Ventral tegmental area (VTA), 52
Veterans Affairs (VA), 72, 270
Victorian Lung Cancer Registry, 270
Video-assisted mediastinoscopic
	lymphadenectomy (VAMLA), 111
Video-assisted mediastinoscopy (VAM),
	106, 110
Video-assisted thoracoscopic surgery (VATS),
	110, 112, 129, 216
Vinorelbine, 231, 240
Vitamin D supplementation, 236
Volume doubling time (VDT), 79
Volumetric analysis, 31
Volumetric measurements, 76

W
Wang™ needle, 106
Wedge resections, 134
White blood cells (WBC), 233
World Health Organization, 6, 256